Antibiotic Resistance

METHODS IN MOLECULAR MEDICINE™

John M. Walker, SERIES EDITOR

60. **Interleukin Protocols,** edited by *Luke A. J. O'Neill and Andrew Bowie,* 2001
59. **Molecular Pathology of the Prions,** edited by *Harry F. Baker,* 2001
58. **Metastasis Research Protocols: *Volume 2, Cell Behavior In Vitro and In Vivo,*** edited by *Susan A. Brooks and Udo Schumacher,* 2001
57. **Metastasis Research Protocols: *Volume 1, Analysis of Cells and Tissues,*** edited by *Susan A. Brooks andUdo Schumacher,* 2001
56. **Human Airway Inflammation:** *Sampling Techniques and Analytical Protocols,* edited by *Duncan F. Rogers and Louise E. Donnelly,* 2001
55. **Hematologic Malignancies:** *Methods and Protocols,* edited by *Guy B. Faguet,* 2001
54. **Mycobacterium Tuberculosis Protocols,** edited by *Tanya Parish and Neil G. Stoker, 2001*
53. **Renal Cancer:** *Methods and Protocols,* edited by *Jack H. Mydlo,* 2001
52. **Atherosclerosis Methods and Protocols,** edited by *Angela F. Drew,* 2001
51. **Angiotensin Protocols,** edited by *Donna H. Wang,* 2001
50. **Colorectal Cancer: *Methods and Protocols*,** edited by *Steven M. Powell,* 2001
49. **Molecular Pathology Protocols,** edited by *Anthony A. Killeen,* 2000
48. **Antibiotic Resistance Methods and Protocols,** edited by *Stephen H. Gillespie,* 2001
47. **Vision Research Protocols,** edited by *P. Elizabeth Rakoczy,* 2000
46. **Angiogenesis: *Reviews and Protocols*,** edited by *J. Clifford Murray,* 2000
45. **Hepatocellular Carcinoma: *Methods and Protocols*, edited by** *Nagy A. Habib,* 2000
44. **Asthma: *Mechanisms and Protocols*, edited by** *K. Fan Chung and Ian Adcock,* 2000
43. **Muscular Dystrophy: *Methods and Protocols,* edited by** *Katherine B. Bushby and Louise Anderson,* 2000
42. **Vaccine Adjuvants: *Preparation Methods and Research Protocols*,** edited by *Derek T. O'Hagan,* 2000
41. **Celiac Disease: *Methods and Protocols*,** edited by *Michael N. Marsh,* 2000
40. **Diagnostic and Therapeutic Antibodies,** edited by *Andrew J. T. George and Catherine E. Urch,* 2000
39. **Ovarian Cancer: *Methods and Protocols*,** edited by *John M. S. Bartlett,* 2000
38. **Aging Methods and Protocols,** edited by *Yvonne A. Barnett and Christopher R. Barnett,* 2000
37. **Electrochemotherapy, Electrogenetherapy, and Transdermal Drug Delivery:** *Electrically Mediated Delivery of Molecules to Cells,* edited by *Mark J. Jaroszeski, Richard Heller, and Richard Gilbert,* 2000
36. **Septic Shock Methods and Protocols,** edited by *Thomas J. Evans,* 2000

METHODS IN MOLECULAR MEDICINE™

Antibiotic Resistance

Methods and Protocols

Edited by

Stephen H. Gillespie

Department of Medical Microbiology,
Royal Free and University College Medical School,
University College London, London, UK

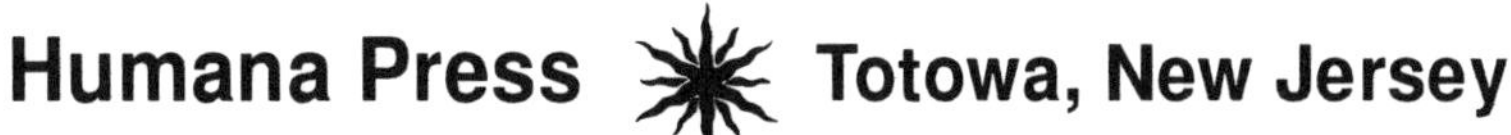
Humana Press Totowa, New Jersey

999 Riverview Drive, Suite 208
Totowa, New Jersey 07512

Cover design by Patricia F. Cleary

Cover illustration: Fig. 2H from Chapter 20, "Atomic Force Microscopy: *Theory and Practice in Bacteria Morphostructural Analysis*" by Pier Carlo Braga and Davide Ricci

This publication is printed on acid-free paper. ∞
ANSI Z39.48-1984 (American Standards Institute) Permanence of Paper for Printed Library Materials.

For additional copies, pricing for bulk purchases, and/or information about other Humana titles, contact Humana at the above address or at any of the following numbers: Tel.: 973-256-1699; Fax: 973-256-8341; E-mail: humana@humanapr.com or visit our Website: http://humanapress.com

Printed in the United States of America. 10 9 8 7 6 5 4 3 2 1

Library of Congress Cataloging in Publication Data

Antibiotic resistance: methods and protocols / edited by Stephen H. Gillespie.
p.; cm.-- (Methods in molecular medicine; 48)
Includes bibliographical references and index.
ISBN 0-89603-777-0 (alk. paper)
1. Drug resistance in microorganisms--laboratory manuals. 2. Antibiotics--Laboratory manuals. I. Gillespie, S. H. II. Series.
[DNLM: 1. Drug Resistance, Microbial--physiology. 2. Anti-Infective Agents--therapeutic use. 3. Antibiotics--therapeutic use. 4. Clinical Protocols. WB 320 A629 2000]
QR17 .A564 2000
616'.01--dc21

00-061334
CIP

Preface

The discovery of antibiotics and their introduction into medical practice was a revolution that has transformed the health of the human race. From its first beginnings under Paul Erhlich, who experimented with arsenical dyes to produce drugs active against trypanosomes and spirochetes, anti-infective chemotherapy is now available against almost all human pathogens. Even viruses, which for 50 years had proved a much more difficult target, are now treatable with chemotherapeutic agents.

From the start of the antibiotic era resistance was noted to be a problem. Erhlich observed that trypanosomes could become resistant to the arsenical dyes that he was using and that the resistant organisms never spontaneously reverted to susceptibility ***(1)***. Fleming carefully identified and listed the bacteria that were not susceptible to the culture filtrate of his *Penicillium* mold ***(2)***. Once antibiotics were introduced into clinical practice, acquired resistance was quickly noted: *Neisseria gonorrhoeae* to sulfonamides being one of the earliest examples. At first, resistance did not appear to be such a problem as the flood of drug discoveries— chloramphenicol, tetracyclines, erythromycin, cephalosporins, and aminoglycosides—appeared in time to widen the number of bacterial species becoming susceptible to antibiotics and to overcome developing resistance problems. Often resistance among bacteria seemed to be limited to organisms isolated in hospitals, mainly from patients with other serious conditions. For example, when resistance to penicillin through the elaboration of a β-lactamase became more common among *Staphylococcus aureus,* the infections were almost exclusively found in hospitals. Indeed the popular name for a *S. aureus* expressing β-lactamase was "the hospital *Staphylococcus*"***(3)***.

The pharmaceutical industry was able to solve the problem of β-lactamase with the discovery and chemical modification of the amido-penicillin nucleus leading to a new range of semisynthetic penicillins including methicillin, flucloxacillin, and ampicillin ***(4)***. The difficulties encountered in overcoming β-lactamase-producing staphylococci were a harbinger of future problems. In succeeding years Gram-negative bacilli developed increasing resistance acquiring and transmitting new resistance determinants with unfailing regularity via plasmids, transposons, and bacteriophages ***(5–7)***. It was only with massive investment in drug discovery and scientific success that kept medicine ahead of the microbes.

In recent years there has been a significant change in the pattern of antimicrobial resistance and public and scientific perceptions of it. Although multiple drug resistance was previously identified in *Salmonella typhi* ***(8)***, multiple drug resistance has emerged in primary respiratory pathogens, such as *Mycobacterium tuberculosis* and *Streptococcus pneumoniae,* spreading widely and rapidly throughout the world ***(9,10)***. This has been coupled with a fall in the number of new compounds coming to the market, at a time when drug development costs have increased dramatically. With the description of glycopeptide intermediate resistant staphylococci, the last vestige of wishful thinking was torn away ***(11)***. Although *S. aureus* had always had a talent for acquiring resistance, it had always remained susceptible to the glycopeptides. The prospect of untreatable tuberculosis and pneumococcal and *S. aureus* infections has generated dramatic and often hysterical headlines in the lay and medical press ***(12)***. In many countries government investigations and reports were commissioned ***(13)***.

At one time antibiotic drug development was considered the cutting edge of science. Erhlich, Fleming, Florey, Chain, and Waxsman all collected Nobel prizes for their efforts in developing successful antibiotics. With increasing success came complacency and research in antibiotics became mere routine and the natural area for industry not academia. All of this has now changed—antibiotic research has returned to the forefront of medical science once again. This volume strives to provide scientists with the critical techniques to enter antibiotic resistance research.

From the point of view of patients and clinicians, rapid diagnosis must be a priority for research. More rapid diagnosis of resistant organisms will allow patients with resistant organisms to be isolated and the correct therapy initiated with minimal delay. This will not only improve treatment outcomes, but will reduce the risk of transmission of resistant organisms. In this volume many different techniques are described that address rapid diagnosis, ranging from DNA amplification techniques to phage display.

It is imperative that scientists be able to plot the transmission of resistant organisms; thus, molecular biological techniques have been harnessed to investigate their epidemiology. For tuberculosis, monitoring treatment has always been problematical and many patients fail to complete an inadequate course of therapy, allowing drug resistant strains to emerge and be transmitted. Several innovative techniques are described and could be readily applied to other organisms.

The complex problems posed by pathogenic microorganisms in causing disease and in developing antibiotic resistance mean that the approach to overcoming them must be sophisticated and multifaceted. We also need to understand the mechanisms of resistance, the biology of resistant organisms, and the way in which they evolve and to quantify the evolutionary barriers to resistance.

In this volume a wide range of techniques have been brought together that will be useful in developing new antibiotic research programs. There is strong emphasis on *M. tuberculosis* and *S. pneumoniae,* and this reflects current research questions and concerns. Although many of the techniques are designed for one organism, they are readily adaptable to other problem organisms. I hope that this volume will be useful to microbiologists developing and implementing new diagnostic and epidemiological techniques, and to basic scientists trying to understand the basic biology of antimicrobial resistance. In whatever sphere of antibiotic research you are in, I hope that you will find this volume of value.

I gratefully acknowledge the assistance provided by Dr. Janet P. Gillespie in managing this project and Ms. Therese Donnelly for her secretarial assistance.

Stephen H. Gillespie

References

1. Erlich P. (1909) Über moderne Chemotherapie. *Beiträge zur experimentallen Pathologie und Chemotherapie* 167–202.
2. Fleming A. (1929) On the antibacterial action of cultures of a *Penicillium*, with special reference to their use in the isolation of *B. influenzae. Brit. J. Exp. Pathol.* **10,** 226–236.
3. Haley RW., Hightower AW., Kabbatz RF., Thornsberry C., Martone WJ., Allen JR., Hughes JM. (1982) The emergence of methicillin resistant *Staphylococcus aureus* infection in United States hospitals. *Ann. Intern. Med.* **97,** 297–308.
4. Batchelor FR., Doyle FP., Naylor JHC., Rolinson GN. (1959) Synthesis of penicillin: 6-amidopenicillanic acid in penicillin fermentations. *Nature* **183,** 257.
5. Lenski RE. Simpson SC. Nguyen TT. (1994) Genetic analysis of a plasmid-encoded, host genotype-specific enhancement of bacterial fitness. *J. Bacteriol.* **176,** 3140–3147.
6. Hyder SL, Steitfeld MM. (1978) Transfer of erythromycin resistance from clinically isolated lysogenic strains of *Streptococcus pyogenes* via their endogenous phage. *J. Infect. Dis.* **138,** 281–286.
7. Poyart C, Pierre C, Quesne G, Pron B, Berche P, Trien-Cust P. (1997) Emergence of vancomycin resistance in the genus *Streptococcus*: characterization of a *vanB* transferable determinant in *Streptococcus bovis. Antimicrob. Agent Chemother.* **41,** 24–29.
8. Goldstein FW., Chumpitaz JC., Guevara JM., Papadopoulou B., Acar JF., Vieu

JF. (1986) Plasmid-mediated resistance to multiple antibioitics in *Salmonella typhi*. *J. Infect. Dis.* **153,** 261–266
9. Muños R., Coffey TJ., Daniels M., et al (1991) Intercontinental spread of serotype 23F *Streptococcus pneumoniae*. *J. Infect. Dis.* **164,** 302–306.
10. The WHO/IUALTD. Anti-tuberculosis drug resistance in the world. World Health Organ, Geneva. **1997**.
11. Hiramatsu K., H. Hanaki, T. Ino, K. Yabuta, T. Oguri , and F. C. Tenover. (1997). Methicillin-resistant *Staphylococcus aureus* clinical strain with reduced vancomycin susceptibility. *J. Antimicrob. Chemother.* **40,** 135–136.
12. Bloom BR, Murray CJL. (1992)Tuberculosis: commentary on a reemergent killer. *Science* **257,** 1055–1064.
13. Standing Medical Advisory Committee. 1998. The Path of Least Resistance. Department of Health. London.

Contents

Contributors

ANA M. AMOROSO • *Laboratorio de Resistencia Microbiologia, Facultad de Farmacia y Bioquimica, Buenas Aires, Argentina*

VICTORIA A. BARCUS • *Department of Biological Sciences, University of Warwick, Coventry, UK*

VICENTE J. BENEDÍ • *Area of Microbiology, Department of Biology, Universitat de les Illes Balears, and IMEDEA (CSIC-UIB), Palma de Mallorca, Spain*

OWEN J. BILLINGTON • *Department of Medical Microbiology, Royal Free and University College Medical School, Royal Free Campus, London, UK*

WILLIAM H. BRABANT • *Seattle Biomedical Research Institute and the Department of Pathobiology, University of Washington, and the Seattle Biomedical Research Institute, Seattle, WA*

PIER CARLO BRAGA • *Department of Pharmacology, School of Medicine, Milano, Italy*

GERARD A. CANGELOSI • *Seattle Biomedical Research Institute and the Department of Pathobiology, University of Washington, Seattle, WA*

FRANKLIN R. COCKERILL, III • *Mayo Clinic, Rochester, MN*

LUCY E. DESJARDIN • *VAMC Research Service, Iowa City, IA*

CHRISTOPHER G. DOWSON • *Department of Biological Sciences, University of Warwick, Coventry, UK*

ANNE-MARIE GASC • *Laboratoire deMicrobiologie et de Genetique Moleculaire CNRS, Toulouse, France*

ELVIRA GARZA-GONZÁLEZ • *Departamento de Bioquimica, Facultad de Medicina, UANL, Nueva Leon, Mexico*

JOHN T. GEORGE • *GR Micro, London, UK*

STEPHEN H. GILLESPIE • *Department of Medical Microbiology, Royal Free and University College Medical School, Royal Free Campus, London, UK*

MARTHA GUERRERO-OLAZARÁN • *Departamento de Bioquimica, Facultad de Medicina, UANL, Nuevo Leon, Mexico*

GABRIEL O. GUTKIND • *Laboratorio de Resistencia Microbiologia, Facultad de Farmacia y Bioquimica, Buenas Aires, Argentina*

REGINE HAKENBECK • *Department of Microbiology, University of Kaiserlautern, Kaiserslautern, Germany*

HEDEAKI HANAKI • *Department of Bacteriology, Juntendo University, Bunkyo-ku, Tokyo, Japan*

GERY L. HEHMAN • *VAMC Research Service, Iowa City, IA*

TOBIN J. HELLYER • *Becton Dickenson Microbiology Systems, Sparks, MD*

PETER W. M. HERMANS • *Department of Paediatrics, Erasmus University Medical Center Rotterdam, Rotterdamdam, The Netherlands*

KEIICHI HIRAMATSU • *Department of Bacteriology, Juntendo University, Bunkyo-ku, Tokyo, Japan*

TERUYO ITO • *Department of Bacteriology, Juntendo University, Bunkyo-ku, Tokyo, Japan*

MARK E. JONES • *MRL Pharmaceutical Services, Utrecht, The Netherlands*

NAINN-TSYR JOU • *Division of Rheumatology, Harbor-UCLA Medical Center, Torrance, CA*

KEITH P. KLUGMAN • *Pneumococcal Disease Research Unit, South African Institute of Medical Research, Johannesburg, South Africa*

KARL KÖHRER • *MRL Pharmaceutical Services, Utrecht, The Netherlands*

MICHAEL R. LIEBLING • *Division of Rheumatology, Harbor-UCLA Medical Center, Torrance, CA*

LUIS MARTÍNEZ-MARTÍNEZ • *Area of Microbiology, Department of Biology, Universitat de les Illes Balears, and IMEDEA (CSIC-UIB), Palma de Mallorca, Spain*

TIMOTHY D. MCHUGH • *Department of Medical Microbiology, Royal Free and University College Medical School, Royal Free Campus, London, UK*

RUTH MCNERNEY • *Department of Infectious and Tropical Diseases, London School of Hygiene and Tropical Medicine, London, UK*

IAN MORRISSEY • *GR Micro, London, UK*

ROBIN PATEL • *Mayo Clinic, Rochester, MN*

MIGNON DU PLESSIS • *Pneumococcal Disease Research Unit, South African Institute of Medical Research, Johannesburg, South Africa*

KEITH POOLE • *Department of Microbiology and Immunology, Queen's University, Kingston, Ontario, Canada*

DAVIDE RICCI • *Department of Biophysical Electronic Engineering, University of Genoa, Italy*

LOUIS B. RICE • *VA Medical Center, Cleveland, OH*

FRANZ-JOSEF SCHMITZ • *Department of Medical Microbiology and Virology, Henrich-Heine University, Düsseldorf, Germany*

MARCEL SLUIJTER • *Department of Paediatrics, Erasmus University Medical Center Rotterdam, Rotterdam, the Netherlands*

Anthony M. Smith • *Pneumococcal Disease Research Unit, South African Institute of Medical Research, Johannesburg, South Africa*

Ramakrishnan Srikumar • *Department of Microbiology and Immunology, Queen's University, Kingston, Ontario, Canada*

J. Keith Struthers • *Coventry Public Health Laboratory and Department of Biological Sciences, University of Warwick, Coventry, UK*

Rolando Tijerina-Menchaca • *Departamento de Bioquimica, Faculdad de Medicina, UANL, Nuevo Leon, Mexico*

James R. Uhl • *Mayo Clinic, Rochester, MN*

Alex van Belkum • *Department of Medical Microbiology and Infectious Diseases, Erasmus University Medical Center Rotterdam, Rotterdam, The Netherlands*

José M. Viader-Salvadó • *Departamento de Bioquimica, Faculdad de Medicina, UANL, Nuevo Leon, Mexico*

Gail C. Whiting • *Department of Medical Microbiology, Royal Free and University College Medical School, Royal Free Campus, London, UK*

I

Diagnosis of Resistance

1

Multiplex Polymerase Chain Reaction Detection of *vanA*, *vanB*, *vanC-1*, and *vanC-2/3* Genes in *Enterococci*

Robin Patel, Jim R. Uhl, and Franklin R. Cockerill, III

1. Introduction

Resistance to the glycopeptide antibiotic vancomycin in enterococci, is phenotypically and genotypically heterogeneous. Three glycopeptide resistance phenotypes, VanA, VanB, and VanC, account for most glycopeptide resistance in enterococci; they can be distinguished on the basis of the level and inducibility of resistance to vancomycin and teicoplanin.

VanA type glycopeptide resistance is characterized by acquired inducible resistance to both vancomycin and teicoplanin and has been described for *Enterococcus faecalis*, *Enterococcus faecium*, *Enterococcus gallinarum*, *Enterococcus casseliflavus*, *Enterococcus durans*, *Enterococcus mundtii*, *Enterococcus raffinosus*, and *Enterococcus avium* (**Table 1**) *(1)*. VanA is the most completely understood type of vancomycin resistance. It is mediated by transposon Tn*1546* or related elements. Tn*1546* was originally described on a plasmid from an *E. faecium* isolate. It consists of a series of genes encoding 9 polypeptides that can be assigned to different functional groups: Transposition functions (ORF1 and ORF2), regulation of vancomycin resistance genes (VanR and VanS), synthesis of the depsipeptide, D-alanyl-D-lactate which when incorporated into the pentapeptide peptidoglycan precursor form a pentapeptide peptidoglycan precursor to which neither vancomycin nor teicoplanin will bind (VanH and VanA), and hydrolysis of normal peptidoglycan (VanX and VanY); the function of VanZ is unknown. The *vanR, vanS, vanH, vanA*, and *vanX* genes are necessary and sufficient for the inducible expression of resistance to glycopeptides. VanY and VanZ are accessory peptides and are not required for resistance. Genetic heterogeneity has been described in *vanA* gene

From: *Methods in Molecular Medicine, vol. 48: Antibiotic Resistance Methods and Protocols*
Edited by: S. H. Gillespie © Humana Press Inc., Totowa, NJ

Table 1
Vancomycin Resistant Enterococci

Phenotype	Genotype	Vancomycin MIC (μg/mL)	Teicoplanin MIC (μg/mL)	Expression	Transfer	Bacterial species
VanA	*vanA*	64–1000	16–512	Inducible	+	*E. faecium* *E. faecalis* *E. avium* *E. gallinarum* *E. durans* *E. mundtii* *E. casseliflavus* *E. raffinosus*
VanB	*vanB*	4–1000	0.5–1	Inducible	+	*E. faecium* *E. faecalis*
VanC	*vanC-1*	2–32	0.5–1	Constitutive/ Inducible	–	*E. gallinarum*
VanC	*vanC-2*	2–32	0.5–1	Constitutive	–	*E. casseliflavus*
VanC	*vanC-3*	2–32	0.5–1	Constitutive	–	*E. flavescens*

clusters of vancomycin resistant enterococci (VRE). The *vanA* gene cluster has been found on the chromosome as well as on plasmids.

VanB type glycopeptide resistance is characterized by acquired inducible resistance to various concentrations of vancomycin but not to teicoplanin and has been described in *E. faecalis* and *E. faecium* (**Table 1**). The *vanB* gene cluster, as described in an *E. faecalis* isolate, has homology to the *vanA* gene cluster but has been less well studied. It appears to be located on the chromosome.

VanC type glycopeptide resistance is a less well characterized type of vancomycin resistance. VanC type glycopeptide resistance is characterized by low level vancomycin resistance but teicoplanin susceptibility and has been described as an intrinsic property of *E. gallinarum*, *E. casseliflavus*, and *Enterococcus flavescens* (**Table 1**) *(2–4)*. The VanC phenotype is felt to be chromosomally encoded and expressed constitutively, although recent data suggest that vancomycin resistance may be inducible in at least some strains of *E. gallinarum*. Pentapeptide peptidoglycan precursors in strains with VanC vancomycin resistance terminate in the D-alanyl-D-serine rather than in D-alanyl-D-alanine. The genes encoding for the synthesis of the depsipeptide D-alanyl-D-serine are referred to as *vanC-1* (in *E. gallinarum*), *vanC-2* (in *E. casseliflavus*) and *vanC-3* (in *E. flavescens)*.

We describe a convenient multiplex polymerase chain reaction (PCR)/ restriction fragment length polymorphism (PCR-RFLP) assay that can be performed directly on isolated colonies of *Enterococcus* spp. to detect and discriminate *vanA*, *vanB*, *vanC-1*, and *vanC-2/3* genes. This multiplex PCR/RFLP assay is a rapid method for determining glycopeptide resistance genotypes for *Enterococcus* spp. Using this procedure, a bacterial colony is inoculated directly into the PCR reaction mixture. Bacterial lysis is achieved by heating the mixture to 95°C for 10 min prior to thermocycling for DNA amplification. Following PCR, amplicon identity and amplicon decontamination is achieved by the addition of a restriction enzyme to the reaction followed by RFLP analysis by gel electrophoresis. The assay provides a more specific and rapid alternative to classical phenotypic methods for the detection of low level glycopeptide resistance (MIC range, 4-8 μg/mL), as occurs with *vanC-1*, *vanC-2*, or *vanC-3* associated resistance in *E. gallinarum*, *E. casseliflavus*, and *E. flavescens*. Current NCCLS breakpoints for susceptibility interpretive categories (susceptible, ≤4 mg/L) do not always allow for discrimination of these genotypes, although the clinical significance of this form of vancomycin resistance is not yet established.

2. Materials

2.1. Growth of Bacterial Colonies

1. Sheep blood agar plates.
2. Platinum loop.
3. Control VRE strains:

   E. faecium B7641 (*vanA*-vancomycin MIC > 256 μg/mL; teicoplanin MIC > 16 μg/mL).

   E. faecalis V583 (*vanB*-vancomycin MIC 64 μg/mL; teicoplanin MIC = 8 μg/mL).

   E. casseliflavus ATCC 25788 (*vanC-2*-vancomycin MIC 4 μg/mL; teicoplanin MIC = 8 μg/mL).

   E. gallinarum GS (*vanC-1*-vancomycin MIC 4 μg/mL; teicoplanin MIC = 8 μg/mL).
4. 37°C incubator.
5. Bunsen burner.

2.2. PCR Amplification

1. *Taq* polymerase (Perkin-Elmer Cetus, Norwalk, CT).
2. dNTP stock (1.25 m*M*) from 100 m*M* concentrates (Roche Molecular Biochemicals, Indianapolis, IN).

   To prepare dNTP stock mix: dATP 10 μL, dGTP 10 μL, dCTP 10 μL, dTTP 10 μL, water 760 μL. Store at –20°C.
3. 50% Glycerol (store at –20°C).

Table 2
Oligonucleotide Primers (Adapted with Permission from Patel et al. [5])

Gene	Primer name	Oligonucleotide sequence (5' to 3')	PCR product size (bp)	Size of *Msp*I restriction fragments (bp)
vanA	vanA-FOR	CATGACGTATCGGTAAAATC	885	231, 184, 163, 131/133
	vanAB-REV	ACCGGGCAGRGTATTGAC		
vanB	vanB-FOR	CATGATGTGTCGGTAAAATC	885	188/189, 160, 136
	vanAB-REV	ACCGGGCAGRGTATTGAC		
vanC-1	vanC123-FOR	GATGGCWGTATCCAAGGA	467	230/237
	vanC1-REV	GTGATCGTGGCGCTG		
vanC-2/3	vanC123-FOR	GATGGCWGTATCCAAGGA	429	338, 91
	vanC23-REV	ATCGAAAAAGCCGTCTAC		

4. 10X PCR buffer (100 m*M* Tris-HCl, pH 8.3, 500 m*M* KCl, 15 m*M* $MgCl_2$).
   To prepare 10X PCR buffer mix: 1 *M* Tris-HCl, pH 8.3 (100 m*M*) 1 mL; 1 *M* KCl (500 m*M*) 0.15 mL; 1 *M* $MgCl_2$ (1 mL) 0.15 mL; 3.85 mL water. Store at 4°C.
5. Thermocycler (DNA Thermal Cycler 480, Perkin Elmer Cetus).
6. 0.5 mL thin walled PCR reaction tubes (Perkin Elmer Cetus).
7. Oligonucleotide primers are synthesized on an Applied Biosystems 394 DNA/RNA synthesizer with the final dimethoxytrityl group removed. The primers are air dried at 60°C and redissolved in distilled water. The absorbance at 260 nm is used to determine the primer concentration, which is then adjusted to 50 µ*M*. Sequences are provided in **Table 2**.
8. 1.5 mL microcentrifuge tubes.
9. Mineral oil.

2.3. Restriction Enzyme Digestion of PCR Product

1. *Msp*I (10 U/µL) and 10X restriction enzyme buffer (Promega Corp., Madison, WI).
2. Microcentrifuge.
3. 37°C incubator.

2.4. Agarose Gel Electrophoresis

1. NuSieve agarose (FMC BioProducts, Rockland, ME).
2. Ethidium bromide stock solution: 5 mg/mL (w/v) in water. Store the solution in a light-proof container at room temperature (*see* **Note 1**).
3. Gel imaging system.
4. Electrophoresis unit, corresponding gel trays and comb bridges.
5. Constant voltage power supply.
6. UV transilluminator, 302 nm.
7. 5X TBE buffer.
8. DNA molecular weight marker: 100 bp DNA ladder (Gibco-BRL, Gaithersburg, MD).

Table 3
Pipeting Scheme for PCR Reaction Master Mix for Six Multiplex PCR Reactions for Detection of *vanA*, *vanB*, *vanC-1*, and *vanC-2/3* Genes in Enterococci*

	Final concentration	μL
Water		138.9
10X PCR buffer	1X	30
dNTP (1.25 m*M*)	200 μ*M*	48
Primers: vanA-FOR	0.2 μ*M*	1.2
vanB-FOR	0.2 μ*M*	1.2
vanAB-REV	0.4 μ*M*	2.4
vanC1-REV	0.2 μ*M*	1.2
vanC23-REV	0.2 μ*M*	1.2
vanC123-FOR	0.4 μ*M*	2.4
Glycerol (50%)	10%	60
Ampli*Taq* (5U/μL)	0.025 U/μL	1.5
Total volume of mix		288

*For greater numbers of PCR reactions, the amounts shown must be adjusted as needed.

9. 56°C water bath.
10. Blue juice: 0.25% Bromophenol blue, 15% (w/v) Ficall-400 (Amersham Pharmacia Biotech, Piscataway, NJ) in water.

3. Methods

3.1. Growth of Bacterial Colonies

Streak a sheep blood agar plate with the bacterial isolate to be tested; incubate at 37°C overnight. One plate of each of the four control isolates should also be prepared and run with each reaction.

3.2 PCR Amplification

Before assembling the amplification mixture, read **Note 1** to get some hints for handling and contamination precautions. Prepare a small surplus of the master mix to avoid pipeting error (*see* **Note 2**).

1. Thaw the components indicated in **Table 3**.
2. Briefly vortex all reagents.
3. Prepare the PCR master mix in a sterile 1.5 mL microcentrifuge tube. A detailed pipeting scheme is given in **Table 3**. Vortex.
4. Aliquot 48 μL of PCR master mix into 0.5 mL PCR tubes. Overlay with 2 drops of mineral oil.

Table 4
Cycling Profile for Multiplex PCR Detection of *vanA*, *vanB*, *vanC-1*, and *vanC-2/3* Genes in Enterococci

1. Lyse bacteria at 95°C for 10 min
2. 36 cycles of amplification:
   i. 94°C for 1 min
   ii. 56°C for 1 min
   iii. 74°C for 1 min
3. Soak at 4°C

5. Inoculate one bacterial colony into the PCR tube underneath the mineral oil.
6. Place the amplification mixture in the thermocycler and start PCR using the cycling conditions shown in **Table 4**.

3.3. Restriction Enzyme Digestion of PCR Product

1. Add one microliter of *Msp*I and 5 µL 10X restriction enzyme buffer to each PCR tube.
2. Centrifuge the tubes at 13,200*g* for 20 s (to drive the restriction enzyme into the PCR reaction).
3. Incubate the tubes at 37°C overnight (*see* **Note 3**).

3.4. Agarose Gel Electrophoresis

1. For a 10 × 15 cm gel, completely dissolve 3.6 g of agarose in 120 mL 1X TBE buffer in a 250-mL Erlenmeyer flask by boiling for several minutes in a microwave oven; then cool the solution to between 50°C and 60°C in a water bath. **Caution:** The hot liquid may bump if shaken too vigorously. Add 6 µL of the ethidium bromide stock solution and gently mix.
2. Seal the edges of the gel tray with autoclave tape and position the corresponding comb 0.5 mm above the plate. Pour the warm agarose into the gel tray and insert the comb. Remove any air bubbles by trapping them in an inverted pipet tip. The gel thickness should be between 5 and 8 mm. After the gel is completely set (30–40 min at room temperature), carefully remove the comb and autoclave tape and mount the gel into the electrophoresis unit. Cover the gel with 1X TBE buffer to a depth above the gel of approx 1 mm.
3. Mix 6 µL of sample with 3 µL of blue juice and place the mixture into a well of the submerged gel using a disposable micropipet. DNA molecular weight markers should be run in parallel.
4. Close the lid of the electrophoresis unit and connect the power supply cables (positive at the bottom of the gel); apply 10V/cm.
5. When the Bromophenol blue dye in the loading buffer has migrated approx 2/3 of the gel length, turn off the power supply and examine the gel with a UV transillu-

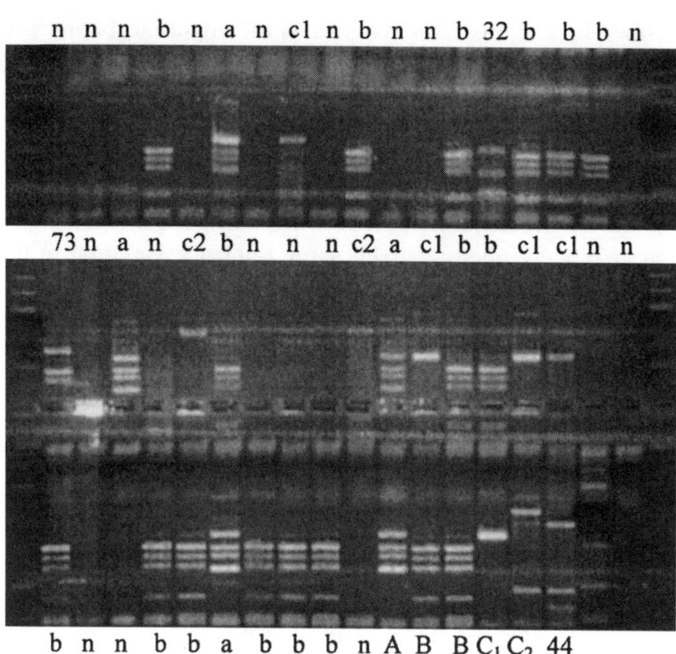

Fig. 1. Restriction fragment length patterns of a collection of enterococcal isolates. a = *vanA*, b = *vanB*, c1 = *vanC-1*, c2 = *vanC-2*, n = no restriction fragment pattern, 32 = isolate 32 (distinct restriction fragment pattern [*see* **Note 4**]), 73 = isolate 73 (vanB3 = distinct restriction fragment pattern—*see* **Note 4**, 44 = isolate 44 (distinct restriction fragment pattern—*see* **Note 4**), A = control *vanA*, isolate B7641, B = control *vanB* isolate V583, C_1 = control *vanC-1* isolate GS, and C_2 = control *vanC-2* isolate ATCC 25788. (Adapted with permission from Patel et al. *[5]*.)

minator. **Caution:** Wear UV protective eyewear and handle the gel with gloves. The pattern of the ethidium bromide-stained DNA fragments is visualized and can be documented by photography.

6. The RFLP may then be interpreted according to the patterns delineated in **Table 2** and shown in **Fig. 1** (*see* **Note 4**).

4. Notes

1. Since ethidium bromide is a powerful mutagen and is toxic, prepare in a fume hood and wear gloves when preparing the solution. Be aware of contaminating sources and apply methods for contamination prevention. Use of physically separated areas and equipment (pipets) for PCR and post-PCR procedures is recommended. Use personal reagent sets and pipets, and disposable bottles and tubes.
2. When setting up PCR, use of a master mix instead of pipeting single reactions is always recommended.

3. As described herein, this assay requires an overnight incubation because of the restriction enzyme digestion step. We have also successfully carried-out this assay using a two hour digestion.
4. We have noted that in some isolates of VRE, a PCR product is produced using our assay but with an amplicon which has a RFLP which differs from those found with the reference *vanA*, *vanB*, *vanC-1*, and *vanC-2* strains ***(5)***. We have detected sequence variability to account for the unique *Msp*I restriction enzyme patterns observed. We have found relatively large sequence variation in the *vanB* and *vanC-2* genes in enterococci, but not, to any great extent, in the *vanA* or *vanC-1* genes, using a PCR sequencing assay ***(6)***. Thus, if an unusual RFLP were detected, we would recommend sequencing the amplicon to confirm the PCR product identity ***(6)***. For example, two of the *vanB* enterococcal isolates which we have studied have a RFLP which differs from those of the reference *vanA*, *vanB*, *vanC-1*, and *vanC-2* strains. We have detected sequence variability to account for the unique *Msp*I restriction pattern observed and we have designated the gene found in these two isolates (one of which is shown as 73 in **Fig. 1**) *vanB3* ***(6)***.
5. This assay will detect DNA sequences of *vanC-2* and *vanC-3*, but because of significant sequence homology between these genes, DNA sequencing of PCR products is required to discriminate between them.
6. Dutka-Malen and colleagues, have also described a multiplex PCR reaction to detect glycopeptide-resistance genes in *Enterococcus* spp.; however our assay distinguishes itself in several ways ***(2)***. First, we inoculate a single bacterial colony from a blood agar plate directly into the PCR reaction mixture. Lysis is carried out by heating the mixture to 95°C for 10 min prior to cycling for amplification. This step saves time. Second, we have added a restriction enzyme digestion step to the assay that confirms the expected PCR product and lessens the chances for contamination or amplicon carryover.

References

1. Clark, N. C., Cooksey, R. C., Hill, B. C., Swenson, J. M., and Tenover, F. C. (1993) Characterization of glycopeptide-resistant enterococci from U.S. hospitals. *Antimicrob. Agent Chemother.* **37,** 2311–2317.
2. Dutka-Malen, S., Evers, S., and Courvalin, P. (1995) Detection of glycopeptide resistance genotypes and identification to the species level of clinically relevant enterococci by PCR. *J. Clin. Microbiol.* **33,** 24–27.
3. Dutka-Malen, S., Molinas, C., Arthur, M., and Courvalin, P. (1992) Sequence of the *vanC* gene of *Enterococcus gallinarum* BM4174 encoding a D-alanine:D-alanine ligase-related protein necessary for vancomycin resistance. *Gene* **112,** 53–58.
4. Navarro, F., and Courvalin, P. (1994) Analysis of genes encoding D-alanine-D-alanine ligase-related enzymes in *Enterococcus casseliflavus* and *Enterococcus flavescens. Antimicrob. Agent Chemother.* **38,** 1788–1793.

5. Patel, R., Uhl, J. R., Kohner, P., Hopkins, M.K., and Cockerill, F. R. (1997) Multiplex PCR detection of *vanA*, *vanB*, *vanC-1* and *vanC-2/3* genes in enterococci. *J. Clin. Microbiol.* **35,** 703–707.
6. Patel, R., Uhl, J. R., Kohner, P., Hopkins, M. K., Steckelberg, J. M., Kline, B., and Cockerill, F. R. (1998) DNA sequence variation within *vanA*, *vanB*, *vanC-1*, and *vanC-2/3* genes of clinical *Enterococcus* spp. isolates. *Antimicrob. Agent Chemother.* **42,** 202–205.

2

Drug Susceptibility of *Mycobacterium tuberculosis* Through the Mycolic Acid Index

José M. Viader-Salvadó, Martha Guerrero-Olazarán, Elvira Garza-González, and Rolando Tijerina-Menchaca

1. Introduction

The methods accepted to determine antimicrobial drug susceptibility of mycobacteria are based on the determination of the microorganisms' growth on solid or liquid medium containing a specified concentration of a single drug.

The development of susceptibility tests of slowly growing mycobacteria that are simple and of low cost is of great importance in order to have rapid access to the ideal patient treatment. With regard to tuberculosis this aim has more importance due to the resurgence of tuberculosis as a public health problem throughout the world and mainly due to the appearance of multidrug resistant strains.

Mycolic acids are α-alkyl-β-hydroxyacids of high molecular weight components of the cellular wall of, for example, genera *Mycobacterium*, *Nocardia*, *Rhodococcus*, and *Corynebacterium* microorganisms. Therefore, the presence of these compounds in a clinical sample or in a microorganism isolated from same indicates the presence of a microorganism that contains mycolic acids in its cellular wall. In 1986, W. R. Butler et al. *(1)* developed a method for the analysis of UV-absorbing p-bromophenacyl derivatives of mycolic acids using high-performance liquid chromatography (HPLC) and were able to differentiate the genera *Corynebacterium*, *Rhodococcus*, *Nocardia* and *Mycobacterium* through their mycolic acid patterns. In 1991, the same group of investigators *(2)* established a differentiation outline of several mycobacterial species through their mycolic acid patterns comparing the relative retention time of chromatographic peaks and their relative heights. In 1995, K. Jost et al. *(3)* proposed the employment of fluorescent 4-bromomethyl-6,7-dimethoxycoumarin

From: *Methods in Molecular Medicine, vol. 48: Antibiotic Resistance Methods and Protocols*
Edited by: S. H. Gillespie © Humana Press Inc., Totowa, NJ

derivatives of mycolic acids to differentiate diverse mycobacterial species in clinical samples and in liquid media increasing 200-fold the sensitivity of the detection. In 1996 the HPLC users group *(3)* published a standardized method for the identification of mycobacteria through p-bromophenacyl derivatives of mycolic acids analyzed by HPLC and later mycolic acid pattern standards for HPLC identification of mycobacteria were established *(5)*. Recently, E. Garza-González et al. *(6)* showed the utility of the Jost derivatization method in clinical isolates and in acid-fast stain-smear positive clinical specimens. The same group of investigators *(7)* described an exponential relationship between the total area of the mycolic acid (TAMA) peaks of a culture of *Mycobacterium tuberculosis* and the viable count obtained through the traditional plate count method after incubating a minimum of three weeks in Middlebrook 7H10 medium. Thus, the amount of mycolic acid in a microorganism suspension or clinical sample is a good indicator of the number of microorganisms present in the bacterial suspension or clinical sample. Thus, TAMA is a good surrogate marker for mycobacterial growth in cultures as the TAMA increases with comparison to the initial value. With this information and using the Jost derivatization method (3), we developed the rapid method to determine the drug susceptibility of *Mycobacterium tuberculosis* that is described here. It is based on the measurement of the mycolic acid index (MAI) defined by the rate of the mycolic acid increase during incubation in presence of a drug and the mycolic acid increase during incubation in absence of the drug. Both of these mycolic acid increases can be measured using the TAMA estimator or by any analytic technique that allows estimating the amount of mycolic acid. This method permits a fast result because the maximum necessary time to carry out the assay is five days. It is very accurate because there is a narrow exponential relationship between the growth of the culture as measured by colony forming units per milliliter and the synthesis of mycolic acids *(7)*.

2. Materials

2.1. Microorganism Suspension Preparation, Inoculation and Culture

All chemicals used in this method must be reagent-grade and all the water distilled.

1. Lowenstein-Jensen slant prepared according to manufacturer's instructions.
2. Tween-80 saline: 0.055% Tween-80 and 0.85% NaCl in water. Store in a refrigerator.
3. Glass beads of 1–2 mm diameter.
4. Isoniazid and rifampin stock solution: According to drug potency, prepare a 0.1-mg/mL isoniazid (isonicotinic acid hydrazide) and 1.0 mg/L rifampin solution in sterile distilled water. Dispense in 0.5-mL aliquots in amber vials, seal and store in a –70°C freezer until used. The day the drug is to be added to the

broth, remove from the freezer thaw to room temperature and use discarding the excess solution. Never refreeze.

5. Control test tube: Suspend 4.7 g of Middlebrook 7H9 powder in 900 mL of 0.055% Tween-80 in water and dispense in 180-mL aliquots in an Erlenmeyer flask of 500 mL. Autoclave at 121°C and 15 psi for 10 min, cool to 45°C and aseptically add 20 mL of Middlebrook OADC enrichment. Dispense the broth in 1-mL aliquots in 13 × 100 mm sterile tubes and incubate for 24 h at 35–37°C for sterility verification.
6. Isoniazid and rifampin test tubes: Add 0.2 mL of the isoniazid or rifampin stock solution into 100 mL of Middlebrook 7H9 broth. Dispense in 1-mL aliquots in 13 × 100 mm sterile tubes and incubate for 24 h at 35–37°C for sterility verification.
7. MacFarland 0.5 standard: Add 0.05 mL of 1% $BaCl_2$ to 9.95 mL of 1% H_2SO_4. Store at room temperature in the dark.

2.2. Mycolic Acid Analysis

All chemicals must be reagent-grade and solvents must be HPLC-grade.

1. 75% aqueous potassium hydroxide. Store at room temperature.
2. 6 *N* hydrochloric acid. Store at room temperature.
3. Potassium bicarbonate reagent: 0.2 *M* in water-methanol (1:1 v/v). Store at room temperature.
4. Derivatization reagent: 1.25 mg/mL of 4-bromomethyl-6,7-dimethoxycoumarin and 0.15 mg/mL of 18-crown-6 ether in CH_2Cl_2. The reagent is stable and can be stored for a long time in a freezer to avoid solvent evaporation.

3. Methods

3.1. Microorganism Suspension Preparation, Inoculation, and Culture

1. Scrape and transfer growth from a Lowenstein-Jensen slant culture to a 13 × 100 mm sterile screw cap tube containing six glass beads and 5 mL of Tween-80 saline (*see* **Note 1**).
2. Homogenize in a vortex for 15 min and allow the large particles to settle.
3. Remove the supernatant and transfer to a 13 × 100 mm sterile tube.
4. Adjust the absorbance at 625 nm of this suspension to a corresponding McFarland 0.5 standard with Tween-80 saline solution, being the microorganism suspension that will be assayed.
5. Inoculate 100 µL of this suspension into 2 control test tubes, 1 isoniazid test tube and 1 rifampin test.
6. After the inoculation, saponify one of the control test tubes (*see* **Note 2**) as below (in **Subheading 3.2., steps 1,2**).
7. Incubate the other control test tube as well as the drug test tubes at 35–37°C for 5 d with constant agitation.
8. After the incubation, determine the amount of mycolic acids through TAMA estimator for each tube.

3.2. Mycolic Acid Analysis

1. Add 0.5 mL of 75% KOH solution to each tube and mix gently.
2. Autoclave at 121°C and 15 psi for 1 h and cool to room temperature.
3. Acidify with 0.7 mL of HCl 6 *N* and add 0.7 mL of CH_2Cl_2 (*see* **Note 3**).
4. Cap the tube tightly, mix vigorously and allow the layers to separate (*see* **Note 4**).
5. Remove the bottom layer with a Pasteur pipet (*see* **Note 5**).
6. Extract the mycolic acids twice more with 0.7 mL of CH_2Cl_2 as described above.
7. Test the aqueous residue with 1% aqueous Congo red indicator for acid pH (blue), if not add 6 *N* HCl drops until acidification and re-extract three times.
8. Collect the organic extracts in a 13 × 100 mm screw-cap tube and evaporate to dryness heating at 60°C in a heating block.
9. Add to the dry mycolic acid extract 0.1 mL of 0.2 *M* $KHCO_3$ and evaporate to dryness heating at 90°C in a heating block and a nitrogen stream (*see* **Note 6**).
10. Cool to room temperature and add 0.5 mL of CH_2Cl_2 and 100 µL of derivatization reagent.
11. Cap the tube tightly, mix in a vortex for 30 s and heat at 90°C for 20 min (*see* **Note 7**).
12. Cool to room temperature and add 1 mL of 12 *N* HCl-methanol-water (1:2:1).
13. Mix thoroughly and remove the bottom organic phase with a Pasteur pipet (*see* **Note 5**).
14. Extract the aqueous phase twice more with 0.7 mL of CH_2Cl_2 as described above.
15. Collect organic extracts in a 2-mL microcentrifuge tube and evaporate to dryness heating at 40ºC in a heating block (*see* **Note 8**).
16. Dissolve the dry residue in 80 µL of freezer-cooled CH_2Cl_2 (*see* **Note 3**), centrifuge the mixture at 16000*g* (14,000 rpm) in a microcentrifuge for 3 s and inject immediately (*see* **Note 9**) a volume at least 3 times the loop volume into the liquid chromatographer (*see* **Note 10**) equipped with a Nova-Pack C18 150X 4.6 mm column (Waters Corporation, Milford, MA), a Nova-Pak C18 20X 3.9 mm guard column (Waters Corporation) and a 157 fluorescence detector (Beckman Instruments, Inc., San Ramon, CA) with an excitation filter of 305–395 nm and an emission filter of 430–470 nm (*see* **Note 11**). A methanol-methylene chloride gradient elution at a flow rate of 2.5 mL/min is used with an initial solvent condition of 98% methanol-2% CH_2Cl_2, concentration of CH_2Cl_2 increased linearly to 20% in 1 min, to 65% in 10 min, to 95% in 5 min, and decreased linearly to 2% in 10 min (*see* **Note 12**). The next injection can be carried out immediately if required (*see* **Note 13**).
17. For each chromatogram, determine TAMA of peaks at retention times between 7 and 10 min (*see* **Note 14**).

3.3. MAI Determination

1. Calculate the MAI of the microorganism suspension according to the following equation:

$$MAI = MA_{D5} - MA_0 / MA_5 - MA_0$$

where MAI represents the mycolic acid index, MA_{D5} represents the total amount of mycolic acids of the microorganism suspension, evaluated by the TAMA estimation, incubated 5 d in the presence of the drug to be evaluated (drug test tube), MA_5 represents the total amount of mycolic acids of the microorganism suspension, evaluated by the TAMA estimation, incubated 5 d in the absence of the drug to be evaluated (incubated control test tube), and MA_0 represents the total amount of mycolic acids of the microorganism suspension, evaluated by the TAMA estimation, before the initial incubation (nonincubated control test tube).

2. Interpret the results as isoniazid-resistant or isoniazid-susceptible strain if MAI to isoniazid is greater or less than 0.15, respectively. Similar interpretation can be done for rifampin.

4. Notes

1. A biological safety cabinet, an isolation room under one-pass negative pressure, approved masks, gloves and eye protection are needed for all the steps in **Subheading 3.1.** following the recommendations of Kent and Kubica *(8)*.
2. If it is not possible to saponify immediately, samples can be frozen at –20°C and processed later with the other tubes.
3. Adding the CH_2Cl_2 with an automatic pipet and passing three times CH_2Cl_2 through the pipet tip before taking the required volume, is recommended.
4. Centrifugation can be used to accelerate the layer separation.
5. Using new Pasteur pipets with a pipet pump to facilitate quantitative extraction is recommended to avoid loss of CH_2Cl_2 drops in the transfer process. When the Pasteur pipet is introduced into the bottom layer, softly expel one or two airdrops. Be careful; do not transfer any of the aqueous layer.
6. It is also possible to use air instead of nitrogen stream.
7. It is convenient to check previously the seal of the screw-cap tubes so that they do not leak methylene chloride in this step. Derivatization yields higher than 95% are easily achieved. The catalyst is a 18-crown-6 ether that enhances the solubility of the potassium ion in the organic solvent and increases the reactivity of the carboxylate.
8. Evaporation temperature must not be higher than 40°C to avoid boiling.
9. Dissolution, centrifugation, and injection must be performed with no delay, because evaporation of methylene chloride will cause the sample to concentrate.
10. A loop of 10 or 20 µL is sufficient, then inject at least 30 or 60 µL, respectively. If an autosampler is used, inject preferably 20 µL. After the injection, clean the syringe at least three times with methylene chloride. Never introduce water into the syringe because of possible blockage. To increase retention time reproducibility a column oven at 30°C can be used.
11. Other similar chromatographic columns as well as other fluorescent detectors can be used. If a spectrofluorometer is used as detector, the excitation and emission wavelengths must be set at 365 and 410 nm, respectively. Never use the column with water because of possible blockage.

12. A gradient of methylene chloride is continued after the retention time of mycolic acids to ensure a complete column wash in every injection, which avoids the possibility of sample carry-over.
13. An extra time is not necessary between injections because the column is equilibrated with the mobile phase at the time that the gradient is returning to initial conditions.
14. The determination of TAMA could be automated, setting the integration software to integrate only between 7 to 10 min; and then, reporting by total addition the total area of all the detected peaks.

Acknowledgments

The authors acknowledge the importance of grant No. 970402004 from "Sistema de Investigación Alfonso Reyes" and No. SA093-98 from "Programa de Apoyo a la Investigacion Cientifica y Tecnologica of the Universidad Autonoma de Nuevo Leon" for this work, Secretaria de Salud del Estado de Nuevo Leon for financial support, Hospital Universitario " Jose Eleuterio Gonzales" and Laboratorio Estatal de Salud in Monterrey, N. L. Mexico for providing samples, María de la Luz Acevedo-Duarte's technical support and Professor R. M. Chandler-Burns' stylistic suggestions in the preparation of this manuscript.

References

1. Butler, W. R. and Ahearn, D. G. (1986) High-performance liquid chromatography of mycolic acids as a tool in the identification of *Corynebacterium*, *Nocardia*, *Rhodococcus*, and *Mycobacterium* species. *J. Clin. Microbiol.* **23,** 182–185.
2. Butler, W. R., Jost, K. C., Jr., and Kilburn, J. O. (1991) Identification of mycobacteria by high-performance liquid chromatography. *J. Clin. Microbiol.* **29,** 2468–2472.
3. Jost, K. C., Jr., Dunbar, D. F., Barth, S. S., Headley, V. L., and Elliott, L. B. (1995) Identification of *Mycobacterium tuberculosis* and *M. avium* complex directly from smear-positive sputum specimens and BACTEC 12B cultures by high-performance liquid chromatography with fluorescence detection and computer-driven pattern recognition models. *J. Clin. Microbiol.* **33,** 1270–1277.
4. Butler, W. R., Floyd, M. M., Silcox, V., Cage, G., Desmond, E., Duffey, P. S., Guthertz, L. S., Gross, W., Jost, K. C., Ramos, L. S., Thibert, L., and Warren, N., eds. Steering Committee, HPLC Users Group (1996) Standardized method for HPLC identification of mycobacteria, U.S. Department of Health and Human Services, Washington, DC.
5. Butler, W. R., Floyd, M. M., Silcox, V., Cage, G., Desmond, E., Duffey, P. S., Guthertz, L. S., Gross, W., Jost, K. C., Ramos, L. S., Thibert, L., and Warren, N., eds. Steering Committee, HPLC Users Group (1999) Mycolic acid pattern standards for HPLC identification of mycobacteria, U.S. Department of Health and Human Services, Washington, DC.

6. Garza-González, E., Guerrero-Olazaran, M., Tijerinα-Menchaca, R., and Viader-Salvado, J. M., (1998) Identification of mycobacteria by mycolic acid pattern. *Arch Med Res* **29,** 303–306.
7. Garza-González, E., Guerrero-Olazaran, M., Tijerinα-Menchaca, R., and Viader-Salvado, J. M., (1997) Determination of drug susceptibility of *Mycobacterium tuberculosis* through mycolic acid analysis. *J. Clin. Microbiol.* **35,** 1287–1289.
8. Kent, P. T. and Kubica, G. P. (1985) Public Health Mycobacteriology: A Guide For The Level III Laboratory. U. S. Department of Health and Human Services publication no. 86–8230. U.S. Department of Health and Human Services, Washington, DC.

3

Micro-Well Phage Replication Assay for Screening Mycobacteria for Resistance to Rifampin and Streptomycin

Ruth McNerney

1. Introduction

Phenotypic methods for screening *Mycobacterium tuberculosis* or *Mycobacterium ulcerans* for susceptibility to therapeutic drugs are necessarily slow due to the protracted growth times of these bacteria. Rapid testing is now possible for the potent antituberculosis drug rifampicin using molecular methods to detect those mutations that confer resistance *(1,2)*. However, the high cost and requirement for specialized equipment may prohibit the application of this technology in resource-poor settings and there is a need for low-cost, rapid tests that are appropriate for use in low-income countries.

One approach that has shown much promise uses bacteriophages to infect the mycobacteria under test. Bacteriophages capable of infecting mycobacteria were first described over fifty years ago and currently more than 250 mycobacteriophages (phages) with a wide range of host specificities are described *(3)*. The construction of luciferase reporter phages by Jacobs and colleagues in 1993 stimulated renewed interest in using phages for rapid susceptibility testing *(4)*. These recombinant phages are able to express the luciferase gene although infecting a mycobacterium and, when the substrate luciferin is added in the presence of adenosine triphosphate (ATP), light is emitted that can be detected by a luminometer or with photosensitive film. Drugs that block phage replication inhibit the production of light and this ingenious technology permits testing of *M. tuberculosis* against rifampin within hours whereas slower acting drugs such as ethambutol, isoniazid, and ciprofloxacin can be tested in two to three days *(5,6)*. Although rapid and simple to perform this technology requires reagents that are not readily avail-

From: *Methods in Molecular Medicine, vol. 48: Antibiotic Resistance Methods and Protocols*
Edited by: S. H. Gillespie © Humana Press Inc., Totowa, NJ

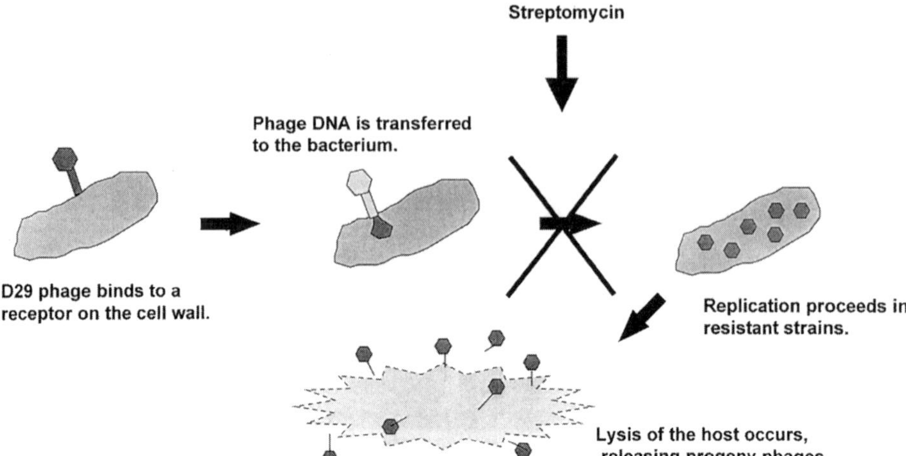

Fig. 1. Streptomycin blocks phage replication in susceptible strains of mycobacteria.

able in developing countries and alternative "low-tech" phages technologies have been developed.

The effect of antituberculosis drugs on the growth of mycobacteriophages was first investigated by Tokunaga and Sellers who, in 1965, demonstrated that streptomycin blocked phage replication in susceptible *M. smegmatis* although not affecting replication in a drug-resistant strain *(7)* (*see* **Fig. 1**). Similar effects were shown with kanamycin *(8)* and rifampicin *(9)* however, when ethambutol was examined it was found to only inhibit phage replication in a proportion of the bacteria. This partial effect was thought to be due to the mode of action of the drug and the unsynchronized nature of the bacterial culture as ethambutol is not active during all phases of the cell cycle *(10)*. In 1980, David and colleagues working at the Institut Pasteur in Paris investigated the inhibitory effects of clofazimine, colistin, rifampicin, streptomycin, dapsone, isoniazid and ethambutol on mycobacteriophage replication *(11)*. As a result of their investigations they concluded that phages could be successfully used to screen for antibacterial agents and that they might be useful when testing mycobacteria that were difficult to grow *(11)*.

The group in Paris worked with Mycobacteriophage D29, a lytic virus that is able to infect and replicate both in slow-growing pathogenic mycobacteria such as *Mycobacterium tuberculosis* and the relatively fast growing saprophytic strains such as *Mycobacterium smegmatis*. Detection of replication and the production of progeny phages was by the traditional method of plating in a lawn of susceptible bacteria where repeated cycles of infection and lysis cause

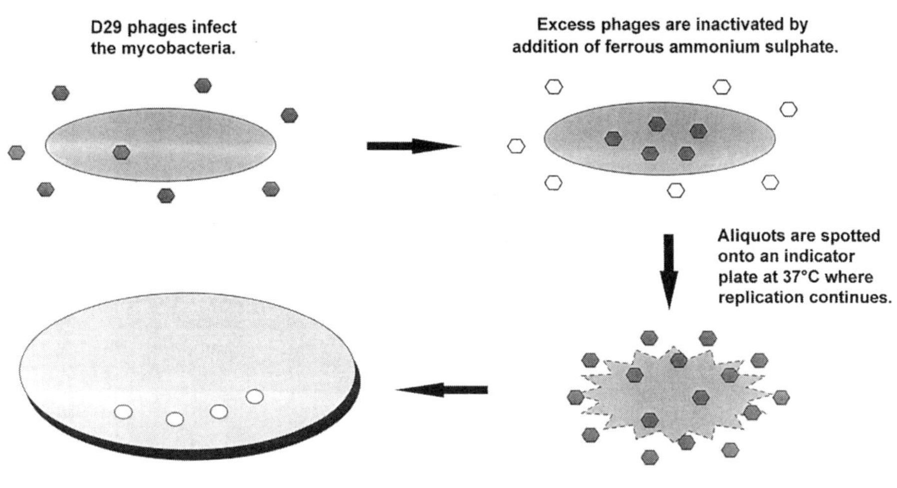

Fig. 2. Outline of phage replication. Inactivation of extra-cellular phages allows simple detection of replication.

clear areas within the bacterial lawn known as plaques. When plating on a lawn of *M. smegmatis*, the plaques were visible following overnight incubation and, by using D29, they were able to adopt *M. smegmatis* as a universal indicator mycobacterium for rapid detection of phages propagated in slow-growing strains ***(12)***.

To facilitate the detection of progeny phages that have resulted from a successful infection it is desirable, following infection of host bacteria, to remove excess free viruses from the culture media. Inactivation of exogenous phages may be achieved using chemical reagents such as acid or sodium hydroxide that destroy the phages but not the more resilient mycobacteria. However, reaction conditions have to be carefully controlled in order to prevent damage to host bacteria by these toxic reagents. The discovery that ferrous salts inactivate D29 phages although not harming mycobacteria or those phages replicating inside them has enabled development of robust methods of detecting phage replication ***(13)*** (*see* **Fig. 2**). Rapid screening for susceptibility to rifampicin and streptomycin may be undertaken and results obtained from isolates of *M. tuberculosis* or *M. ulcerans* growing on Lowenstein-Jensen in less than 48 h. A convenient micro-well plate format has been adopted to speed the process and enable the screening of large numbers of isolates.

Phages can only replicate in bacteria that are metabolically active and when working with slow-growing mycobacteria isolated on solid media it is necessary to incubate the bacteria in broth for at least 18 h before use if efficient rates of infection are to be achieved. Bacteria taken from the slope are suspended in broth and mixed with the appropriate concentration of the drug under test in the wells of a sterile microtiter plate. Each isolate is exposed to zero, 2 mg/L, and 10 mg/L of the drug under test and incubated at 37°C. Test wells of a reference susceptible strain of bacteria are also included for comparison. The next day D29 phages are added to each well and the plate incubated at 37°C, to permit infection. During the latent period of infection, prior to lysis of the host bacteria, excess phages are inactivated by addition of ferrous ammonium sulphate to a final concentration of 10 m*M*. Small (10–15 µL) aliquots of this mixture are then spotted onto pre-prepared *M. smegmatis* indicator plates.

Following overnight incubation at 37°C any viable phages in the mixture will have formed visible plaques in the bacterial lawn, each plaque representing a single infected colony forming unit of mycobacteria. Large numbers of plaques should be visible from those samples of bacteria incubated at zero drug concentration. If the bacteria are susceptible to the drug under test then no plaques will be seen in those samples incubated with concentrations of drug above the breakpoint whereas plaques will be produced by resistant strains. Those strains able to support phage replication at drug concentrations above those tolerated by the wild-type reference strain are classed as resistant (*see* **Fig. 3**). The assay described here has been optimized for slow-growing *M. tuberculosis* and *M. ulcerans* isolates grown of Lowenstein-Jensen slopes but D29 phages are able to infect other species of mycobacteria and the test can be adapted to screen fast-growing species. However, for accurate results incubation times need to be adjusted due to the more rapid cycle of infection in these organisms. Similarly, when testing drugs such as ethambutol and isoniazid that do not directly block phage replication longer drug exposures are required and stains cannot be tested directly from the slope ***(14)***.

Stocks of the phages and *M. smegmatis* indicator bacteria may be maintained "in-house" and indicator plates may be prepared in advance and stored at 4°C. The method requires no specialized equipment other than that utilized in the routine microbiology laboratory; however, when handling *M. tuberculosis* or *M. ulcerans* all work should be performed in a bio-safety containment facility.

2. Materials

2.1. Production of D29 Phage Stocks

1. Bacteriophage D29 ***(15)***.
2. *M. smegmatis* stains including *M. smegmatis* 607 (American Type Culture Collection) for propagation of phage D29 (*see* **Note 1**). Prepared stocks of phages should remain viable for several months when stored at 4°C and for over 12 months if lyophilized (*see* **Note 6**).

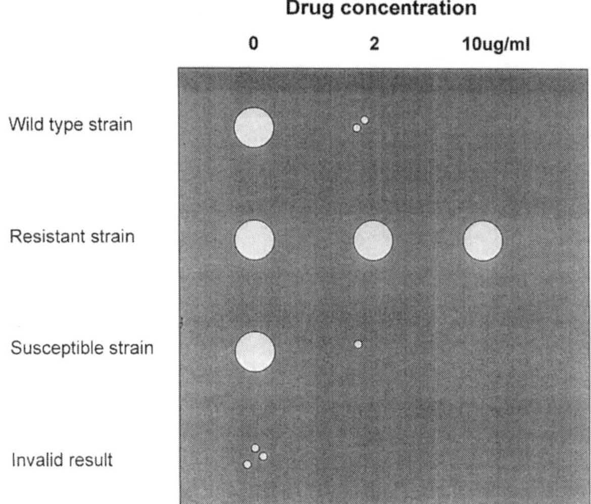

Fig 3.

3. Middlebrook 7H9 or Luria-Bertani broth may be used to perform the assay and should be prepared according to the manufacturers instructions (*see* **Note 3**). Middlebrook 7H9 requires supplementation with 10 v/v OADC and 1 m*M* calcium chloride. Luria-Bertani broth requires supplementation with 0.2% glucose and 1 m*M* calcium chloride.
4. 1.5% Bacto agar.
5. Triple vented 90 mm Petri dishes.
6. Disposable 1 µL plastic inoculation loops are used to inoculate cultures with *M. tuberculosis* or *M. ulcerans*.

2.2. Phage Assay

1. *M. tuberculosis* isolates (*see* **Note 9**).
2. *M. ulcerans* isolates .
3. Lowenstein-Jensen slopes
4. Sterile flat bottom 96-well microtiter plates with lids.
5. Stock drug solutions of 50 mg/mL rifampicin in dimethyl formamide and 10 mg/mL streptomycin sulphate in water may be stored at –20°C for up to six months.

3. Method

3.1. Production of Mycobacteriophage D29 Stocks

1. Dilute phage stock to approx 4×10^3 pfu/mL in Middlebrook 7H9 broth with 10% OADC. Spread 100 µL over the surface of a 90 mm agar plate prepared with 1.5% Bacto agar in Middlebrook 7H9 with 10% OADC and a 10% vol of

stationary phase *M. smegmatis* culture. Place in 37°C incubator and leave overnight.

2. The next day examine for bacterial growth, large numbers of plaques should be visible, but lysis of the bacterial lawn should not be complete. If lysis is 100% with none of the bacterial lawn visible repeat plating with a more dilute suspension of phages.
3. Add 10 mL of broth to the plate and return to 37°C incubator.
4. Aliquot and store at 4°C. Do not freeze. Do not expose to UV light or leave in the sun. Sodium azide may be added to a final concentration of 0.1% as a preservative (*see* **Notes 5** and **6**).
5. Quantify the concentration of the phage stock by making 10-fold dilutions to 10^{10} and spotting 10 μL aliquots of each dilution onto an indicator plate. Count the number of pfu visible after overnight incubation at 37°C. Always use a fresh pipet tip for each dilution. The stock produced should contain between 10^9 and 10^{10} pfu/mL.

3.2. Production of Indicator Plates

1. Streak *M. smegmatis* on 1.5% agar in Middlebrook 7H9 with 10% OADC and grow at 37°C for 3 days. Store sealed at 4°C for up to 3 wk.
2. Take a single colony and inoculate 300 mL Middlebrook 7H9 broth with 10% OADC in a 500 mL bottle.
3. Incubate at 37°C with shaking for 2 d until stationary phase is reached.
4. Store at 4°C until required (up to one month). Before using, gently mix the suspension and leave to stand for a few minutes to allow any large clumps to settle.
5. Prepare molten 1.5% agar in Luria-Bertani broth cooled to approx 45°C. Add a 10–15% vol of *M. smegmatis* culture. Mix by inversion and pour into 90 mm Petri dishes (*see* Note 7).
6. Allow to set and store at 4°C for up to 2 wk. Seal the plates to prevent drying. If necessary before using, dry the indicator plates by placing in an incubator for up to 30 min to remove any surface liquid. Label plates with a marker pen.

3.3. Micro-Well Phage Replication Assay

Mycobacterium tuberculosis and *Mycobacterium ulcerans* are class III pathogens and *M. tuberculosis* is highly infectious via the respiratory route. All work with these organisms should take place within P3 containment facilities including use of a Class I microbiological safety cabinet. Disposal is by phenol-based disinfectants and autoclaving.

1. Prepare dilutions of the drug at 2X the test concentration in assay broth (Middlebrook 7H9 broth with 10% OADC and 1 m*M* calcium chloride) (*see* **Note 8**). Place 75 μL aliquots of zero, 4 mg/L and 20 mg/L drug in the wells of a sterile microtiter plate.
2. Prepare bacteria by adding a 1 μL loop of culture from the LJ slope to 2 mL assay broth in a bijou bottle with 4–8 3 mm diameter glass beads.

3. Vortex for 20 s to disperse the bacteria and leave to stand for a 3 min to allow aerosols to settle.
4. Process a reference susceptible strain of the species of mycobacteria under test.
5. Place 75 μL of the bacterial suspension in each well containing the appropriate concentration of drug (*see* **Note 9**).
6. Cover plate and seal in a plastic bag before incubating at 37°C for 24 h (*see* **Note 10**).
7. Dilute phages in assay broth to 10^8/mL with the appropriate concentration of drug (0, 2, or 10 mg/L) and add 50 μL to the appropriate wells. Reseal plate and replace in 37°C incubator for between 60 and 90 min.
8. Prepare indicator plates by labeling and if necessary place in the incubator to dry surface moisture.
9. Shortly before required prepare 30 m*M* ferrous ammonium sulphate hexahydrate solution in Middlebrook 7H9 broth. Add 100 μL to each well.
10. Mix the contents of each well using a fresh pipet tip before placing a 10 μL drop on the surface of the indicator plate (*see* **Note 11**). When the drops have been absorbed plates may be sealed in plastic bags and placed in the incubator. If care is taken up to 12 samples (four strains) may be spotted on a single 90 mm plate.
11. Next morning examine the plates for lysis and record results (*see* **Note 12**). Strains are classed as resistant if plaques continue to be produced in samples incubated with higher concentrations of drug than for the wild-type as shown in **Fig. 3**. If a strain fails to produce a high degree of lysis in the zero drug sample (i.e., so few pfu that individual plaques can be easily discerned) then the result is invalid and the test should be repeated. If no plaques are seen in the zero drug sample then those bacteria are either dead, dormant, or not susceptible to infection by the phage. Repeat with a fresh culture and confirm that the correct species has been used. If plaques are seen in all wells, including drug treated wild-type stains then inactivation of phages failed. Repeat assay using fresh ferrous ammonium sulphate (*see* **Note 13**).

4. Notes

1. I use a derivative of *M. smegmatis* 607, *M. smegmatis* mc^{2}155 ***(16)***, that was obtained from William R. Jacobs Jr., Howard Hughes Medical Institute, Albert Einstein College of Medicine, New York.
2. When testing susceptibility to streptomycin a resistant strain should be used for the indicator plate and *M. smegmatis* SMR5 ***(17)*** used in this work was obtained from Peter Sander, Institut fur Medizinische Mikrobiologie, Hanover, Germany. Stocks of bacteria may be maintained in-house as described.
3. Middlebrook 7H9 or Luria-Bertani broth (LB) (Difco Laboratories, Detriot, MI) may be used to perform the assay and should be prepared according to the manufacturers instructions. LB may also be prepared from its constituents: bactrotrypone (1%), yeast extract (0.5%), and sodium chloride (1%). Middlebrook broth requires supplementation with OADC (Difco, Detriot, MI). A supplement of 0.2% glucose is added when LB is used as assay broth. Infection by D29 is

enhanced by the addition of 1 m*M* calcium to the culture media. The detergent polyoxyethylenesorbitan (Tween) may not be included as it blocks adsorption of phages to the cell wall.

4. It is important to avoid contamination of mycobacterial cultures with phages. In the event of accidental spillage work surfaces and instruments may be cleaned with bleach and 70% alcohol.
5. Sodium azide is toxic and may cause explosive mixtures in the presence of copper. Manufacturers safety data sheets and local safety regulations should be consulted before handling this substance.
6. For long term storage of phages or shipping under difficult conditions freeze dry with 10% 0.75M trehalose. Following lyophilization store at room temperature, avoid exposure to UV light. Rehydrate by adding sterile water to the original volume.
7. When mixing indicator bacteria with molten agar take care not to let the agar mix get too cool; if the mix starts to gel the smegmatis bacteria will not blend sufficiently to provide a uniform lawn. Take care not to damage the bacteria by mixing while the media is too hot. It is convenient to pour 40 mL of the melted agar mix into sterile 50 mL centrifuge tubes, let them cool before adding 5 mL of supplement and top up with 5–10 mL of smegmatis. Use a water bath at 45°C when handling large volumes.
8. Drug stocks are stored frozen, dilution to the appropriate drug concentration are made in assay broth and should be prepared daily.
9. Optimum results are obtained from young healthy cultures. It is recommend that cultures of *M. tuberculosis* over 12-wk-old, those that are contaminated, and those stored at 4°C be subcultured before testing. Cultures of *M. ulcerans* should be maintained at 32°C.
10. Plates are sealed in plastic bags to prevent drying by evaporation and to enhance safety. For additional protection plates or tubes containing infectious material should be placed in sealed plastic boxes.
11. When testing rifampin bacterial strains such as *M. smegmatis* 607 or mc^{2}155 may be used as the indicator bacteria as they are naturally resistant to this drug. However, when testing susceptibility to streptomycin a resistant strain such as *M. smegmatis* SMR5 ***(17)*** should be used as the indicator strain. Plates are prepared in the same manner as for mc^{2}155; however stocks of this bacteria should be maintained in 20 μg/mL streptomycin.
12. If plaques on the indicator plate are indistinct because of poor growth of the *M. smegmatis* lawn leave at 37°C for longer. Use a fresh batch of *M. smegmatis* or increase the volume added when preparing the plates. Check the indicator bacteria are not added when the temperature of the molten agar is above 50°C.
13. If plaques are indistinct check that calcium was added to the assay broth. Checks on the viability of phage stocks should be performed. If a precipitate is observed on the indicator plates following spotting then the concentration of ferrous ammonium sulphate or calcium chloride was too high, less precipitation is observed when using Luria broth than with Middlebrook 7H9. For enhanced visualization of plaques add 20 μL/mL yellow food coloring (Egg yellow, Supercook, Leeds, UK) to the molten agar mix.

Acknowledgments

The work described here was funded by the Department for International Development, U.K.

References

1. Telenti, A., Imboden, P., Marchesi, F., Lowrie, D., Cole, S., Colston, M. J., Matter, L., Schopfer, K., and Bodmer, T. (1993) Detection of rifampicin-resistance mutations in *Mycobacterium tuberculosis. Lancet* **341,** 647–650
2. De Beenhouwer, H., Lhiang, Z., Jannes, G., Mijs, W., Machtelinckx, L., Rossau, R., Traore, H., and Portaels, F. (1995) Rapid detection of rifampicin resistance in sputum and biopsy specimens from tuberculosis patients by PCR and line probe assay. *Tuber. Lung Dis.* **76,** 425–430.
3. McNerney, R. (1999) TB: the return of the phage. A review of fifty years of mycobacteriophage research. *Int. J. Tuberc. Lung Dis.* **3,** 179–184.
4. Jacobs, W. R., Jr., Barletta, R. G., Udani, R., Chan, J., Kalkut, G., Sosne, G., Kieser, T., Sarkis, G. J., Hatfull, G. F., and Bloom, B. R. (1993). Rapid assessment of drug susceptibilities of *Mycobacterium tuberculosis* by means of luciferase reporter phages. *Science* **260,** 819–822.
5. Riska, P. F. and Jacobs, W. R., Jr. (1998) The use of luciferase-reporter phage for antibiotic-susceptibility testing of mycobacteria, in *Methods in Molecular Biology* (Parish, T. and Stoker, N. G., eds.), Humana, Totowa, NJ, pp. 431–455.
6. Riska, P. F., Su, Y., Bardarov, S., Freundlich, L., Sarkis, G., Hatfull, G., Carriere, C., Kumar, V., Chan, J., and Jacobs, W. R., Jr. (1999) Rapid film-based determination of antibiotic susceptibilities of *Mycobacterium tuberculosis* strains by using a luciferase reporter phage and the Bronx Box. *J. Clin. Microbiol.* **37,** 1144–1149.
7. Tokunaga, T. and Sellers, M. I. (1965) Streptomycin induction of premature lysis of bacteriophage-infected mycobacteria. *J. Bacteriol.* **89,** 37–538.
8. Nakamura, R. M., Tokunaga, T., and Murohashi, T. (1967) Premature lysis of bacteriophage-infected mycobacteria induced by kanamycin. *Am. Rev. Respir. Dis.* **96,** 542–544.
9. Jones, W. D., Jr. and David, H. L. (1971) Inhibition by rifampin of mycobacteriophage D29 replication in its drug-resistant host, *Mycobacterium smegmatis* ATCC 607. *Am Rev Respir Dis* **103,** 618–624.
10. Phillips, L. M. and Sellers, M. I. (1970) Effects of ethambutol, actinomycin D and mitomycin C on the biosynthesis of D29-infected *Mycobacterium smegmatis*, in *Host-virus Relationships in Mycobacterium, Nocardia and Actinomyces* (Juhasz, S. E. and Plummer, G., eds.), Charles C. Thomas, Springfield, IL, pp. 80–102.
11. David, H. L., Clavel, S., Clement, F., Moniz, and Pereira, J. (1980) Effects of antituberculosis and antileprosy drugs on mycobacteriophage D29 growth. *Antimicrob. Agents Chemother.* **18,** 357–359.
12. David, H. L., Clavel, S., and Clement, F. (1980) Adsorption and growth of the bacteriophage D29 in selected mycobacteria. *Ann. Virol.* **13,** 167–184.
13. McNerney, R., Wilson, S. M., Sidhu, A. M., Harley, V. S., al Suwaidi, Z., Nye, P. M., Parish, T., and Stoker, N. G. (1998) Inactivation of mycobacteriophage D29

using ferrous ammonium sulphate as a tool for the detection of viable *Mycobacterium smegmatis* and *M. tuberculosis*. *Res. Microbiol.* **149,** 487–495.

14. Wilson, S. M., al Suwaidi, Z., McNerney, R., Porter, J., and Drobniewski, F. (1997) Evaluation of a new rapid bacteriophage-based method for the drug susceptibility testing of *Mycobacterium tuberculosis*. *Nat. Med.* **3,** 465–468.
15. Froman, S., Will, D. W., and Bogen, E. (1954). Bacteriophage active against virulent *Mycobacterium tuberculosis*. I. Isolation and activity. *Am. J. Publ. Hlth.* **44,** 1326.
16. Snapper, S. B., Melton, R. E., Mustafa, S., Kieser, T., and Jacobs, W. R., Jr. (1990) Isolation and characterization of efficient plasmid transformation mutants of *Mycobacterium smegmatis*. *Mol. Microbiol.* **4,** 1911–1919.
17. Sander, P., Meier, A., and Bottger, E. C. (1995) rspL+: a dominant selectable marker for gene replacement in mycobacteria. *Mol Microbiol* **16,** 991–1000.

4

Application of SSCP to Identification of Resistance Mutations

Timothy D. McHugh

1. Introduction

There has been a significant increase in the number of genes associated with antibiotic resistance that have been described. For many antimicrobials all of the principal genes associated with their action have been identified *(1)*. There is increasing interest in the epidemiological distribution of resistance mutations of these genes and research into their origin and routes of transmission. At the more fundamental level, there is interest in the impact of such mutations on the fitness/survivability of the pathogen *(2)*. We have described the strategies for selection of mutants in the mycobacteria *(3)* and also a polymerase chain reaction—single-stranded conformational polymorphism (PCR-SSCP) approach to investigation of the distribution of such mutants. In this method PCR amplimers are denatured to form single-stranded nucleic acids and then submitted to gel electrophoresis to identify sequence polymorphisms. Sequencing of clones remains relatively expensive and time consuming for investigating a large number of isolates from clinical practice or strains from mutation experiments. This chapter outlines a method for screening large numbers of PCR amplimers, which can then inform rational selection for cloning and sequence analysis, or for identifying novel mutations for detailed sequence. Alternatively, this approach can be used for rapid screening where the SSCP profile relating to each mutation is already known.

1.2. Single-Stranded Conformational Polymorphism (SSCP)

Gel electrophoresis separates nucleic acids on the basis of mobility through a matrix. In agarose gel electrophoresis it is the size of the molecule that is most important and in polyacrylamide electrophoresis, as used in a sequencing

From: *Methods in Molecular Medicine, vol. 48: Antibiotic Resistance Methods and Protocols*
Edited by: S. H. Gillespie © Humana Press Inc., Totowa, NJ

gel, the factors with the most influence on mobility are the molecular mass and the net charge of the molecule. By adjusting the gel running conditions it is possible to refine these variables further, so that the shape or conformation of the molecule has a consistent and reproducible effect on the mobility of the molecule. This is the principle underlying SSCP, in which polymorphism in the conformation of single-stranded nucleic acid (usually DNA PCR amplimers) is demonstrated on a polyacrylamide gel format. In the first instance polyacrylamide gels were used and the running temperature was held at a constant predetermined level, routinely 20°C or 30°C, to demonstrate polymorphism in PCR amplimers of the genes of interest. This approach has proved successful in many genome screening projects ***(4–6)*** and with visualization using radiolabeled PCR amplimers, is said to achieve a sensitivity of 1 base pair change/400 nucleotides ***(7)***.

In order to achieve reproducible results using temperature controlled SSCP, careful and precise monitoring of the gel temperature is essential. This requires either expensive equipment or the undivided attention of the experimenter over the gel running time. This problem is overcome with the use of the commercially available acrylamide analog MDE® (Flowgen). Use of this matrix removes the need for temperature regulation beyond that of routine manual sequencing but retains the same degree of sensitivity.

Visualization of bands on the gel is often achieved by incorporation of either ^{35}S or ^{32}P nucleotides in the initial PCR reactions. In an attempt to reduce the risks associated with ionizing radiation silver staining protocols optimized for sequencing gels are a practical alternative and are readily available in a commercial kit (Promega). These have proved to be satisfactory in routine use in our laboratory. The inconvenience of the extra stages incorporated in gel manipulation is easily outweighed by the expense and hazards of use and disposal of radioactive materials.

1.3. Polymorphism in the rpo*B of* Mycobacterium tuberculosis

We have successfully used the MDE gel format with silver staining in a variety of applications including analysis of the polymorphism in the *lyt*A gene of *Streptococcus pneumoniae* ***(8)*** and extensively in the analysis of drug resistance mutations in *Mycobacterium tuberculosis*, particularly in reference to the pyrazinamidase gene (*pza*) ***(9)*** and RNA polymerase (*rpo*B) ***(3)***. To illustrate the use of this methodology in identification of drug resistance mutations, PCR-SSCP of *rpo*B is described here, but the method is readily adaptable to genes from other bacterial species.

Approximately 95% of rifampin resistance in *M. tuberculosis* can be ascribed to an 81 base pair hot-spot in the RNA polymerase B gene ***(1)***. The range of mutations observed in clinical practice has been defined and although more than 36 mutations have been recorded, 3 mutations account for 74% of those observed. Telenti et al. *(6)* first used a SSCP format to identify the *rpo*B mutations observed in their clinical practice. The methodology described here was established as a tool for the rapid screening of large numbers in vitro selected mutants, although it has proven useful in the analysis of clinical isolates.

Using published data relating to the resistance hot spot a PCR amplification protocol was designed to create an amplimer spanning the hot spot and giving a fragment size of 120 bp. A simple DNA extraction protocol is described using boiling of colony picks. The PCR product is processed directly for SSCP without prior purification steps. These two features reduce the workload markedly and make the approach efficient for screening of large numbers of single colonies. Following PCR amplification, the PCR product is sampled, denatured with SSCP buffer and loaded directly to the vertical format gel. The gel is run overnight and then developed using the silver staining technology. Permanent images can be produced by direct exposure of the gel to photographic film, by scanning the gel into a computer package or by photography.

2. Materials

2.1. Organisms and DNA Extraction

1. Sterile deionized water.
2. Microcentrifuge.

2.2. RNA Polymerase B (rpoB) PCR

1. Sterile deionized water.
2. 10X PCR buffer: 500 m*M* KCl, 100 m*M* Tris-HCl (pH 8.8 at 25°C), 15 m*M* $MgCl_2$, 1% Triton X-100.
3. Nucleotide mix containing: 10 m*M* each dATP, dCTP, dGTP, and dTTP.
4. Primers at a concentration of 10 µ*M* each:
   5'-AGT TCT TCG GCA CCA GC-3' and
   5'-CGC TCA CGT GAC AGA CC-3'
5. BIOTAQ® DNA polymerase 5 U/µL (Bioline London, UK).
6. Positive control DNA, 10 ng/µL genomic DNA prepared from *M. tuberculosis* H37Rv.
7. Mineral oil.
8. Thermal cycler (Hybaid Omnigene III London, UK).

2.3. SSCP

1. Vertical electrophoresis apparatus with a well-forming comb (e.g. Life Technologies model S2).
2. Silane.
3. Sigmacote (Sigma Chemical Co).
4. MDE® (Flowgen).

5. 5X TBE buffer (stock): 54 g Tris base, 27.5 g boric acid, 20 mL 0.5 *M* EDTA (pH 8.0). Dilute in deionized water (120 mL in 880 mL) to 0.6X.
6. SSCP loading buffer: 0.1% SDS, 10 m*M* EDTA.
7. SSCP stop dye: 95% formamide and a few grains bromophenol blue.

2.4. Visualization

1. Plastic trays large enough to immerse the electrophoresis plate.
2. Rotary shaker (e.g., Luckham R100/TW Rotatest shaker).
3. Fix/stop solution 10% acetic acid: 200 mL glacial acetic acid in 1 800 mL deionized water.
4. Staining solution: combine 2 g $AgNO_3$ with 3 mL 37% formaldehyde in 2 L deionized water.
5. Developing solution: dissolve 60 g Na_2CO_3 in 2 L deionized water. Chill to 10°C. Immediately before use add 3 mL 37% formaldehyde and 400 µL sodium thiosulphate (10 mg/mL).

3. Method

3.1. Organisms and DNA Extraction

M. tuberculosis colonies are picked from Löwenstein Jensen slopes following culture at 37°C for 3 wk (*see* **Notes 1** and **2**).

1. Using a sterile bacteriological loop, transfer a well grown colony to 100 µL sterile distilled water (*see* **Note 3**) in a 1 mL sterile microcentrifuge tube.
2. Heat to 100°C for 20 min (*see* **Note 4**).
3. Microcentifuge at 12,000*g* for 1 min.
4. Transfer the supernatant which contains DNA and is used as the template for PCR (*see* **Note 5**).

3.1. rpo*B PCR*

1. Prepare a PCR master mix (**Note 6**) containing 10 µL X10 PCR buffer, 3 µL deoxynucleoside triphosphate stock, 1 µL *Taq* polymerase and 10 µL primers in a total volume of 90 µL for each PCR reaction.
2. For each PCR run include a positive control (10 ng genomic *M. tuberculosis* DNA) and a negative control (sterile distilled water).
3. Aliquot the master mix into thin walled PCR reaction tubes (*see* **Note 7**).
5. Add an aliquot of 10 µL template DNA (sample, genomic DNA or sterile distilled water) to each tube and mixed (*see* **Note 8**).
6. Overlay the reaction mix with 3 drops (approx 50 µL) mineral oil.
7. Transfer the reaction tubes to a thermal cycler and perform the amplification under the following conditions: one cycle of 95°C for 1 min; thirty cycles of 94°C for 1 min, 65°C for 2 min, 72°C for 3 min; one cycle of 72°C for 7 min.
8. Process the 120 bp amplimer by SSCP.

3.3. SSCP

1. Prepare a 0.5% MDE gel using 0.6X TBE and a 0.4 mm thickness gel poured in a vertical format gel-rig (*see* **Notes 9** and **10**) and a well forming rather than a sharkstooth comb.
2. Denature 6 µL of the PCR amplimer at 95°C for 10 min with 3 µL SSCP loading buffer and 3 µL stop dye.
3. Quench the samples on ice and 10 µL loaded directly to the gel.
4. Run the gel for 6 h at 6 W at room temperature (*see* **Notes 11** and **12**).

3.4. Visualization

1. After electrophoresis carefully separate the glass plates. The gel should be bound to the shorter plate (*see* **Note 13**).
2. Gel fixing: place the plate in a shallow plastic tray, cover with fix/stop solution and agitate for 20 min at room temperature (*see* **Note 14**). The fix/stop solution is saved to terminate the developing reaction.
3. Wash the gel three times for 2 min each in ultrapure water with agitation. The gel plate is carefully drained after each wash (*see* **Note 15**).
4. Transfer the gel to staining solution and agitate for 30 min at room temperature.
5. Rinse the gel by dipping briefly (>5 s) into ultrapure water, draining and then place immediately into a tray of prechilled developing solution (*see* **Note 16**).
6. Developing: agitate the gel until the bands start to appear, this may take several minutes depending on the temperature of the developer.
7. Terminate the reaction is terminated by addition of the fix/stop solution to the developing solution with agitation (*see* **Note 16**).
8. Rinse the gel twice in ultrapure water, 2 min each. Drain.
9. Dry the gel in air by standing it vertically.
10. Permanent images can be created by photography, scanning or by photocopying. Photography provides the most durable record and is universally acceptable for publication purposes.

4. Notes

1. *Mycobacterium tuberculosis* is an ADCP Category III organism and must be handled under appropriate containment conditions.
2. Larger numbers of mycobacteria may be prepared by culture for 3–4 wk in Middlebrooks 7H9 broth medium at 37°C.
3. Extraction from broth culture is as follows: an aliquot of broth culture is pelleted in a 1.5 mL microcentrifuge tube (12,000*g* for 5 min) and the supernatant discarded. The deposit is heated to 80°C for 20 min in a waterbath. 100 µL of chloroform is added and the tube vortexed for 30 s. The sample is microcentrifuged (12,000*g* for 1 min) and the aqueous layer used as the PCR sample.
4. Samples must be heat killed (80°C for a minimum of 20 min) before leaving the Category III (P3) facility.

5. This method of DNA preparation yields DNA in adequate quantity and quality for PCR. As this DNA preparation is not pure it is likely to deteriorate rapidly on storage. If further manipulations of the DNA are proposed than a more thorough isolation may be required.
6. For ease of handling and to control reagent preparation a PCR mastermix is prepared containing all the reagents but not the template DNA. The mastermix volume is calculated as the number of test reactions + positive control + negative control + 1 (e.g., for 4 tests the mastermix would be 4 + 1 + 1 + 1 = 7 vol).
7. A strict four room strategy is applied for all PCR protocols. Reagents and equipment must only be moved from room 2 to 4 and never the reverse:
   Room 1 - DNA template preparation
   Room 2 - PCR clean room; preparation of the mastermix
   Room 3 - PCR grey room; mixing of DNA template and mastermix
   Room 4 - all handling of amplimers.
8. Thorough mixing is essential for efficient PCR reactions, this is best achieved by gentle pumping of the pipet 2–3 times.
9. The gel is bound to the shorter plate using silane and for ease of separation the remaining plate is coated with Sigmacote.
10. In our experience, problems associated with smiling or frowning gels can be minimized by use of a wide format vertical gel rig (e.g., Life Technologies S2) with the wells formed in the center of the rig.
11. The precise time for optimal separation of the fragments will vary with a host of factors, particularly ambient temperature and gel rig design. Thus, there will always be an element of trial and error for setting run times. This is minimized by running amplimers with known sequences as standards for reference purposes.
12. As soon as the gel is running then the developing sodium carbonate should be prepared and placed at 4°C to ensure that it is thoroughly chilled prior to use.
13. When coating the gel plate with bind silane, remember that the plate will be immersed in developing solutions, thus the plate with the gel on it should not have integral seals, cooling tanks, or other attachments.
14. The best results are obtained with rapid fixing with agitation, however, it is acceptable to fix overnight with no agitation to achieve similar results.
15. Poor quality water will result in high background staining, water of purity of at least 18 $M\Omega$ is required.
16. The rinse steps must be as brief as possible or the signal deteriorates. On addition of the fix/stop the image may continue to develop for a short period time.

References

1. Ramaswamy, S. and Musser, J. M. (1998) Molecular genetic basis of antimicrobial agent resistance in *Mycobacterium tuberculosis*: 1998 update. *Tubercle Lung. Dis.* **79,** 3–29
2. Gillespie, S. H. and McHugh, T. D. (1997) The biological cost of resistance. *Trends Microbiol.* **5,** 337–339.

3. Billington, O. J., McHugh, T. D. and Gillespie, S. H. (1999) The physiological cost of rifampin resistance induced *in vitro* in *Mycobacterum tuberculosis. Antimicrob. Agents. Chemother.* **43,** 1866–1869.
4. Suzuki Y, Orita M, Shiraishi M, Hayashi K & Sekiya T. (1990) Detection of ras gene mutations in human lung cancers by single-strand conformation polymorphism analysis of polymerase chain reaction products. *Oncogene* **5,** 1037–1043.
5. Rowe, P. S., Oudet, C. L., Francis, F., et al. (1997) Distribution of mutations in the PEX gene in families with X-linked hypophosphataemic rickets (HYP). *Human. Mol. Gen.* **6,** 539–549.
6. Telenti, A., Imboden, P., Marchesi, F., et al. (1993) Detection of rifampin-resistance mutations in *Mycobacterium tuberculosis. Lancet* **341,** 647–650.
7. Orita, M., Iwahana, H., Kanazawa, H., Hayashi, K., and Sekiya, T. (1989) Detection of polymorphisms of human DNA by gel electrophoresis as single-strand conformation polymorphisms. *Proc. Natl. Acad. Sci.* **86,** 2766–2770 .
8. Gillespie, S. H., McHugh, T. D., Ayes, H., Dickens, A., Estradiou, A., and Whiting, G. C. (1997) Allelic variation of the *lytA* gene of *Streptococcus pneumoniae. Infect. Immun.* **65,** 3936–3938.
9. Hannan, M. M., McHugh, T. D., Billington, O., Gazzard, B., and Gillespie, S. H. (1997). Variation in *pnc*A gene: molecular biology and clinical significance. *Span. J. Chemoth.* **10(Suppl. 2),** 140.

5

Quantitative, Single-Tube, Nested, PCR (QSTN-PCR) for Determining the Antibiotic Susceptibility of *Mycobacterium tuberculosis*

Nainn-Tsyr Jou and Michael R. Liebling

1. Introduction

Rapid drug susceptibility testing for *Mycobacterium tuberculosis* (Mtb) is imperative in an age when drug resistance is not rare and up to one-third of the world's population may be infected with this organism *(1)*. A sensitive, PCR-based system to test mycobacterial antibiotic susceptibility is one approach to this problem. We reasoned that a quantitative PCR could detect the growth of bacilli by detecting an increase in the amount of mycobacterial DNA. Inclusion of an effective antibiotic in the culture media would prevent bacterial growth and concomitant increase in target DNA, thus distinguishing cultures which were susceptible to an antibiotic from those which were not.

To test this hypothesis, we developed a sensitive, competitive, quantitative, single-tube, nested PCR (QSTN-PCR) using primers which targeted the multiple insertion element, *IS6110 (2)*. This format detects attomole quantities of DNA from less than 100 bacilli. By examining growth slopes and using a proportional method for assessing drug susceptibility, the assay can distinguish strains of *M. tuberculosis* which are sensitive to isoniazid or rifampin from strains which are not with only 4-7 d of incubation. Most importantly, the initial numbers of bacilli required for the assay theoretically permit direct testing from samples which are only marginally smear positive e.g., 10^3 organisms. This compares favorably with radiometric techniques that may require more than 10^8 mycobacteria and frequently average 31 d from sample processing to susceptibility reporting according to recent data *(3)*.

From: *Methods in Molecular Medicine, vol. 48: Antibiotic Resistance Methods and Protocols*
Edited by: S. H. Gillespie © Humana Press Inc., Totowa, NJ

2. Materials

1. Incubator, 37°C.
2. Colorimeter (Viteck).
3. Exhaust protective biological safety cabinet (NuAire, Plymounth, MN).
4. *Mycobacterium tuberculosis* (Mtb), antibiotic sensitive strain H37Rv ATCC 27294 (American Type Culture Collection).
5. Mtb, rifampin resistant strain ATCC 35838 (American Type Culture Collection).
6. Mtb, isoniazid resistant strain, CAP E-05, 1995, Set E-A (College of American Pathology).
7. Middlebrook 7H9 broth.
8. Lowenstein-Jensen slants.
9. BBL® MycoPrep™ Specimen Digestion/Decontamination Kit (Becton Dickinson, Sparks, MD).
10. Penicillin-phosphate buffer. Prepare 5000 mg/mL of penicillin G as a stock solution and store in small aliquots at –20°C. Then, add 1 mL of penicillin G stock solution into a bottle of 40 mL phosphate buffer. Make fresh solution for each time.
11. 4 µg/mL isoniazid and 80 µg/mL rifampin in H_2O. Store in small aliquots at –70°C for up to six mo.
12. 50 mg/mL lysozyme in H_2O. Store in aliquots at –20°C. Discard each aliquot after use. The final working solution is 10 mg/mL lysozyme in 50 m*M* glucose, 25 m*M* Tris-HCl (pH 8.0), and 10 m*M* EDTA (pH 8.0).
13. 20 mg/mL proteinase K (Amresco, Solon, OH) in H_2O. Store in aliquots at –20°C. The final working solution is 2 mg/mL proteinase K in 0.2 *M* NaCl and 1% SDS.
14. 1 *M* glucose. Sterilize by filtration through 0.45 µm filter.
15. 1 *M* Tris-HCl, pH 8.0.
16. 0.5 *M* EDTA, pH 8.0.
17. 4 *M* NaCl.
18. 9% SDS.
19. Sonicated salmon sperm DNA, 1 mg/mL in TE buffer. Store in aliquots at –20°C.
20. Buffer-saturated phenol (pH 7.4 ± 0.1) (Amresco). Store at 4°C.
21. Chloroform/isoamyl alcohol (24:1) (Amresco). Store at room temperature.
22. 70% ethanol.
23. 1X Tris-EDTA buffer (1X TE): 10 m*M* Tris-HCl (pH 8.0), 1 m*M* EDTA (pH 8.0).
24. PCR MIMIC™ Construction kit (Clontech Laboratories, Inc., Palo Alto, CA). This kit includes: MIMIC DNA fragment (0.5 ng/µL in TE buffer), CHROMA SPIN+TE-100 Columns, 100 ng/µL ϕX174/*Hae* III digest for estimating yield of PCR MIMIC, 5 µg/µL Ultrapure glycogen solution (MIMIC Dilution Solution). Dilute this stock solution in TE buffer to give a 10 µg/mL working solution. Store CHROMA SPIN Columns at 4°C and all other components at –20°C.
25. GeneAmp® thin-walled reaction tubes (Perkin Elmer, Foster City, CA).
26. GeneAmp® dNTPs (Perkin Elmer).
27. AmpliTaq® DNA Polymerase (5 U/µL) and 10X PCR Buffer: 100 m*M* Tris-HCl, (pH 8.3; 500 m*M* KCl; 15 m*M* $MgCl_2$; 0.01% gelatin). Store at –20°C in a constant temperature freezer.

28. Sterile H_2O.
29. 6X dye; 0.25% bromophenol blue, 0.25% xylene cyanol FF, and 30% glycerol. Store at 4°C.
30. Oligonucleotide primers.
31. DNA Thermal Cycler.
32. 100 bp DNA Ladder.
33. Model GS-700 Imaging Desitometer (Bio-Rad, Hercules, CA).
34. 18% sodium sulfite solution. Store solution in a well-capped brown bottle.
35. Polaroid® type 667 B&W film.
36. Polaroid® type 665 positive/negative film.
37. Ethidium bromide, 0.625 mg/mL solution in a dropper bottle. Shield the solution from light. Add one drop of the solution per 50 mL gel or staining solution to give a final concentration of 0.5 μg/mL. Store at room temperature.
38. Agarose I (Amresco).
39. Agarose 3:1, High Resolution Blend (Midwest Scientific, St. Louis, MO).
40. Electrophoresis buffer: Prepare 5X Tris-borate buffer (TBE) stock solution and store at room temperature. Mix 54 g Tris, 27.5 g boric acid, and 20 mL of 0.5 *M* EDTA (pH 8.0) in one liter water. Dilute to 1X TBE for use.
41. Horizontal Gel Electrophoresis Apparatus. Make a 5.7 × 8.3-cm mini gel.
42. Power supply.
43. Photo-Documentation Camera (e.g., FB-PDC-34 Fisher Scientific, Pittsburgh, PA).
44. UV transilluminator.

3. Methods

3.1. Control Cultures

1. Grow *M. tuberculosis* (Mtb) H37Rv, isoniazid (INH) resistant, and rifampin (RIF) resistant organisms are grown on Lowenstein-Jensen slants for 10 to 14 d.
2. Suspend one colony of each organism in 3 mL Middlebrook 7H9 broth and incubate for 6 d.
3. After 6 d, adjust a suspension to 10^8 organisms/mL. Make a concentration of 10^4 organisms/mL by diluting the suspension 10,000-fold in Middlebrook 7H9 broth, then incubate at 37°C and harvest on days 0, 4, and 7.
4. Set up six 4 mL control cultures on day 0:
   a. 10^2 organisms/mL of Mtb H37Rv (1% Mtb control culture),
   b. 10^4 organisms/mL of Mtb H37Rv without antibiotic,
   c. a culture of 10^4 organisms/mL of Mtb H37Rv containing 0.3 μg/mL of INH,
   d. a culture of 10^4 organisms/mL of Mtb H37Rv containing 4 μg/mL of RIF,
   e. a culture of 10^4 organisms/mL of INH resistant Mtb containing 0.3 μg/mL of INH, and
   f. a culture of 10^4 organisms/mL RIF resistant Mtb containing 4 μg/mL of RIF.
   Immediately, remove 1 mL aliquot of each control culture for DNA extraction.
5. Continue to cultivate the remaining control cultures at 37°C. On day 4 and day 7 of incubation, remove 1 mL aliquot for DNA extraction.

3.2. Sputum Processing

1. Collect and handle sputum specimens according to Centers for Disease Control and Prevention/National Institutes of Health (CDC/NIH) guidelines or equivalent for any potentially biohazardous contamination.
2. Use BBL® MycoPrep™ Specimen Digestion/Decontamination Kit for the digestion and decontamination of sputums. Follow the instructions provided in the kit.
3. Resuspend the final sputum pellet in 2 mL of the penicillin-phosphate buffer. The samples are now ready for DNA extraction.

3.3. DNA Extraction

1. To minimize the loss of *M. tuberculosis* DNA during precipitation by ethanol in the final step, add 80 µg of salmon sperm carrier DNA into the samples.
2. Spin down cells for 20 min in a microcentrifuge at 12,000*g*.
3. Discard the supernatant and resuspend the pellet in 200 µL of the lysozyme working solution.
4. Incubate for 30 min on ice.
5. Add 200 µL of the Proteinase K working solution. Mix the sample by pipeting up and down and incubate for two hours at 55°C. Mix the reaction by inverting the tube every 30 min.
6. After incubation, add 400 µL of buffer-saturated phenol (pH 7.4 ± 0.1), vortex thoroughly, and spin for 10 min at 4°C.
7. Remove the upper aqueous supernatant containing mycobacterial DNA to a sterile microcentrifuge tube, being careful not to disturb the interface.
8. Add an equal volume of chloroform/isoamyl alcohol (24:1), vortex thoroughly, and spin for 10 min at 4°C.
9. Remove the upper phase to a sterile tube and repeat **step 8**.
10. Transfer the upper supernatant to a sterile tube, add an equal volume isopropanol at room temperature. Mix gently by inverting the tube several times. Incubate the reaction for one hour at –20°C.
11. Spin the tube for 15 min in a microcentrifuge at 4°C.
12. Pipet off the supernatant slowly and leave a little at the bottom of the tube.
13. Wash the DNA pellet with ice-cold 70% ethanol and spin for 15 min at 4°C.
14. Remove the ethanol with a pipet.
15. Dry the DNA pellet under vacuum for 5–10 min and then dissolve in 50 µL TE buffer. Store the DNA at –20°C for further analysis by competitive, quantitative, single-tube, nested PCR assay.

3.4. Competitive, Quantitative, Single-Tube, Nested PCR (QSTN-PCR)

It is important to understand the composite nature of this form of PCR. Essentially, it is a combination of a single-tube, nested PCR (STN-PCR) and a competitive, quantitative PCR. Our modification of the STN-PCR using primers that are specific for the *IS6110* insertion element of Mtb has been described previously, as have the advantages of this methodology *(4,5)*. Briefly, the single-tube, nested PCR was designed to avoid the inherent contamination potential of standard nested PCR, without relinquishing the extremely powerful amplification of the nested format (**Fig. 1**).

To perform this assay in a competitive and quantitative manner (QSTN-PCR), a PCR MIMIC™ Construction kit and composite primers are used to generate a nonhomologous internal standard called a PCR MIMIC. Ultimately, this PCR MIMIC is used to compete with, and quantify, sample Mtb DNA in the QSTN-PCR.

3.4.1. Preparation of Mtb-Specific PCR MIMIC

The MIMIC DNA provided in the PCR MIMIC Construction kit consists of a 574-bp fragment of the v-*erb*B gene (**Fig. 2**). It is a template from which the Mtb-specific PCR MIMIC is constructed. In addition, three sets of the primers are required for construction of the Mtb-specific PCR MIMIC:

1. a set of outer primers specific for *IS6110* insertion element of Mtb,
2. a set of inner primers specific for *IS6110*, and
3. a set of composite primers (MRL71 and MRL72). The composite primers are produced by attaching the outer and inner *IS6110*-specific primers to 20-bp sequences that are complementary to lateral portions of the v-*erb*B fragment, underlined in **Fig. 2**. **Figure 3** illustrates the design of these composite primers.

3.4.1.1. Primer Design

1. Outer and Inner Primers Specific for *IS6110*: The outer primers for the *IS6110* target and their sequences are MRL29 (5'-GGACAACGCCGAATTGCGAAG GGC-3') and MRL30 (5'-TAGGCGTCGGTGACAAAGGCCACG-3'). The inner primers and their sequences are MRL31 (5'-CCATCGACCTACTACGACC-3') and MRL32 (5'-CCGAGTTTGGTCATCAGCC-3'). For the principles involved in the design of these primers, *see* **Note 1**.
2. Composite Primers: The sequence of the upstream composite primer, MRL71, is 5'-GGACAACGCCGAATTGCGAAGGGCCCATCGACCTACTACGACCC GCAAGTGAAATCTCCTACG-3'. The sequence of the downstream composite primer, MRL72, is 5'-TAGGCGTCGGTGACAAAGGCCACGCCGAGTTT GGTCATCAGCCTCTGTCAATGCAGTTTGTAG-3'. To easily distinguish the amplification product of the PCR MIMIC from that of the target DNA after gel electrophoresis, the composite primers are designed to produce at least a 150- bp difference in the size of these products (*see* **Note 2**).

3.4.1.2. Primary PCR Amplification for the Production of Mtb-Specific PCR MIMIC

1. In a 0.5-mL thin-wall microcentrifuge tube, make up the following reaction mixture: sterile H_2O, 17.3 µL; 10X PCR Reaction buffer, 2.5 µL; dNTP mix (10 m*M* each), 2.0 µL; MIMIC DNA (0.5 ng/µL), 2.0 µL; upstream composite primer,

I. FIRST STAGE - High Annealing Temperature (70^{0}C)

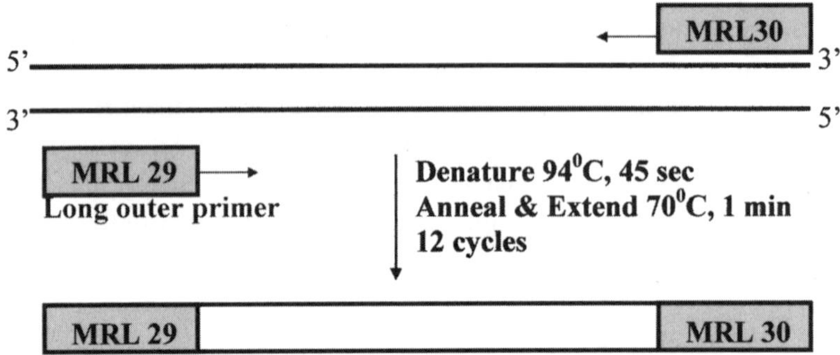

II. SECOND STAGE - Low Annealing Temperature (60^{0}C)

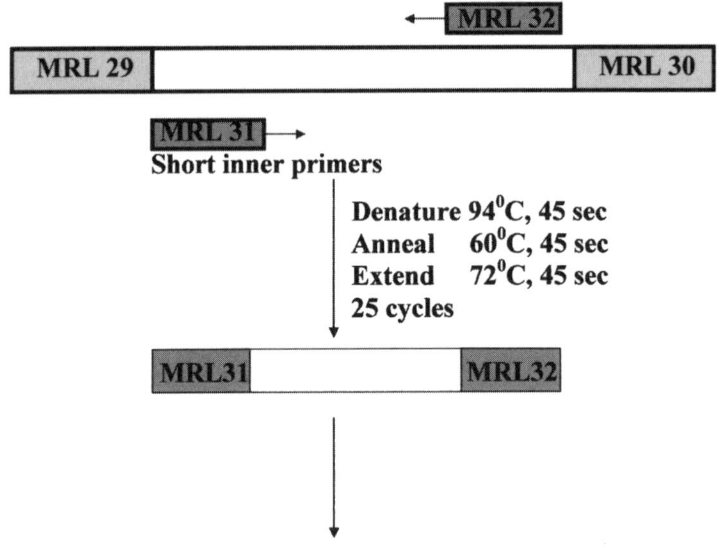

4% Agarose Gel Electrophoresis

Fig. 1. Diagram of the Single-Tube, Nested PCR. Long outer primers allow initial amplification of a large product using a high annealing temperature that does not permit amplification by short inner primers. When the annealing temperature is lowered after the initial few cycles, the inner primers use the initial large product to produce a predominant smaller product that can then be detected by a variety of methods, such as gel electrophoresis.

GGATCCC CGCAAGTCAA ATCTCCTCCG TCTTGGAGAA GGGAGAGCGT
TTGCCCCAGC CACCCATTTG TACCATTGAT GTGTACATGA TCATGGTCAA
ATGCTGGATG ATTGATGCAG ACAGCCGTCC CAAGTTTCGT GAGCTGATTG
CAGAGTTCTC CAAAATGGCT CGTGACCCTC CCCGCTATCT TGTTATACAG
GGAGATGAAA GGATGCACTT GCCTAGCCCT ACAGATTCCA AGTTTTATCG
CACCCTGATG GAGGAGGAGG ACATGGAAGA CATTGTGGAT GCAGATGAGT
ATCTTGTCCC ACACCAGGGC TTTTTCAACA TGCCCTCTAC ATCTCGGACT
CCTCTTCTGA GTTCATTGAG CGCTACTAGC AACAATTCTG CTACAAACTG
CATTGACAGA AATGGGCAGG GGCACCCTGT GAGGGAAGAG GCTTCCTGCC
TGCTCCAGAG TATGTAAACC AGCTGATGCC CAAGAAACCA TCTACTGCCA
TGGTCCAGAA TCAAATCTAC AACTTCATCT CTCTCACAGC AATCTCAAAG
CTCCCCATGG ACTCAAGATA CCAGAATTC

Fig. 2. The sequence of the MIMIC DNA fragment. This fragment is a 574 bp, *Bam*H1/*Eco*R1 fragment of the v-*erb*B gene. The underlined 20 base sequences are used to design composite primers for PCR MIMIC construction (*see* **Subheading 3.4.1.1.**).

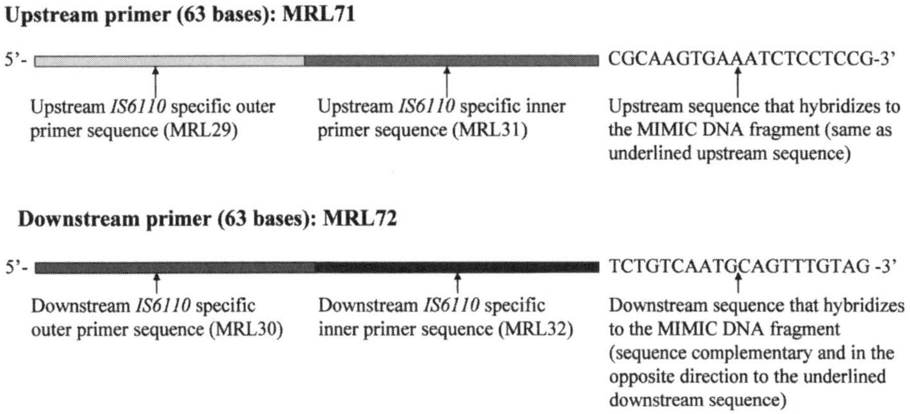

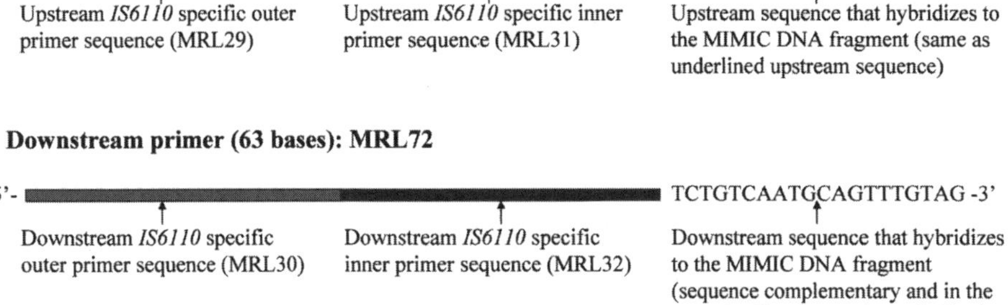

Fig. 3. Composite primer design.

MRL71 (20 μ*M*), 0.5 μL; downstream composite primer, MRL72 (20 μ*M*), 0.5 μL; and AmpliTaq DNA polymerase (5 U/μL), 0.2 μL. Thus, the final reaction volume is 25 μL.

2, Overlay the reaction mixture with 25 μL light mineral oil.
3. Carry out 25 PCR cycles using the following parameters: denature at 94°C for 45 s, anneal at 50°C for 45 s, and extend at 72°C for 90 s (*see* **Note 3**).
4. Electrophorese 5 μL of the first PCR product on an 1% agarose gel using a 100 bp ladder marker to confirm the size of the expected 486-bp product.

3.4.1.3. Secondary PCR Amplification for the Production of Mtb-Specific PCR MIMIC

1. Dilute 2 µL of the primary PCR product to 200 µL in H_2O.
2. Set up secondary PCR reaction as follows: sterile H_2O, 75.4 µL; 10X PCR Reaction buffer, 10 µL; dNTP mix (10 m*M* each), 8 µL; 100X dilution of primary PCR product, 2 µL; upstream *IS6110* outer primer, MRL29 (20 µ*M*), 2 µL; downstream *IS6110* outer primer, MRL30 (20 µ*M*), 2 µL; and Ampli*Taq* DNA polymerase (5 U/µL), 0.6 µL. Thus, the final reaction volume for this PCR is 100 µL.
3. Overlay the reaction mixture with 100 µL light mineral oil.
4. Carry out 25 PCR cycles, using the same cycling parameters described above for the primary PCR.
5. Electrophorese 5 µL of the secondary PCR product on an 1% agarose gel. Again, a 486-bp band should be observed.

3.4.1.4. Purification of the Mtb-Specific PCR MIMIC

1. Add equal amount of chloroform to the secondary PCR reaction. Mix well and spin for 1 min at maximum speed in a microcentrifuge. Save the top aqueous phase that contains the PCR product for further purification on a CHROMA SPIN Column.
2. Invert two CHROMA SPIN Columns several times to thoroughly resuspend the gel matrix.
3. Place the columns into the 17 × 100 mm polypropylene tubes, centrifuge for 3 min at 700*g* in a swing bucket rotor and discard the supernatant.
4. Place the columns in the clean microcentrifuge tubes and carefully pipet 45 µL of the PCR product to the center of the gel bed. Apply the remaining PCR product to another spin column.
5. Centrifuge the columns for 5 min at 700*g* in a swing bucket rotor.
6. Combine the eluate from each spin column.
7. Add 0.1 vol of 10X PCR buffer to the purified PCR MIMIC DNA.
8. Check the quality of the PCR MIMIC DNA by gel electrophoresis.

3.4.1.5. Quantification of Mtb-Specific PCR MIMIC

The quantity of the PCR MIMIC can be determined by comparing the intensity of the electrophoretic bands produced by the PCR MIMIC with the intensity of bands generated by known quantities of ϕX174/*Hae* III size markers, provided in the PCR MIMIC™ Construction kit.

1. Set up three dilutions of ϕX174/*Hae* III digest size markers (100 ng, 200 ng, and 400 ng) and one dilution of the purified Mtb-specific PCR MIMIC DNA (1 µL of the total purified products) using sterile H_2O, 10X PCR buffer, and 6X dye in a final volume of 15 µL.
2. Load the ϕX174 DNA/*Hae* III size markers and Mtb-specific PCR MIMIC samples on a 4% agarose gel.
3. Electrophorese at 100 V until the xylene cyanol (green dye) travels two-thirds of the length of the gel.

4. Stain the gel in 0.5 µg/mL of ethidium bromide solution for 20 min and destain in H_2O for another 20 min.
5. View the gel on a UV transilluminator and photograph using a Polaroid® type 665 positive/negative film to record the result (*see* **Note 4**).
6. Use the GS-700 Imaging Densitometer to scan the negative, focusing on the 603-bp bands of the three ϕX174 DNA dilutions and the 486-bp band of the PCR MIMIC. The intensity and the nanogram quantity of the 603-bp fragment for each dilution are used to produce a standard curve from which the quantity of the Mtb-specific PCR MIMIC can be derived.
7. To calculate the amount of the 603-bp ϕX174 DNA fragment, use the following equation: ng of ϕX174 DNA fragment = (size of ϕX174 DNA fragment) (ng of ϕX174 DNA)/(sum of all ϕX174 DNA fragments). For instance, to determine the amount of DNA present in the 603-bp band when 100 ng of ϕX174 DNA was electrophoresed, the equation would be : ng of ϕX174 DNA fragment = (603 bp) (100 ng)/(5386 bp) = 11.19 ng. Thus, when 200 ng and 400 ng of the ϕX174 DNA fragment are electrophoresed the intensity of the 603-bp band detected by the densitometer represents the equivalent of 22.39 ng and 44.78 ng of DNA, respectively.
8. By knowing the amount of the ϕX174 DNA fragment, the yield in nanogram per microliter of Mtb-specific PCR MIMIC can be derived using a GS-700 Imaging Densitometer Molecular Analyst® software/PC, Version 1.4 (*see* **Subheading 3.4.2.4.** under Densitometry for details).
9. Convert nanograms to molar quantities and calculate the concentration of the Mtb-specific PCR MIMIC in attomoles/µL (*see* **Note 5**).
10. Dilute the concentrated Mtb-specific PCR MIMIC solution to 100 attomoles/µL with the MIMIC Dilution Solution. Store the diluted and concentrated Mtb-specific PCR MIMIC DNA solutions at –20°C in a frost-free freezer.

3.4.2. Protocol for the Competitive, Quantitative, Single-Tube, Nested PCR (QSTN-PCR)

3.4.2.1. Overview

In this procedure a constant amount of purified Mtb DNA samples from the control cultures on days, 0, 4, and 7 is first titrated against 10-fold dilutions of the Mtb-specific PCR MIMIC DNA. Based on the result of this preliminary competitive PCR, a second, fine-tuned, QSTN-PCR is set up using a two- or fourfold dilution of one of the previous 10-fold dilutions. Both of these PCR reactions are performed in two different stages. In the first stage of 12 cycles, the long outer primers, MRL29 and MRL30, generate a 580-bp *IS6110* DNA and a 486-bp Mtb-specific PCR MIMIC DNA using a higher Ta of 70°C. Then, in the second stage, 25 cycles in length, the short inner primers, MRL31 and MRL32, generate a 198-bp *IS6110* target DNA and a 438-bp Mtb-specific PCR MIMIC DNA products at a lower Ta of 60°C.

3.4.2.2. Preliminary QSTN-PCR Amplification

1. Use Mtb-specific PCR MIMIC stock solution (100 attomoles/μL) to prepare eight 10-fold serial dilutions of the PCR MIMIC (M_1 through M_8, 10 through 10^{-6} attomoles/μL, respectively), using MIMIC Dilution solution as diluent. The dilution series can be stored at –20°C and discarded after three uses.
2. Prepare PCR master mix as follows: sterile H_2O, 33 μL; 10X PCR Reaction buffer, 5 μL; dNTP mix (10 m*M* each), 4 μL; purified Mtb DNA solution in TE buffer, 1 μL (*see* **Note 6**); MRL29 (1 μ*M*), 0.3 μL; MRL30 (1 μ*M*), 0.3 μL; MRL31 (20 μ*M*), 2 μL; MRL32 (20 μ*M*), 2 μL; and Ampli*Taq* DNA polymerase (5 U/μL), 0.4 μL. Multiply the amount of each ingredient by the total number of the QSTN-PCR reactions, combine the solutions, and mix them gently by pipeting. Aliquot 48 μL of the master mix to each labeled PCR tube.
3. Add 2 μL of each dilution of the Mtb-specific PCR MIMIC (M_3–M_7) to a tube containing 48 μL of the master mix (*see* **Note 7**).
4. Overlay the reaction mixture with 50 μL light mineral oil.
5. Begin the thermal cycling using the following parameters: perform 12 cycles of denaturation at 94°C for 45 s, annealing and extension at 70°C for 1 min followed by another 25 cycles of denaturation at 94°C for 45 s, annealing at 60°C for 45 s, and extension at 70°C for 45 s.
6. Electrophorese 5 μL PCR products on a 4% agarose gel.
7. Stain the gel in ethidium bromide solution and photograph to record the result. Use Polaroid® type 667 B&W films.

3.4.2.3. Fine-Tuned QSTN-PCR

1. Assess by visual comparison which 10-fold dilution produced Mtb-specific PCR MIMIC and target *IS6110* DNA bands of approximately equal intensity. Then use the 10-fold less PCR MIMIC dilution to make a two- or fourfold dilution series.
2. Make 6 two- or fourfold serial dilutions.
3. Prepare the PCR master mix as above. Add 2 μL of each dilution to a tube containing 48 μL of the PCR master mix. Overlay the reaction mixture with 50 μL mineral oil.
4. Initiate the PCR cycling using the same parameters as in the preliminary QSTN-PCR.
5. Electrophoreses 5 μL of the PCR products on 4% agarose gel, stain the gel in ethidium bromide solution and photograph to record the result using Polaroid® type 665 positive/negative film.

3.4.2.4. Densitometry

1. Use the Molecular Analyst® Software for Bio-Rad's Image Analysis System (Version 1.4) to analyze the results. Place the negative on the densitometer and set the gel resolution and pixel depth to 600 dpi and 12, respectively.
2. Define the area of the PCR MIMIC and target DNA bands (438- and 198-bp, respectively). Then, scan the negative and save the image as .img.
3. Modify the background contrast of the image by adjusting the light intensity to maximize the contrast between the bands and the background.

4. Click Analyze Vol Object or use shortcut key, "ctl+E". Then, click Local Background Subtraction.
5. Print out the results. The values for the band density appear in the column, "Adj Volume OD × mm^2".
6. Export data to Microsoft Excel™ for curve plotting and statistical analysis.

3.4.2.5. Product Quantification

The results of QSTN-PCR on triplicate samples from a culture are used to determine the amount of *IS6110* target DNA present in the culture on that day. By plotting, Log (intensity of Mtb *IS6110* DNA/intensity of PCR MIMIC DNA) versus Log (attomoles of added PCR MIMIC DNA) for each of the triplicates, three linear regression lines can be generated using Microsoft Excel™ (**Fig. 4**). The x-intercept for each of these lines represents the point at which the quantity of the target DNA is equal to PCR MIMIC DNA, i.e., the point at which Log (intensity of Mtb *IS6110* DNA/intensity of PCR MIMIC DNA) = 0 and (Mtb *IS6110* DNA/PCR MIMIC DNA) = 1.

The total quantity of *IS6100* target DNA in a culture can then be calculated using the following equation: attomoles of Mtb *IS6110* DNA in a culture = (total volume of Mtb DNA sample/volume of added Mtb DNA sample in QSTN-PCR) × (attomoles of Mtb *IS6110* DNA in QSTN-PCR reaction sample).

3.5. Determination of Growth, Drug Susceptibility, and Drug Resistance

3.5.1. Growth Slopes

Using the amount of Mtb *IS6110* target DNA in cultures on Days 0, 4, and 7, "growth slopes" can be constructed by plotting target DNA in attomoles versus time and using linear regression analysis in Microsoft Excel™ to determine the slope of the line.

Tradition has defined the clinically significant number of resistant mycobacteria in a culture at 1% *(6,7)*. Therefore, antibiotic resistance is defined in the assay by a growth slope that is not significantly lower in the presence of antibiotic than the growth slope of a 1% control culture grown in the absence of antibiotic (**Figs. 5A** and **B**). Similarly, antibiotic susceptibility is defined by a growth slope that is significantly lower in the presence of antibiotic than the growth slope of a 1% control culture grown in the absence of antibiotic (**Fig. 6**).

For each set of sample runs, controls include simultaneous cultures of:

1. a known multi-antibiotic susceptible strain,
2. standard strains known to be resistant to the individual antibiotics to be tested,
3. a 1% dilution of the multi-antibiotic susceptible strain.

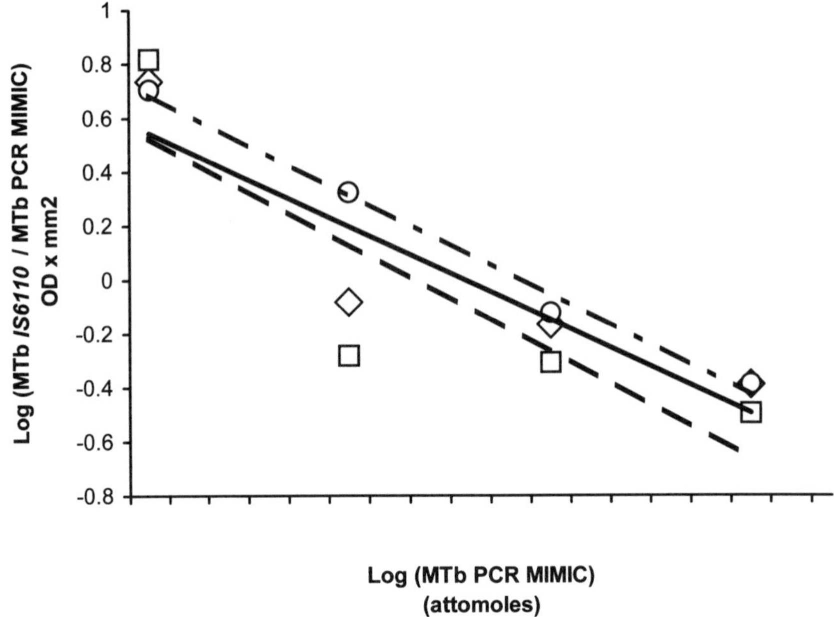

Fig. 4. Graphic analysis of QSTN-PCR to determine the quantity of Mtb *IS6110* DNA in a day 4 culture of Mtb H37Rv. *See* **Subheading 3.4.2.5.** for details of the analysis.

These cultures control for culture conditions, antibiotic effectiveness and sensitivity of the assay.

3.5.2. Statistical Determination of Drugs Susceptibility of M. tuberculosis

1. To assess the drug susceptibility or resistance of an Mtb specimen, first determine the 95% confidence interval around the mean of the three growth slopes for that specimen.
2. To determine 95% confidence intervals, use the formula: $X - ZSx \leq \mu \leq X + ZSx$, where X = mean of triplicate growth slopes; Sx = standard error of the mean, X; Z = 1.96; μ = true mean.
3. If two confidence intervals do not overlap, they define growth slopes that are significantly different. Examine a specimen's mean and confidence interval to determine if the specimen's slope is significantly lower than that of the 1% control. For instance, the multi-antibiotic sensitive strain, H37Rv in the presence of isoniazid or rifampin, had a negative slope whose 95% confidence interval did not overlap the confidence interval of the 1% control (**Fig. 6**). This meets the definition for antibiotic susceptibility (**Subheading 3.5.1.**). Similarly, the isoniazid resistant strain, CAP E-05, had a mildly positive growth slope and its 95% confidence interval did not overlap that of the 1% control (**Fig. 5A**). However,

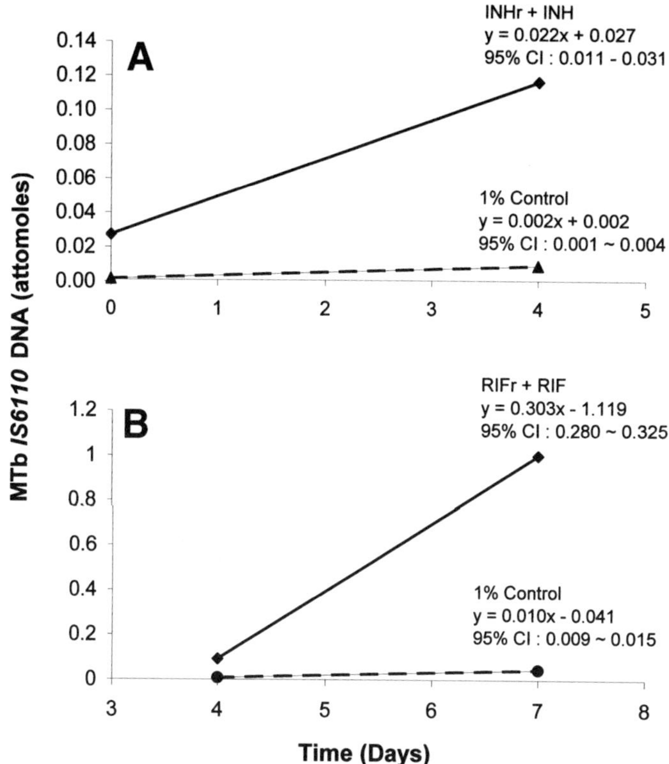

Fig. 5. Growth slope analysis of resistant organisms. **(A)** Day 0 to day 4 growth slopes for an isoniazid resistant strain cultured in the presence of isoniazid (INHr + INH) and a 1% control cultured in the absence of antibiotics. **(B)** Day 4 to day 7 growth slopes for a rifampin resistant strain cultured in the presence of rifampin (RIFr + RIF) and a 1% control cultured in the absence of antibiotics. Occasionally, there will be an early lag phase in the growth of a mycobacterial sample that makes early analysis difficult. By analyzing the growth slope from day 4 to day 7, this problem may be circumvented. 95% CI = 95% confidence interval around the mean value of the indicated slope. *See* **Subheadings 3.5.1.** and **3.5.2.** for the statistical definition of resistance used in this assay and represented in this figure.

this strain's growth slope was not significantly lower that the growth slope of the 1% control. Therefore, this result fulfilled criteria for the antibiotic resistance. (**Subheading 3.5.1.**) (*see* **Note 8**).

4. Notes

1. The annealing temperature (Ta) of the outer primers should be kept between 70°C and 75°C and the Ta of the inner primers between 45°C and 55°C. To achieve the

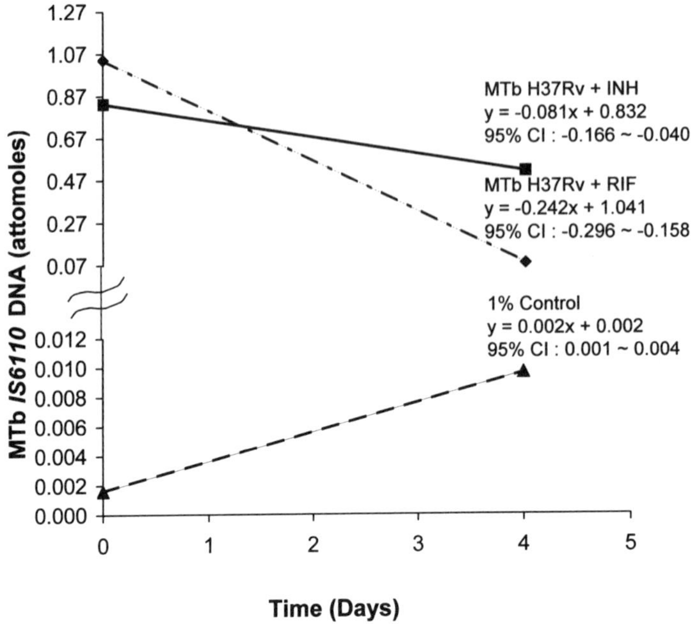

Fig. 6. Day 0 to day 4 growth slopes for the multi-antibiotic susceptible strain, Mtb H37Rv, cultured in the presence of isoniazid (Mtb H37Rv + INH) or rifampin (Mtb H37Rv + RIF) and 1% control cultured in the absence of antibiotics. 95% CI = 95% confidence interval around the mean value of the identified slope. *See* **Subheadings 3.5.1.** and **3.5.2.** for the statistical definition of susceptibility used in this assay and represented in this figure.

appropriate temperatures, the outer primers are made much longer than the inner primers. For instance, the outer primers, MRL 29 and MRL30, are 24 bases long with Ta = 73°C, whereas the inner primers, MRL31 and MRL32, are 19 bases with Ta = 55°C.

2. In this case, the PCR MIMIC DNA is 438 bp and the target DNA is 198 bp long when amplified by both outer (MRL29 and MRL30) and inner (MRL31 and MRL32) primers. The high resolving capacity of the 4% agarose allows differentiation of the PCR products. Under certain circumstance, up to four different sized bands can be seen, because of the four possible pairings of four primers used in the STN-PCR. In our experience, only one band is observed when 6 n*M* of the IS*6110* specific outer primers and 800 n*M* of the *IS6110* specific inner primers are used in the STN-PCR reaction. Also, the first PCR stage should not be more than 12 cycles or the initial PCR products may be visualized on the agarose gel.
3. The cycling parameters have been optimized using a Perkin-Elmer DNA Thermal Cycler 480. They may be different using other models or other Thermal cyclers.

4. Polaroid® type 665 positive/negative film is used to obtain a high quality photographic negative for densitometric scanning. Set the aperture and shutter speed settings at less than f4.5 and 30 s, respectively (Fisher Biotech Photo-Documentation Camera, FB-PDC-34). Use #15 Orange Tiffen filter for photography of ethidium bromide-stained gels. Camera settings vary depending upon the gel; use these parameters as a starting point. The processing time of the film is 30 s at 18°C and above. The positive requires coating and the negative requires a clearing procedure. Prepare 18% sodium sulfite clearing solution before exposing and developing the film. Mix 440 g of anhydrous desiccated sodium sulfite in 2 liters warm water. Stir continuously until all powder is dissolved. Allow the solution cool to ~21°C before use. Store the solution in amber bottles at room temperature. Immerse the negative in the clearing solution within 3 min after development. Agitate the film for at least 60 s or longer until all the residual developer layer and opaque backcoat are gone. A negative can be kept in the solution for up to 72 h. Then wash the negative in running water for 5 min. Hang dry the negative using the clamps. Avoid excessive heat or dusty areas.
5. $$\text{\# of attomoles} = \frac{(\text{ng of PCR MIMIC per microliter}) \times (1\ \text{g}/10^{9}\ \text{ng}) \times (10^{18}\ \text{attomole})}{(660\ \text{g/mole}) \times (\text{bp of the PCR MIMIC})}$$

   where 660 g/mole = molecular weight per bp.
6. To determine how much DNA solution is required for the QSTN-PCR, run a STN-PCR assay first to screen the yield of your purified DNA products. Follow the protocol described in **Subheading 3.4.2.2.** to perform the STN-PCR assay excluding the Mtb-specific PCR MIMIC DNA in the reaction mixtures. Electrophorese the STN-PCR products on a 4% agarose gel. If the bands are visible or strong, use half of the amount in the preliminary QSTN-PCR. If the bands are faint or absent, repeat the STN-PCR assay by increasing the amount of DNA to obtain satisfactory visibility of the bands before performing the preliminary QSTN-PCR.
7. Use Mtb-specific PCR MIMIC M_3 through M_7 dilutions for the preliminary QSTN-PCR. If the target DNA is too abundant, it may be necessary to use a higher concentration of the M_1 dilution or decrease the volume of experimental DNA added to the QSTN-PCR reaction. If too little target DNA is present, it may be necessary to increase the volume of experimental DNA added to the QSTN-PCR or use M_8.
8. Limitations of QSTN-PCR. This is a labor-intensive method that could benefit from automation. In addition to the 4–7 d of culture for marginally smear-positive sputums containing 1000–5000 Mtb, the extraction, QSTN-PCR, and analysis take another 3 d. This still compares favorably to approx 30 d from sample acquisition using radiometric techniques *(1)*. However, the gel electrophoresis required for this technique tend to become a bottle neck and limit increases in through-put. Using real-time fluorescent quantitation such as that available in the ABI 7700 (*Taq*Man) might decrease the PCR and analysis steps to 1 d (*see* **Chapter 13**). The lower limits of this assay may depend on the number of *IS6110* insertion elements present in the strain to be tested. For example, *M. bovis* con-

tains only 1 copy of *IS6110*, whereas strains of Mtb have as many as 16. Unfortunately, some strains have been identified that have no copies of *IS6110* and this technique would not be capable of assessing their drug susceptibility ***(8)***.

Finally, if the 1% control fails to grow, the assay cannot be run. In our experience this is a rare event.

Acknowledgments

This work was supported by a Meyer Young Investigator Award from Southern California Chapter of the Arthritis Foundation and Grant No R95-RE1-169.

References

1. Snider, G. L. (1997) Tuberculosis then and now: a personal perspective on the last 50 years. *Ann. Intern. Med.* **126,** 237–243.
2. Thierry, D., Cave, M. D., Eisenach, K. D., Crawford, J. T., Bates, J. H., Gicquel, B., and Guesdon, J. L. (1990) *IS6110*, an IS-like element of Mycobacterium tuberculosis complex. *Nucleic Acids Res.* **18,** 188.
3. Huebner, R. E., Good, R. C., and Tokars, J. T. (1993) Current practices in Mycobacteriology: results of a survey of state public health laboratories. *J. Clin. Microbiol.* **31,** 771–775.
4. Jou, N. T., Yoshimori, R. B., Mason, G. R., Louie, J. S., and Liebling, M. R. (1997) Single-tube, nested, reverse transcriptase PCR for detection of viable *Mycobacterium tuberculosis. J. Clin. Microbiol.* **35,** 1161–1165.
5. Wilson, S. M., McNerney, R., Nye, P. M., Godfrey-Faussett, P. D., Stoker, N. G., and Voller, A. (1993) Progress toward a Simplified Polymerase Chain Reaction and Its Application to Diagnosis of Tuberculosis. *J Clin Microbiol* **31,** 776–782.
6. Inderleid, C. (1991) Antimycobacterial agents: in vitro susceptibility testing, spectrums of activity, mechanisms of action and resistance and assays for activity in biologic fluids, in *Antibiotics in Laboratory Medicine, Second edition* (Lorian, V., ed.), Williams and Wilkins, Baltimore, pp. 141–148.
7. Siddiqi, S. H. (1992) Radiometric (BACTEC) tests for slowly growing mycobacteria, in *Clinical Microbiology Procedures Handbook* (Isenberg, H. D., ed.), American Society for Microbiology, Washington, DC, pp. 5.14.1–5.14.25.
8. Yuen, .L. K. W., Ross, B. C., Jackson, K. M., and Dwyer, B. (1993) Characterization of *Mycobacterium tuberculosis* strains from Vietnamese patients by southern blot hybridization. *J. Clin. Microbiol.* **31,** 1615–1618.

6

Rapid Rifamycin Susceptibility Testing of Small-Volume *Mycrobacterium tuberculosis* Cultures by Detection of Precursor rRNA

William H. Brabant and Gerard A. Cangelosi

1. Introduction

Clinical laboratory identification of *Mycobacterium tuberculosis* and the *Mycobacterium avium-intracellulare* complex (MAC) has been facilitated in recent years by new DNA and RNA amplification tests *(1–4)*. However, drug susceptibility testing of slowly-growing mycobacteria remains time-consuming and costly, and the need for more rapid tests remains acute *(5)*.

Methods for detecting drug-resistant mycobacteria can be divided into phenotypic and genotypic categories *(4,5)*. Phenotypic methods, including plate, broth, and radiometric tests, measure the bacteriostatic or bacteriocidal effects of drugs on pathogen cells. Such methods detect drug resistance regardless of its genetic basis, but they typically require a long delay due to the slow growth of the organisms. Proposed mycobacteriophage-based phenotypic tests may overcome this problem *(6–8)*. Genotypic methods include polymerase chain reaction (PCR) assays for the genetic determinants of resistance *(4,5,9,10)*. These methods are rapid and specific, but they are unable to provide a complete diagnosis because of the complex genetics of drug resistance. The best-case example for the genotypic approach is the detection of resistance to rifamycin-derived drugs. Most rifampin-resistant *M. tuberculosis* isolates have mutations within an 81-base region of the *rpoB* gene coding for the β-subunit of DNA-dependent RNA polymerase. However, 1% to 10% of rifampin-resistant *M. tuberculosis* isolates, and a much greater percentage of MAC isolates, have wild-type sequences within this region *(5,9–11)*. An additional complication encountered in some nontuberculous mycobacteria is extensive sequence polymorphism among the *rpoB* genes of rifamycin-susceptible strains *(10,11)*.

From: *Methods in Molecular Medicine, vol. 48: Antibiotic Resistance Methods and Protocols*
Edited by: S. H. Gillespie © Humana Press Inc., Totowa, NJ

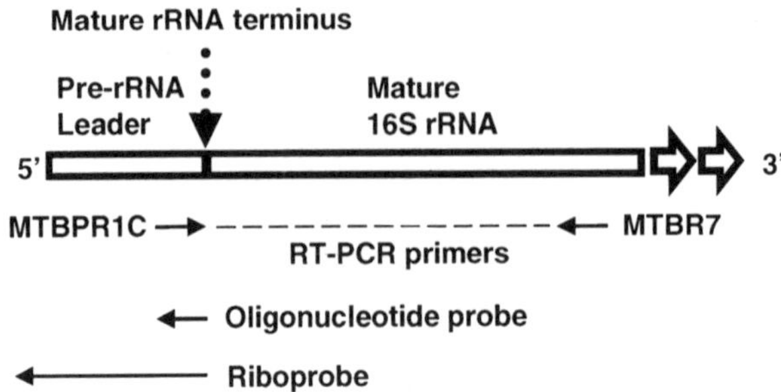

Fig. 1. Probes and RT-PCR primers specific for intact pre-16S rRNA in *M. tuberculosis*. The pre-rRNA leader, thought to be about 160 bases long ***(18)***, is removed in the final steps of ribosome assembly to form the mature 16S rRNA subunit. RT-PCR primers MTBPR1C and MTBR7 recognize sites that straddle the mature rRNA terminus, so that only intact pre-rRNA molecules are amplified. A 26-mer oligonucleotide probe complementary to MTBPR1C has been used to detect pre-rRNA in slot blot hybridization assays ***(13)***. A 174-base RNA probe generated by T7 RNA polymerase transcription with incorporation of multiple radiolabeled ribonucleotides ***(13,14)*** is much more sensitive than the 26-mer.

In order to combine the advantages of genotypic methods (speed, species-specificity, and compatibility with molecular pathogen detection) and phenotypic methods (detection of drug resistance regardless of genetic basis), we developed phenotypic assays that detect mycobacterial ribosomal RNA precursors (pre-rRNA). Pools of pre-rRNA are large, robust, and readily detectable in dividing bacterial cells, but are rapidly drained under conditions that directly or indirectly inhibit RNA synthesis ***(12)***. Such conditions include exposure of susceptible cells to rifamycin or fluoroquinolone drugs ***(13,14)*** (*see* **Note 1**). Pre-rRNA sequences have excellent phylogenetic specificity, which may make them detectable in unpurified samples. Most nucleic acid hybridization methods used to detect mature rRNA can, with appropriate probes or primers, be used to detect pre-rRNA. **Figure 1** shows several direct hybridization probes and reverse-transcriptase PCR primers that are useful for detecting mycobacterial pre-rRNA

We describe here a simple reverse transcriptase-PCR (RT-PCR) assay for *M. tuberculosis* pre-rRNA in cells briefly exposed to rifampin. This procedure was chosen for its speed and low cost. It can be divided into three phases: Exposure of cells to rifampin (steps 1–5), cell lysis and nucleic acid extraction (steps 6–23), and RT-PCR detection of pre-rRNA (steps 24–33). Starting with colonies or broth cultures, phenotypic rifampin susceptibility results can be obtained over the course of 2 normal working days.

2. Materials

1. Slant, plate, or broth cultures of test isolates.
2. Slant, plate, or broth cultures of known rifampin-resistant and rifampin-susceptible *M. tuberculosis* complex strains, preferably attenuated-virulence strains such as *M. tuberculosis* H37Ra or *M. bovis* BCG.
3. Dubos broth with albumin enrichment and glycerol, prepared according to manufacturer's instructions, or equivalent *M. tuberculosis* culture medium such as Middlebrook 7H9.
4. Sterile capped plastic 10 mL culture tubes.
5. Sterile 100 mg/mL rifampin. Concentrated stocks of rifampin (10 mg/mL) can be prepared in dimethyl sulfoxide, sterilized by filtration through 0.2 µm Acrodiscs, and stored frozen.
6. CO_2 incubator.
7. Autoclaved plastic 2 mL and 1.7 mL microcentrifuge tubes.
8. Sterile plastic PCR tubes.
9. 10 mg/mL lysozyme (Sigma Chemical Co.) in TE (10 m*M* Tris pH 7.5, 1 m*M* EDTA), stored in small aliquots at –20°C.
10. 10 mg/mL Proteinase K (Boehringer Mannheim) in TE, stored in small aliquots at –20°C.
11. Lysis solution: 100 m*M* Tris pH 7.5, 50 m*M* EDTA, 2% (w/v) N-lauryl sarcosine, 1% (w/v) sodium dodecyl sulfate, 30 mg/L dithiothreitol, stored at room temperature.
12. GnSCN solution: 100 m*M* Tris pH 7.5, 4.5 *M* guanidine thiocyanate, 10% formamide, 2.1% N-lauryl sarcosine. Gentle heating may be required to dissolve the guanidine thiocyanate. This solution is stable at room temperature, however precipitates may form in cool rooms. Precipitates redissolve rapidly with gentle heating.
13. A water bath set at 37°C.
14. A heating block set at 85°C.
15. Extraction buffer: 50 m*M* Tris-HCl, 10 m*M* EDTA, 100 m*M* NaCl, and 0.5% w/v SDS, pH adjusted to 7.6 using NaOH.
16. 1-methyl-2-pyrrolidinone (Aldrich Chemical, Milwaukee, WI). **Warning:** corrosive.
17. Phenol-Water-Chloroform (Applied Biosystems, catalog #400765). **Warning:** corrosive.
18. Chloroform. **Warning:** corrosive.
19. 3 *M* sodium acetate (NaOAc).
20. 100% ethanol.
21. Deionized water treated with 0.1% (v/v) diethyl pyrocarbonate for 12 h, autoclaved, and stored in small aliquots (DEPC-treated water).
22. 40 U/µL RNasin, (Promega, Madison, WI).
23. RNase-free DNase I, 10 U/µL (Boehringer-Mannheim).
24. Superscript II RNase H Reverse Transcriptase (RT), 200 U/µL (Gibco-BRL Products, catalog #18064-014).
25. 5X first strand buffer (supplied with Gibco-BRL RT).

26. 25 m*M* $MgCl_2$.
27. 15 µ*M* RT primer MTBR7 (5'- GAG AGA ACC CGG ACC TTC GTC GAT G 3'). This primer, which is nearly specific to the *M. tuberculosis* complex, recognizes a region of the mature small-subunit rRNA that begins 441 bases downstream from the 5' mature rRNA terminus (**Fig. 1**).
28. 15 µ*M* PCR primer MTBPR1C (5'-CCC TTT TCC AAA GGG AGT GTT TGG GT 3'). This primer, which is specific to the *M. tuberculosis* complex ***(13)***, hybridizes to cDNA complementary to the 5' pre-rRNA leader region, immediately upstream of the mature rRNA terminus (**Fig. 1**).
29. *Taq* polymerase, 5 U/µL (Fisher Biotech, catalog #FB-6000-15).
30. 10X PCR Buffer A, which contains 15 m*M* $MgCl_2$ (supplied with Fisher Biotech *Taq* polymerase).
31. Deoxyribonucleotide (dNTP) mixture, 10 m*M* each (supplied with Fisher Biotech *Taq* polymerase).
32. 0.1 *M* dithiothreitol.
33. PCR Thermocycler.
34. 2% agarose with 0.05% ethidium bromide (**Warning:** possible carcinogen).
35. Electrophoresis equipment: Gel casting tray, comb, and power supply.

3. Methods

1. ***Biosafety note: Steps 1–13 must be conducted under Biosafety Level 3 guidelines for safe handling of airborne pathogens.***

   Prepare and label three culture tubes for the rifampin-susceptible control strain H37Ra, three for the rifampin-resistant control strain, and three for each additional unknown strain to be tested.
2. To each set of three tubes, add 100 µg/mL rifampin stock as follows: None to tube A; 5 µL (0.5 µg) to tube B; and 20 µL (2.0 µg) to tube C. These "break-point concentrations" can be modified as desired.
3. Suspend one or several colonies (depending on colony size) of each isolate in 3 mL of culture broth. Suspend enough cells to obtain slight visual turbidity (OD_{660} = 0.05 to 0.2). If inocula come from broth cultures, dilute them at least 1:4 into fresh broth to the same turbidity range. This manipulation will stimulate pre-rRNA synthesis in any stationary-phase cells that are present in the samples (*see* **Note 2**).
4. Vortex vigorously to suspend cells as evenly as possible (*see* **Note 3**), and distribute each suspension to culture tubes A–C, 1 mL per tube.
5. Incubate tubes for 24 ± 2 h at 37°C under 5% CO_2. We conduct this incubation on a rotary shaker, however that may not be necessary given the small culture volume.
6. Immediately before beginning the lysis procedure, prepare the enzyme mixture by mixing 10 µL of 10 mg/mL proteinase K per 1 mL of 10 mg/mL lysozyme. You will need 3 mL of enzyme mixture for each strain being tested. The enzyme mixture should be used within one hour of when the two components are thawed

and combined (*see* **Notes 4**, **5**, and **6**) for alternative lysis protocols that do not require enzymes or heat).

7. Transfer the 1-mL cultures to prelabeled screw-cap microcentrifuge tubes and spin at 13,000*g* in an aerosol-proof microcentrifuge for 2 min. Decant supernatant into disinfectant.
8. Resuspend each pellet in 1 mL of enzyme mixture and incubate at 37°C for 30 min.
9. Vortex briefly, centrifuge, and decant supernatant as above.
10. Resuspend each pellet in 0.4 mL lysis solution, and incubate in an 85°C heat block for 5 min.
11. Add 0.6 mL GnSCN solution to each sample and mix. If lysates are not to be analyzed immediately, they can be stored at –20°C for at least several months.
12. To a 2.0 mL microcentrifuge tube add 100 mL lysate, 100 mL 1-methyl-2-pyrrolidinone, 350 mL extraction buffer, and 550 mL phenol-chloroform
13. Vortex briefly and heat at 85°C for 12 min.

    Biosafety note: The samples are no longer infectious after this step. Tubes can now be surface-sterilized and safely removed from the BSL3 lab for completion of the procedure.
14. Centrifuge at 13,000*g* for 8 min.
15. Transfer the aqueous layer (~400 µL) to an autoclaved 2.0 mL microcentrifuge tube.
16. Add 600 µL chloroform, vortex briefly, and centrifuge at 13,000*g* for 5 min.
17. Transfer the aqueous layer (~300 µL) to a new autoclaved 1.7 mL microcentrifuge tube (*see* **Note 5**).
18. Add 30 µL 3 *M* NaOAc and 1 mL 100% ethanol.
19. Store at –20°C for ≥1 h. If analysis is not to proceed immediately, this storage step can be extended indefinitely.
20. Vortex briefly, centrifuge at 13,000*g* for 15 min, and carefully decant supernatant.
21 Wash the pellet once in 70% ethanol and once in 100% ethanol.
22. Carefully air-dry the inverted tube on a paper towel for 1 to 5 min.
23. Redissolve dried pellet in 100 µL of DEPC-treated water and 1 µL of RNasin.
24. The remaining steps are conducted using a preprogrammed PCR thermocycler (*see* **Note 6**). Prepare a master mix containing, per sample, 0.84 µL of RNasin, 0.56 µL of 25 m*M* $MgCl_2$, and 0.6 µL of RNase-free DNase. Be sure to prepare extra master mix for the two control reactions in the next step (*see* **Notes 7** and **8**).
25. Mix 2 µL of this master mix with 5 µL of each sample from **step 23** in a PCR tube. Prepare the following two negative control tubes in the same fashion: A no-sample control tube containing 5 µL of DEPC-treated water instead of nucleic acid sample, and a no-RT control tube containing nucleic acid from one of the "A" (no-rifampin) culture tubes (*see* **step 28**).
26. Place the tubes in the thermocycler and run the DNase program (37°C for 1 h to digest DNA, 90°C for 5 min to denature the enzyme, and 4°C to hold the samples).
27. Prepare a second master mix containing, per sample (plus controls), 4 µL 5X first strand buffer, 1 µL of 15 µ*M* primer MTBR7, 4 µL of DEPC-treated water, and 2 µL of 0.1 *M* dithiothreitol. Add 11 µL of this second master mix to each tube and incubate for 5 min at 70°C in the thermocycler.

28. Prepare a third master mix containing, per sample (plus controls), 1.5 μL dNTP mixture, 0.375 μL DEPC-treated water, and 0.125 μL RT. Remove the tubes from the thermocycler and add 2 μL of this third master mix to each tube except the no-RT control, which instead receives 1.5 μL dNTP mixture and 0.5 μL of DEPC-treated water (the no-RT control assures that DNase treatment was effective and positive signals come from amplification of pre-rRNA, rather than of the chromosomal DNA sequence encoding it).
29. Return the tubes to the thermocycler and incubate at 70°C for a further 10 min.
30. Prepare a fourth master mix containing, per sample (plus controls), 10 μL 10X PCR buffer A, 2 μL dNTP mixture, 1 μL each of primers MTBR7 and MTBPR1C (both 15 μ*M*), 0.5 μL *Taq* polymerase, and 83.5 μL DEPC-treated water. Add 98 μL of this fourth master mix to new labeled 0.2 μL PCR tubes, followed by 2 μL of each RT reaction.
31. Run the RT-PCR program on these tubes, as follows: One cycle of 94°C for 2 min. Five cycles of 94°C for 2 min, 50°C for 1 min, 72°C for 3 min. Fifteen cycles of 94°C for 1 min, 50°C for 1 min, 72°C for 2 min. Fifteen cycles of 94°C for 1 min, 50°C for 1 min, 72°C for 3.5 min. One cycle of 72°C for 7 min. Hold at 4°C.
32. Visualize results by 2% agarose gel electrophoresis.
33. Interpret results as follows. Low-level (0.5 μg/mL) or high-level (2.0 μg/mL) resistance to rifampin is indicated by 491-base pair RT-PCR amplification products derived from culture tubes B or C, respectively (*see* **Note 9**). In order for the test to be considered valid, all strains should yield amplification products from culture tube A (the no-rifampin control). The no-sample and no-RT controls should be negative. The inclusion of rifampin-resistant and rifampin-susceptible control strains in the test provides additional confidence in results.

Pre-rRNA pools can be measured as indicators of ongoing rRNA synthesis, and therefore of ongoing cell growth, for purposes other than drug susceptibility testing. Such measurements could be useful in a variety of microbiological investigations on the growth of individual microbial species in complex samples. The caveat is that pre-rRNA pools are stabilized (or partially stabilized) under some nongrowth conditions in some cells ***(12,17)***.

4. Notes

1. Some drugs (e.g., isoniazid) appear to inhibit pre-rRNA processing simultaneously with synthesis, thereby stabilizing pre-rRNA pools in susceptible cells. Pre-rRNA pools are not good indicators of susceptibility to such drugs.
2. Natural fluctuations in pre-rRNA pools between active growth and stationary phase ***(12)*** are effectively controlled by diluting samples into fresh medium at the outset of the assay. Immediately upon such a nutritional shift-up, stationary-phase *M. tuberculosis* complex cells with depleted pre-rRNA pools initiate pre-rRNA synthesis, resulting in large pre-rRNA pools within 24 hours (unless pre-rRNA synthesis is inhibited by rifampin). We have never failed to observe this in

repeated experiments on *M. bovis* BCG cells held in stationary phase for ≥4 months under both aerobic and anaerobic conditions.

3. It is often difficult to evenly distribute flocculent *M. tuberculosis* cell suspensions between the three culture tubes. This problem is common to all diagnostic procedures that require division of *M. tuberculosis* samples. However, the quantitative error introduced by this problem is negligible relative to the total depletion of pre-rRNA that occurs in susceptible *M. tuberculosis* complex cells exposed to rifampin ***(13)***.
4. Because of its abundance and its complex secondary and tertiary structure, pre-rRNA is significantly more robust than bacterial messenger RNA. Nonetheless, it is prudent to take standard precautions to protect samples from RNase contamination, especially in the steps that come after phenol-chloroform extraction (**steps 17–31**). Such precautions include the use of latex gloves and dedicated reagents and supplies.
5. Given the stability and abundance of pre-rRNA, it is likely that most published methods for lysing mycobacterial cells and extracting their RNA would work as well, if not better, than the lysis and extraction protocols described above. In some experiments, we have successfully replaced **steps 6–11** with a more simple mechanical lysis protocol modified from Stahl and Urbance ***(15)***. Cultures are centrifuged and cell pellets are resuspended in 1 mL of breakage buffer (50 m*M* Tris, 20 m*M* $MgCl_2$, 50 m*M* KCl, 5 m*M* 2-mercaptoethanol, pH 7.5), transferred to screw-top microcentrifuge tubes containing 0.1 mm diameter glass beads, and disrupted for 3 min on a BioSpec Mini-Bead Beater 8 (fast setting). The lysates are cleared by centrifugation for 2 min at 13,000*g*, then transferred to sterile microcentrifuge tubes for further processing or storage as in **step 11**. We have not determined if such lysates work well in the RT-PCR assay described here, but we have had no problems with them in other PCR amplification reactions. Very simple and widely-used alternative protocols employing FastPrep equipment and reagents (Bio 101, La Jolla, CA) may also work well ***(16)***.
6. The complex series of incubations required for RT-PCR are simplified by running all of them in a thermocycler with a program for each individual step.
7. Always make 10% more master mix than needed to make up for pipeting error.
8. When mixing of small-volume reactions, use brief microcentrifugation to force droplets to the bottoms of tubes, and mix by pipeting gently up and down a couple of times.
9. The MAC differs from the *M. tuberculosis* complex in that most MAC isolates are heterogeneous with regard to drug susceptibility, and most MAC cell populations have small subpopulations drug-resistant (SmT) colony variants which are usually detectable in the sensitive RT-PCR assay. We have described a more useful slot-blot hybridization assay for pre-rRNA in the MAC ***(14)***.

References

1. Heifets, L. (1997) Mycobacteriology laboratory. *Clin. Chest Med.* **18,** 35–53.
2. Kennedy, N., Gillespie, S. H., Saruni, A.,O., Kisyombe, G., McNerney, R., Ngowi, F. I., and Wilson, S. (1994) Polymerase chain reaction for assessing treatment response in patients with pulmonary tuberculosis. *J. Infect. Dis.* **170,** 713–716.

3. Roth, A., Schaberg, T., and Mauch, H. (1997) Molecular diagnosis of tuberculosis: current clinical validity and future perspectives. *Eur. Respir. J.* **10,** 1877–1891.
4. Shinnick, T. M. and Jonas, V. (1994) Molecular approaches to the diagnosis of tuberculosis, in *Tuberculosis: Pathogenesis, Protection, and Control* (Bloom, B. R., ed.), ASM, Washington, DC
5. Heifets, L. and Cangelosi, G. A. (1999) Drug susceptibility testing of *Mycobacterium tuberculosis*—A neglected problem at the turn of the century. *Intl. J. Tuberc. Lung Dis.,* **3,** 564–581.
6. Carriere, C., Riska, P. F., Zimhony, O., Kriakov, J., Bardarov, S., Burns, J., Chan, J., and Jacobs, W. R., Jr. (1997) Conditionally replicating luciferase reporter phages: improved sensitivity for rapid detection and assessment of drug susceptibility of *Mycobacterium tuberculosis*. *J. Clin. Microbiol.* **35,** 3232–3239.
7. Riska, P. F., Jacobs, W. R., Jr., Bloom, B. R., McKitrick, J., and Chan, J. (1997) Specific identification of *Mycobacterium tuberculosis* with the luciferase reporter mycobacteriophage: use of p-Nitro-a-Acetylamino-b-Hydroxy propiophenone. *J. Clin. Microbiol.* **35,** 3225–3231.
8. Wilson, S., Al-Suwaidi, Z., McNerney, R., Porter, J., and Drobniewski, F. (1997) Evaluation of a new rapid bacteriophage-based method for the drug susceptibility testing of *Mycobacterium tuberculosis*. *Nature Med.* **3,** 465–468.
9. Telenti, A., Honore, N., Bernasconi, C., March, J., Ortega, A., Heym, B., Takiff, H. E., and Cole, S. T. (1997) Genotypic assessment of isoniazid and rifampicin resistance in *Mycobacterium tuberculosis:* a blind study at reference laboratory level. *J. Clin. Microbiol.* **35,** 719–723.
10. Gingeras, T. R., Ghandour, G., Wang, E., Berno, A., Small, P. M., Drobniewski, F., Alland, D., Desmond, E., Holodniy, M., and Drenkow, J. (1998) Simultaneous genotyping and species identification using hybridization pattern recognition analysis of generic *Mycobacterium* DNA arrays. *Genome Res.* **8,** 435–448.
11. Inderlied, C. B., Kemper, C. A., and Bermudez, L. E. M. (1993). The *Mycobacterium avium* complex. *Clin. Microbiol. Rev.* **6,** 236–310.
12. Cangelosi, G. A., and Brabant, W. H. (1997) Depletion of pre–16S rRNA in starved *Escherichia coli* cells. *J. Bacteriol.* **179,** 4457–4463.
13. Cangelosi, G. A., Brabant, W. H., Britschgi, T. B., and Wallis, C. W. (1996) Detection of rifampicin- and ciprofloxacin-resistant *Mycobacterium tuberculosis* by using species-specific assays for precursor rRNA. *Antimicrob. Agents Chemother.* **40,** 1790–1795.
14. Cangelosi,G. A., Palermo, C. O., Laurent, J. -P., Hamlin, A. M., and Brabant, W. H. (1999). Colony morphotypes on Congo Red agar segregate along species and drug susceptibility lines in the *Mycobacterium avium-intracellulare* complex. *Microbiology*, **145,** 1317–1324.
15. Stahl, D. A. and Urbance, J. W. (1990) The division between fast- and slow-growing species corresponds to natural relationships among the mycobacteria. *J. Bacteriol.* **172,** 116–124
16. Hellyer, T. J., DesJardin, L. E., Hehman, G. L., Cave, M. D., and Eisenach, K. D. (1999) Quantitative analysis of mRNA as a marker for viability of *Mycobacterium tuberculosis*. *J. Clin. Microbiol.* **37,** 290–295.

17. Cangelosi, G. A., Hamlin, A. M, Buck, K. R., and Scholin, C. A. (1997) Detection of stable pre-rRNA in toxigenic *Pseudo-nitzschia* species. *Appl. Environm. Microbiol.* **63,** 4859–4865.
18. Ji, Y., Colston, J. M., and Cox, R. A. (1994). Nucleotide sequence and secondary structures of precursor 16S rRNA of slow-growing mycobacteria. *Microbiology* **140,** 123–132.

7

Detection of Penicillin Resistance in *Streptococcus pneumoniae* by a Seminested PCR Strategy

Mignon du Plessis, Anthony M. Smith, and Keith P. Klugman

1. Introduction

The first appearance of clinically significant penicillin-resistant *Streptococcus pneumoniae* (pneumococcus) occurred in 1967 in Australia *(1)* and penicillin-resistant and multiresistant pneumococci have subsequently spread globally and reached high prevalence in many countries *(2)*.

Effective treatment of pneumococcal infections requires rapid detection of both the organism and its susceptibility pattern. Presently, culture of the causative organism and susceptibility testing require at least 48 h. However, owing to the development of molecular techniques, it is now possible to detect penicillin-resistant pneumococci in a CSF specimen, using a seminested PCR strategy *(3,4)*. This method is rapid, specific and sensitive and, since it does not depend on the presence of viable organisms, it may be applicable in cases of prior antibiotic treatment.

The targets for β-lactam antibiotics are cell wall-synthesizing enzymes known as penicillin-binding proteins (PBPs). Penicillin-resistant pneumococci produce altered PBPs that have reduced affinities for β-lactam drugs. Studies have shown that alterations in PBP 2X result in low-level penicillin resistance, whereas high-level penicillin resistance requires alterations in PBPs 2B and 1A *(5,6)*. This led us to develop two PCR assays which, not only detect penicillin resistance in the pneumococcus (PBP 2B assay), but also distinguish between higher and low-level resistance (PBP 1A assay). The design of the primers, used for detecting penicillin-resistance, is based on common alterations which are present in the *pbp2b* and *1a* genes of all penicillin-resistant pneumococci *(7–10)*. Nucleotide sequence analysis of the pneumococcal *pbp2b*

From: *Methods in Molecular Medicine, vol. 48: Antibiotic Resistance Methods and Protocols*
Edited by: S. H. Gillespie © Humana Press Inc., Totowa, NJ

gene from penicillin-resistant isolates has shown extensive alterations in the gene compared with the *pbp2b* gene of susceptible strains ***(11)***. Smith and Klugman showed that all penicillin-resistant pneumococci evaluated in their study had nucleotide sequence divergence within a 300-bp area at the center of the *pbp2b* transpeptidase-encoding region ***(10)***. They also revealed that amino acid substitutions occurring within this area could be grouped into five different profiles. For the PBP 2B PCR diagnosis of penicillin resistance, four primers are used which encompass these multiple mutational pathways in the *pbp2b* gene (2B-R1, 2B-R2, 2B-R3, and 2B-R4). In the analysis of the pneumococcal *pbp1a* gene, Smith and Klugman described four amino acid substitutions common to all penicillin-resistant isolates with MICs of ≥0.25 μg/mL ***(8)***. The design of resistance primer 1A-R1 is based on these four consecutive mutations. Resistance primer 1A-R2 is designed to bind to an area downstream of the conserved Ser-428-Arg-Asn motif. Since mutations in this area of the gene were found to occur in isolates for which penicillin MICs are ≥1 μg/mL, only DNA from higher level resistant isolates will be amplified with this primer.

2. Materials

2.1. Preparation of DNA template for PCR

1. Tris-EDTA buffer: 10 m*M* Tris-HCl, 1.0 m*M* EDTA, pH 8.0 (autoclave at 15 psi, 121°C for 15 min and store at room temperature).
2. 10% SDS: store at room temperature.
3. 20 mg/mL proteinase K: prepare in sterile, deionized H_2O and store at –20°C.
4. 5 *M* NaCl: store at room temperature.
5. 10% CTAB in 0.7 *M* NaCl: heat to 65°C to dissolve and store at room temperature (do not autoclave).
6. Phenol: chloroform: isoamyl (25:24:1): store at 4°C. (**CAUTION:** phenol burns when it comes into contact with the skin so use gloves when handling this chemical.)
7. Chloroform: store at room temperature.
8. Isopropanol: store at room temperature or 4°C.
9. 70% ethanol: store at 4°C or –20°C.

2.2. Buffers and Stock Solutions for PCR

All PCR components are available commercially. All components should be diluted in sterile, deionized H_2O and stored at –20°C, unless otherwise stated.

1. Geneamp® 10X PCR buffer (Perkin-Elmer, Blanchburg, NJ): 20 m*M* Tris-HCl, pH 9.0, 100 m*M* KCl, 0.1 m*M* EDTA, 1.0 m*M* DTT, 0.5% Tween-20, 50% (v/v) glycerol.
2. 25 m*M* $MgCl_2$.
3. dNTPs: a mixture of all four (dATP, dCTP, dGTP, dTTP) at a concentration of 1.25 m*M* each. Dispense into 100–200 μL aliquots.

Table 1
Sequences of Oligonucleotide Primers Used in the PCR Diagnosis of Penicillin Resistance in *Streptococcus pneumoniae*

		Position in pbp gene	
Primer	Sequence (5' → 3')	2B	1A
2B-R1	GCCTTTTCTAGGCCAATGCCGATTAC	697-722	
2B-R2	GCCTACGATTCATTCCCGATT	700-720	
2B-R3	AAATTGGCATATGGATCTTTTCCT	694-717	
2B-R4	GTTTTAACTAACAATTTAGAATCC	814-837	
2B-U	CTGACCATTGATTTGGCTTTCCAA	346-369	
2B-D	TTTGCAATAGTTGCTACATACTG	1006-1028	
1A-R1	AAGAACACTGGTTATGTA		2662-2679
1A-R2	AGCATGCATTATGCAAAC		2317-2334
1A-U	ACAAATGTAGACCAAGAAGCTCAA		1843-1866
1A-D	TACGAATTCTCCATTTCTGTAGAG		2863-2886

4. Primers: 10 μ*M* stock solutions.
5. Ampli*Taq* Gold DNA polymerase: 5 U/mL (e.g., Perkin-Elmer, Roche Molecular Systems, Inc., Branchburg, NJ) (*see* **Note 1**).
6. Agarose: use molecular biology grade suitable for preparation of high concentration gels on which to separate fragments ranging from 100 bp–5 kb.
7. Tris/acetic acid/EDTA electrophoresis buffer: prepare a 10X stock (400 m*M* Tris, 400 m*M* acetic acid, and 20 m*M* EDTA), store at 4°C.
8. Sample loading buffer (5X): 0.25% bromophenol blue, 40% sucrose.
9. DNA molecular weight markers.
10. Ethidium bromide: 10 mg/mL, wrap in aluminum foil and store at 4°C. (**CAUTION:** a powerful mutagen and potential carcinogen so use gloves when handling this chemical.)

2.3. Primers

The selection of the *pbp2b* and *1a* primers is based on the published sequence data of penicillin-resistant, wild-type *Streptococcus pneumoniae* strains *(8,10)* (*see* **Table 1**).

3. Methods

3.1. Preparation of CSF Specimens for PCR

Aliquot 20 μL of the CSF specimen into a 0.5 mL microcentrifuge tube and boil for 5–10 min. This can be carried out by placing tubes in a polystyrene float in a beaker of water and heating with a Bunsen burner. Centrifuge briefly (5 s) to pellet heavy debris and use 3–5 μL of supernatant as template for PCR (*see* **Note 2**).

3.2. Preparation of DNA Template for PCR

1. Harvest bacterial cells from an overnight plate culture into a 1.5 mL microcentrifuge tube and pellet by centrifugation at 4800*g* for 3 min.
2. Resuspend pellet in 567 µL TE buffer.
3. Add 30 µL SDS and 3 µL proteinase K.
4. Incubate at 37°C for 1 h or until solution goes clear (*see* **Note 3**).
5. Add 100 µL NaCl and mix by inverting the tube.
6. Add 80 µL CTAB/NaCl, mix, and incubate at 65°C for 10 min.
7. Add an equal volume phenol: chloroform: isoamyl, mix, and centrifuge at 4800*g* for 5 min.
8. Remove aqueous phase (top phase) and transfer to a fresh tube (*see* **Note 4**).
9. Add equal volume chloroform, mix, and centrifuge at 4800*g* for 5 min.
10. Remove top phase and transfer to a fresh tube.
11. Add 0.6 vol isopropanol, mix and centrifuge at 4800*g* for 10 min.
12. Pour off supernatant and wash pellet with 70% ethanol.
13. Dry pellet in a heating block (37–45°C) for 15–30 min.
14. Resuspend pellet in 50 µL TE buffer (*see* **Note 5**).
15. DNA can further be diluted 1:10 and 1–2 µL used for PCR (*see* **Note 6**).

3.3. Polymerase Chain Reaction

3.3.1. Primer Combinations

The PBP 2B PCR assay requires 6 primers in total, in a single reaction:

2B-U and 2B-D are external primers specific for amplifying pneumococcal DNA. 2B-R1, 2B-R2, 2B-R3, and 2B-R4 are internal primers which, together with the downstream primer 2B-D, amplify products which indicate penicillin resistance (*see* **Fig. 1**).

The PBP 1A PCR assay requires 3 primers in two separate reactions (*see* **Note 7**):

1. Primers 1A-U, 1A-D, and 1A-R1
2. Primers 1A-U, 1A-D, and 1A-R2

1A-U and 1A-D are external primers specific for amplifying pneumococcal DNA. 1A-R1 and 1A-R2 are internal primers which, together with primer 1A-D, amplify products which indicate penicillin resistance (*see* **Fig. 2**).

3.3.2. Preparation of Reaction Mixes

1. Prepare PCR reaction mixes in 50 µL vol in 0.5 mL microcentrifuge tubes.
2. Prepare a master mix for the PCR reaction (calculate the volume according to the number of individual reactions to be prepared).
3. An individual reaction contains the following: 5 µL 10X reaction buffer, 4 µL 25 m*M* $MgCl_2$, 5 µL dNTPs (1.25 m*M* stock), 1 µL of each primer (10 µ*M* stock), 0.5 µL (2.5 U) Ampli*Taq* Gold DNA polymerase. Make up to volume with sterile, deionized H_2O, taking into account that template still has to be added.

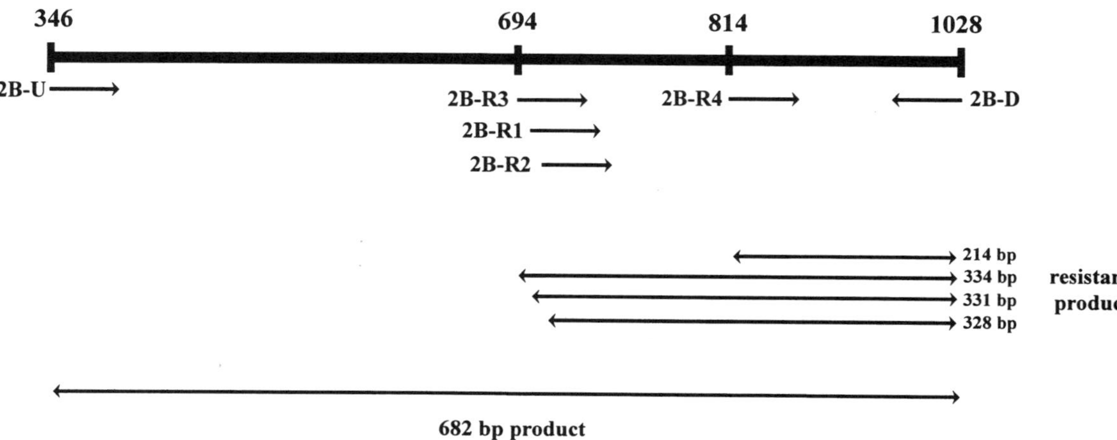

Fig. 1. Primer binding sites in the streptococcus pneumoniae *pbp2b* gene.

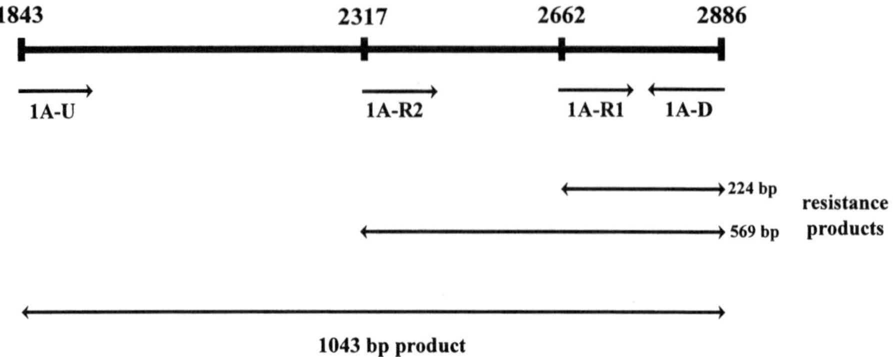

Fig. 2. Primer binding sites in the streptococcus *pbp1a* gene.

4. Mix well by inversion, centrifuge briefly and aliquot the reaction mix into each tube.
5. Add template (50 ng DNA or 3–5 µL boiled CSF) taking care to avoid cross contamination (use separate tips for each transfer) (*see* **Note 8**).
6. Overlay each tube with mineral oil if necessary.

3.3.3. Positive and Negative Controls

It is essential to include controls to ensure that the PCR results obtained are true positives and negatives (*see* **Note 9**).

The positive controls are:

1. pneumococcal genomic DNA isolated from an organism of known MIC.
2. a known culture positive CSF.

The negative controls are:

1. a tube containing all PCR reagents except template.
2. a known culture negative CSF.

3.3.4. Thermal Cycling

The PCR process includes an initial 10 min incubation at 93°C to activate the Ampli*Taq* Gold DNA polymerase and denature the target DNA. This is followed by: 25 cycles at 93°C for 45 s, 50°C or 55°C for 45 s (*see* **Note 7**) and 72°C for 45 s. A 5 min extension at 72°C is required at the end of the final cycle.

3.3.5. Analysis of PCR Products

1. Prepare a 2% agarose gel containing 1X TAE buffer and 6% ethidium bromide.
2. Add 5 µL loading dye to the amplification product.

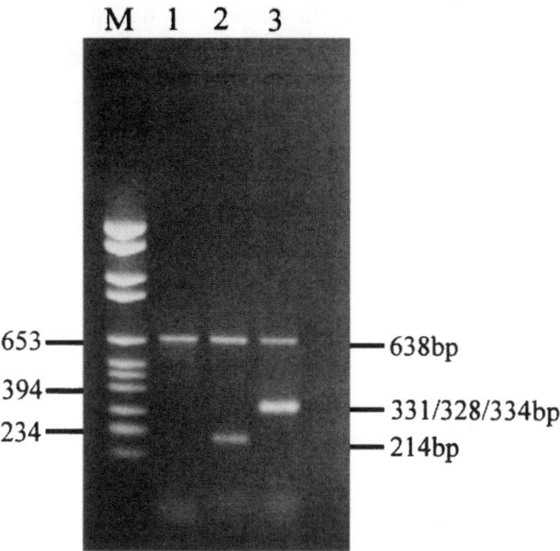

Fig. 3. Agarose gel electrophoresis of PCR-amplified DNA fragments of the *pbp2b* gene from *S. pneumoniae*. Lane M, molecular weight marker (in base pairs). Lane 1, isolates whose penicillin MICs are 0.03/0.06 µg/mL produce a single 638- bp pneumococcal specific product. Isolates whose MICS are ≥0.12 µg/mL produce an additional resistance product: either a 214-bp product arising from amplification with primers 2B-R4 + 2B-D (lane 2), a 331- bp product arising from amplification with primers 2B-R1 + 2B-D (lane 3), a 328- bp product arising from amplification with primers 2B-R2 + 2B-D (lane 3), OR a 334- bp product arising from amplification with primers 2B-R3 + 2B-D (lane 3).

3. Load 5 µL sample into the well of the gel.
4. Load a DNA marker into one of the flanking wells.
5. Run the gel at 10 V/cm until the bromophenol blue has migrated approx 1/3 the length of the gel.
6. Visualize the DNA bands by placing the gel on a UV transilluminator.
7. Photograph the gel.

3.3.6. Interpretation of Results

1. PBP 2B Assay (*see* **Fig. 3**).

   The resistance primers 2B-R1, 2B-R2, 2B-R3, and 2B-R4, together with downstream primer 2B-D, amplify products of 331-bp, 328-bp, 334-bp, and 214-bp, respectively. The presence of any of these bands implies that the organism has a penicillin MIC of ≥0.12 µg/mL. Primers 2B-U and 2B-D produce a 638-bp species specific product which confirms the identification of the organism as *S. pneumoniae*.
2. PBP 1A Assay (*see* **Fig. 4**).

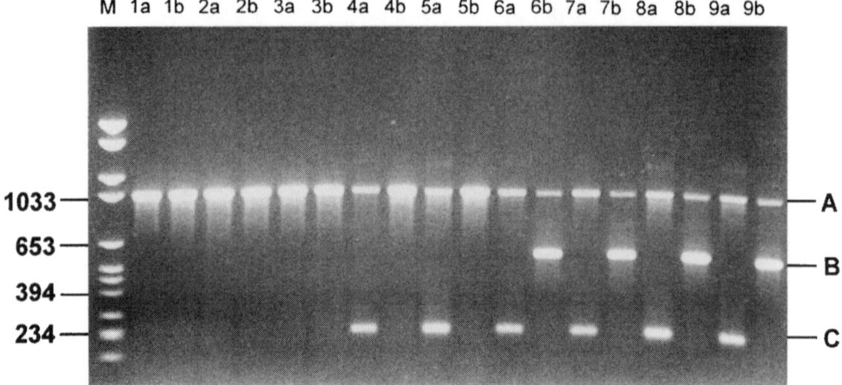

Fig. 4. Agarose gel electrophoresis of PCR-amplified DNA fragments of the *pbp1a* gene from *S. pneumoniae*. Lane M, molecular weight marker (in base pairs). Primer combinations are as follows: 1A-U + 1A-D + 1A-R1 (lanes a); 1A-U + 1A-D + 1A-R2 (lanes b). The penicillin MICs for the isolates are as follows: 0.03 μg/mL (lanes 1), 0.06 μg/mL (lanes 2), 0.125 μg/mL (lanes 3), 0.25 μg/mL (lanes 4), 0.5 μg/mL (lanes 5), 1 μg/mL (lanes 6), 2 μg/mL (lanes 7), 4 μg/mL (lanes 8), 8 μg/mL (lanes 9). **A,** a 1043-bp arising from amplification with primers 1A-U and 1A-D; **B,** a 569-bp product arising from amplification with primers 1A-D and 1A-R2; **C,** a 224-bp product arising from amplification with primers 1A-D and 1A-R1.

Those isolates for which penicillin MICs are 0.03–0.06 μg/mL produce only one amplification product, the 1043-bp product which identifies the organism as *S. pneumoniae*. Isolates with intermediate levels of resistance (MICs, 0.25–0.5 μg/mL) produce an additional amplification product of 224-bp (primers 1A-R1 and 1A-D), whereas isolates whose MICs are ≥1 μg/mL produce two resistance products of 224-bp and 569-bp (primers 1A-R2 and 1A-D). The 569-bp product is indicative of higher-level penicillin resistance.

3.4. Sensitivity and Specificity of the PCR Assays

When optimizing a PCR assay, sensitivity and specificity are critical factors. The sensitivity of the assay is determined by the smallest amount of DNA that can be detected in the shortest possible time. The assay should also be specific in that the primers should not amplify DNA from bacterial species other than *S. pneumoniae*.

3.4.1. Sensitivity

3.4.1.1. Colony Forming Units (CFUs)

1. Pick off a single colony from an overnight culture of *S. pneumoniae* and transfer into 50 μL H_2O or culture negative CSF (*see* **Note 10**).

2. Prepare a series of 10-fold dilutions using either H_2O or culture negative CSF as a diluent (dependent on whether the colony was originally resuspended in H_2O or CSF).
3. For each dilution, plate 25 µL onto Columbia blood agar plates and incubate overnight at 37°C in 5% CO_2.
4. Boil diluted samples for 5–10 min and analyze 5 µL by PCR for 20 and 25 cycles.
5. Do colony counts and determine the CFUs present in the 5 µL suspensions used for PCR.
6. The sensitivity is determined by the number of CFUs present in the lowest dilution detected by PCR, i.e., the least number of CFUs which will give a positive PCR result.

3.4.1.2. Genomic DNA

1. Measure the concentration of the genomic DNA using a spectrophotometer (260 nm). For double-stranded DNA, an optical density of 1 (at 260 nm) is roughly equivalent to 50 µg/mL.
2. Dilute DNA 10-fold in sterile, deionized H_2O and use 1 µL of each dilution per PCR reaction for 20 and 25 cycles.
3. The sensitivity is determined by the amount of DNA present in the lowest dilution detected by PCR, i.e., the smallest amount of genomic DNA which will give a positive PCR result.

3.4.2. Specificity

This is determined by testing the PCR assays using a variety of bacterial species, in particular other streptococcal species as well as organisms which are likely to be found in a CSF specimen, e.g., *Neisseria meningitidis, Haemophilus influenzae, Listeria monocytogenes*, coagulase negative staphylococcus, *Moraxella catarrhalis, Mycobacterium tuberculosis*, and *Enterococcus faecalis*. Bacterial DNA is isolated according to the aforementioned protocol and PCR carried out exactly the same as for *Streptococcus pneumoniae* for 20 and 25 cycles (*see* **Note 11**).

4. Notes

1. Ampli*Taq* Gold DNA polymerase is useful for the development and optimization of multiplex amplification systems, particularly those in which primers are not well designed and/or the reaction conditions are not optimal. Ampli*Taq* Gold reduces background, significantly enhances yield and improves specificity by eliminating mispriming because it remains inactive until heated. This feature allows flexibility in reaction setup, including premixing of PCR reagents at room temperature.
2. PCR is able to detect the presence of pneumococcal DNA, equally as efficiently, in both the supernatant and deposit fractions of a CSF specimen, however, since the pellet is likely to contain inhibitors it is advisable to use the supernatant.

3. When the bacterial cell wall lyses the solution becomes viscous and turns clear. If the solution remains turbid after the 1 h incubation, add more sodium dodecyl sulfate (SDS) and/or proteinase K and incubate at 45°C.
4. If lots of white precipitate is present at the interface, it is advisable to repeat this step.
5. Avoid vortexing as this tends to shear the DNA. Resuspend by gentle pipeting or incubation at 65°C for 5 min (for large quantities).
6. PCR has been shown to adequately detect as little as 10fg DNA and 3×10^3 cfu/mL *(3,12)*. Too much DNA is likely to inhibit the PCR reaction rather than increase the sensitivity.
7. An annealing temperature of 55°C is optimal for all the primers except for primer 1A-R1 which appears to anneal better at 50°C. Primers 1A-U and 1A-D anneal equally well at both 50°C and 55°C.
8. For multiple PCR reactions encompassing a variety of primers and DNA templates, it is essential to use separate tips when adding different components together, in particular the PCR reagents and primers. Contamination of a single component will result in false positives and/or negatives. Ensure that sterile, deionized water is used throughout and that this water is used for PCR only, i.e., not for general use in the laboratory.
9. Application of this PCR assay to a clinical specimen requires two controls, namely, one for the specimen processing stage and one for the PCR stage.
10. When developing a PCR assay for detecting DNA directly from a clinical specimen, it is advisable to evaluate the sensitivity and specificity by spiking culture negative specimen rather than using H_2O. The presence of inhibitors in the specimen may produce false negatives.
11. *Taq* DNA polymerase lacks a proofreading activity and thus does not correct any mismatches should the primer not match the target DNA identically at the 3' end. Primer mismatches can result in nonspecific product formation. It has been demonstrated that during the first few cycles of a PCR, extension from mismatched primers can occur, albeit very inefficiently *(13)*. Only later in the PCR, when perfectly matched products of these initial extensions serve as templates, will exponential amplification commence. After approx 25 cycles of PCR, similar amounts of DNA (for matched and mismatched target DNA) will be visualized on an agarose gel. Analysis of amplification products after 15–20 cycles, effectively eliminates the probability of nonspecific DNA fragments being amplified to the degree that they will be visible by gel electrophoresis. We therefore suggest that the minimum number of PCR cycles be run such that nonspecific amplification is reduced without compromising efficient amplification of the target DNA.

References

1. Hansman, D. and Bullen, M. M. (1967) A resistant pneumococcus. *Lancet* **ii,** 264–265.
2. Appelbaum, P. C. (1992) Antimicrobial resistance in *Streptococcus pneumoniae*: an overview. *Clin. Infect. Dis.* **15,** 77–83.

3. du Plessis, M., Smith, A. M., and Klugman, K. P. (1998) Rapid detection of penicillin-resistant *Streptococcus pneumoniae* in cerebrospinal fluid by a seminested PCR strategy. *J. Clin. Microbiol.* **36,** 453–457.
4. du Plessis, M., Smith, A.M., and Klugman, K. P. (1999) Application of *pbp1a* PCR in identification of penicillin-resistant *Streptococcus pneumoniae. J. Clin. Microbiol.* **37,** 628–632.
5. Barcus, V. A., Ghanekar, K., Yeo, M., Coffey, T. J., and Dowson, C. G. (1995) Genetics of high-level penicillin resistance in clinical isolates of *Streptococcus pneumoniae. FEMS Microbiol. Lett.* **126,** 299–304.
6. Smith, A. M., Klugman, K. P., Coffey, T. J., and Spratt, B. G. (1993) Genetic diversity of penicillin-binding protein 2B and 2X genes from *Streptococcus pneumoniae* in South Africa. *Antimicrob. Agents. Chemother.* **37,** 1938–1944.
7. Martin, C., Sibold, C., and Hakenbeck, R. (1992) Relatedness of penicillin-binding 1a genes from different clones of penicillin-resistant *Streptococcus pneumoniae* isolated in South Africa and Spain. *EMBO J.* **11,** 3831–3836.
8. Smith, A. M. and Klugman, K. P. (1998) Alterations in PBP 1A essential for high-level penicillin resistance in *Streptococcus pneumoniae. Antimicrob. Agents Chemother.* **42,** 1329–1333.
9. Asahi, C. and Ubukata, K. (1998) Association of a Thr–371 substitution in a conserved amino acid motif of penicillin-binding protein 1A with penicillin-resistance of *Streptococcus pneumoniae. J. Clin. Microbiol.* **42,** 2267–2273.
10. Smith, A. M. and Klugman, K. P. (1995) Alterations in penicillin-binding protein 2B from penicillin-resistant wild-type strains of *Streptococcus pneumoniae. Antimicrob. Agents Chemother.* **39,** 859–867.
11. Dowson, C. G., Hutchinson, A., Brannigan, J. A., George, R. C., Hansman, D., Linares J., Tomasz, A., Maynard Smith, A., and Spratt, B. G. (1989) Horizontal transfer of penicillin-binding protein genes in penicillin-resistant clinical isolates of *Streptococcus pneumoniae. Proc. Natl. Acad. Sci. USA* **86,** 8842–8846.
12. Rudolph, K. M., Parkinson, A. J., Black, C. M., and Mayer, L. W. (1993) Evaluation of polymerase chain reaction for diagnosis of pneumococcal pneumonia. *J. Clin. Microbiol.* **31,** 2661–2666.
13. Kaltenböck, B. and Schneider, R. (1998) Differential amplification kinetics for point mutation analysis by PCR. *Biotechniques* **24,** 202–206.

8

Diagnosis of Penicillin Resistance by PCR-RFLP

Gail C. Whiting

1. Introduction

Streptococcus pneumoniae is an important human pathogen causing a wide spectrum of disease including pneumonia, otitis media, bacteraemia, and meningitis. It is a significant cause of morbidity and mortality worldwide and now penicillin resistance is becoming an ever increasing problem ***(1–3)***. Initially, all *S. pneumoniae* isolates were exquisitely sensitive to penicillin and thus it was the drug of choice. However, the increase in resistance to penicillin seen in *S. pneumoniae* throughout the world has complicated treatment protocols. Penicillin resistance in *S. pneumoniae* also leads to some degree of cross resistance to other β-lactams, including the third generation cephalosporins and the carbapenems.

Penicillin resistance in *S. pneumoniae* results from multiple alterations in the penicillin binding proteins (PBPs) which are required during the final stages of the biosynthesis of peptidoglycan, an essential structural component of the cell wall. In penicillin-resistant strains, alterations in these PBPs lead to a reduced affinity for the antibiotic ***(4)***. Penicillin-resistant clinical isolates of *S. pneumoniae* have modifications in three of the five high molecular weight penicillin-sensitive PBPs, PBP1a, PBP2x, and PBP2b ***(5,6)***. The altered proteins have arisen due to interspecies recombination events that have occurred between pneumococcal *pbp* genes and those of related streptococci, *S. mitis*, *S. oralis*, and *S. sanguis*. The interspersed sections of DNA have given these altered genes the name "mosaic genes." There is wide variation in the sequence of resistant *pbp* genes ***(7,8)***. In contrast, *pbp* genes of penicillin-sensitive strains show very little variation. The amino acid substitutions that result from gene mosaicism are found mainly to occur in the carboxy-terminal transpeptidase domain and cause a reduction in the affinity of PBP proteins for penicillin ***(9,10)***.

From: *Methods in Molecular Medicine, vol. 48: Antibiotic Resistance Methods and Protocols*
Edited by: S. H. Gillespie © Humana Press Inc., Totowa, NJ

In clinical practice, *S. pneumoniae* is defined as penicillin susceptible with an MIC of <0.1 mg/L, intermediately resistant with an MIC of 0.1 to <2 mg/L, and resistant with an MIC of >2 mg/L. The time taken to determine penicillin susceptibility may be critical for choosing the therapy for bacteraemia and meningitis. Culture methods for the identification of *S. pneumoniae* currently require 16 to 24 h to perform and the conventional culture-based susceptibility testing requires a further 24 h. Recently a number of PCR amplification-based techniques have been reported for the identification of penicillin resistant strains although all of these methods rely on multiple PCR amplifications and may in addition require culture-based identification prior to susceptibility testing ***(11–13)***.

Alterations in the *pbp2b* gene may lead to resistant strains with MICs of ≥0.1 mg/L and this suggests that *pbp2b* may be appropriate to be used as a single target for diagnosing penicillin resistance ***(10)***. We have used a combination of PCR amplification and restriction fragment length polymorphism analysis (RFLP) of the *pbp2b* gene, using the restriction enzyme *Hin*fI, to identify penicillin susceptibility successfully ***(14)***. A similar method has recently been described using *Hae*III and *Rsa*I profiling that confirms the utility of this approach in identifying penicillin susceptible organisms ***(15)***.

This chapter describes the protocol for the determination of penicillin resistance by PCR-RFLP (**Table 1**). The primers used for the PCR amplification, PBP2B1 and PBP2B2, are directed to the 3' 486 codons of the *pbp2b* transpeptidase domain ***(9,16)***. Susceptible isolates (MIC <0.1 mg/L) invariably demonstrate a single RFLP profile, pattern A. Isolates with an MIC >1 mg/L have characteristic RFLP profiles of patterns H, J, or K. Intermediate resistant strains with an MIC of 0.1 to <1 mg/L have a wider range of profiles. The PCR primers are specific for the pneumococcal *pbp2b* gene and so this method is appropriate for the rapid detection of penicillin-sensitive and penicillin-resistant *S. pneumoniae* isolates from sterile clinical specimens such as CSF ***(14)***.

2. Materials

2.1. DNA Preparation

1. Blood agar plates.
2. Sterile 0.5 mL microcentrifuge tubes.
3. Sterile distilled water.

2.2. PCR Amplification

1. *Taq* DNA polymerase: 5 U/µL in 20 m*M* Tris-HCl (pH 7.5), 100 m*M* NaCl, 0.1 m*M* EDTA, 2 m*M* DTT, 50% glycerol, 0.1% Tween-20 (Bioline, London, UK), store at –20°C.
2. 10X PCR buffer: 160 m*M* $(NH_4)_2SO_4$, 670 m*M* Tris-HCl (pH 8.8 at 25°C) 0.1% Tween-20 (Bioline), store at –20°C.

Table 1
Performance of the pbp2b PCR-RFLP to Determine Penicillin Resistance

Susceptibility (MIC)[a]	Sensitivity	Specificity	PPV[b]	NPV[b]
Susceptible (<0.1 mg/L)	100%	93.1%	97.5%	100%
Intermediate (0.1–<1 mg/L)	72.0%	98.9%	88.9%	96.9%
Resistant (>1 mg/L)	94.4%	98.9%	94.4%	98.9%

[a]Data from 106 U.K. isolates.
[b]PPV, positive predictive value; NPV, negative predictive value.

3. $MgCl_2$: 50 m*M* stock (Bioline), store at –20°C.
4. Nucleotides: 5 m*M* stock prepared by adding 10 µL of each of 100 m*M* dATP, dCTP, dGTP and dTTP (Promega, Southampton, UK) to 160 µL distilled water, store at –20°C in 40 µL aliquots.
5. Primers: PBP2B1 5' GAT CCT CTA AAT GAT TCT CAG GTG G 3' and PBP2B2 5' CAA TTA GCT TAG CAA TAG GTG TTG G 3'. Aliquot supplied oligonucleotides into smaller volumes and store at –20°C. Immediately prior to use add distilled water to appropriate volumes of PBP2B1 and PBP2B2 in a microcentrifuge tube to give a 0.1 m*M* solution.
6. Mineral oil: light white.
7. Sterile distilled water.
8. Sterile 0.5 mL thin walled PCR thermal reactor tubes.
9. Sterile, plugged micropipet tips (0.5–10 µL, 1–40 µL, 1–160 µL, 1–1000 µL) (*see* **Note 1**).

2.3. Electrophoretic detection of pbp2b

1. Agarose: Ultrapure, low EEO (Life Technologies, Paisley, UK).
2. 5X Tris-borate (TBE) buffer: 54 g Tris base, 27.5 g boric acid, 20 mL 0.5 *M* EDTA (pH 8.0). Store at room temperature. Discard if a precipitate forms. Dilute 1:10 for use.
3. Ethidium bromide: 10 mg/mL (*see* **Note 2**).
4. 6X gel electrophoresis loading buffer: 0.25% bromophenol blue, 40% (w/v) sucrose in water, store at 4°C.
5. Size marker: pGEM (Promega), for use dilute 1:10 to 100 ng/µL with 6X electrophoresis gel loading buffer and store at –20°C in 20 µL aliquots.

2.4. Digestion with Hin*fI*

1. *Hin*fI: 10 U/µL (Promega), store at –20°C.
2. 10X Restriction enzyme buffer: 60 m*M* Tris-HCl, 60 m*M* $MgCl_2$, 1 *M* NaCl, 10 m*M* DTT (pH 7.5) (Promega), store at –20°C.
3. Sterile 0.5 mL microcentrifuge tubes.
4. Sterile distilled water.

2.5. Data Analysis

1. Flat-bed digital scanner.
2. Personal Computer.
3. Band analysis software (e.g., Gel Compar).

3. Method

3.1. DNA Preparation

To release DNA from bacterial cells the following direct lysis procedure can be used.

1. Cultivate *S. pneumoniae* on blood agar plates in a 5 to 10% carbon dioxide atmosphere at 37°C overnight.
2. Pick up a single bacterial colony with a sterile inoculating loop and place in 50 µL of sterile distilled water in a microcentrifuge tube.
3. Emulsify the colony by vortexing or pipeting up and down.
4. Heat treat the sample at 95°C for 5 min to lyse the cells.
5. Centrifuge the sample at 13,000*g* for 2 min in a microcentrifuge to remove cell debris.
6. Use the supernatant containing the DNA for the PCR reaction.

3.2. PCR Amplification (see Note 3)

1. Prepare the PCR mastermix containing the following in a microcentrifuge tube: 1X PCR buffer, 1.5 m*M* $MgCl_2$, 0.2 m*M* dNTPs, 4 µ*M* of oligonucleotide primers and 1 U Taq DNA polymerase (*see* **Note 4**).
2. After each addition mix well by gently stirring with the pipet tip.
3. Briefly centrifuge the mastermix.
4. Transfer 95 µL of mastermix to each reaction tube and overlay with 100 µL of mineral oil (*see* **Note 5**).
5. Add 5 µL of DNA template to each reaction tube to give a final volume of 100 µL and briefly centrifuge the reactions (*see* **Note 6**).
6. Place tubes in a programmed thermocycler and initiate cycling conditions with an denaturation step at 95°C for 5 min followed by 30 cycles of denaturation at 94°C for 1 min, annealing at 55°C for 2 min and extension at 72°C for 3 min. Finally incubate the samples at 72°C for 7 min to ensure that DNA extension is complete (*see* **Note 7**).
7. Remove the completed PCR reactions from the machine and store at 4°C until required (*see* **Note 8**).

3.3. Electrophoretic Detection of pbp2b

PCR with primers PBP2B1 and 2 should yield a single product of approx 1.5 kb (*see* **Note 9**).

1. Prepare a 1.8% agarose gel in 0.5X TBE by microwaving or boiling until the agarose is dissolved.

2. Allow the gel to cool and add ethidium bromide to 0.5 µg/mL. Swirl the gel gently in the flask to mix without generating air bubbles and pour into a 13 × 13 cm gel tray with a 16- or 18-well comb. Allow to set for approx 30 min.
3. Extract 10 mL of PCR reaction mixture from below the mineral oil layer.
4. Combine with 2 µL of 6X electrophoresis gel-loading buffer and mix by pipeting.
5. Apply the sample to each well (*see* **Note 10**).
6. Load 2 µL of stock pGEM DNA marker as a size standard.
7. Perform electrophoresis in 0.5X TBE at 100–150 mA. The bromophenol blue indicator in the loading buffer should migrate approx 2/3 the length of the gel.
8. Visualize the gel under transmitted UV light. The gel may by photographed with Polaroid type 667 film or recorded with an appropriate digital imaging system.

3.4. Digestion with *HinfI*

1. Extract 17 µL of unpurified PCR product from below the mineral oil layer.
2. On ice, add the PCR product to a tube containing 2 µL of 10X restriction enzyme buffer and 10 U *Hin*fI to give a total reaction volume of 20 µL. Ensure that the restriction enzyme is kept on ice at all times.
3. Briefly centrifuge the digests and incubate at 37°C for up to 16 h.

3.5. Electrophoretic Detection of pbp2b *HinfI* Restriction Patterns (see Note 11)

1. Prepare a 1.8% agarose gel in 0.5X TBE as described previously.
2. Briefly centrifuge the digests, combine with 4 µL of 6X loading buffer and mix by pipeting.
3. Apply the sample to each well. For a size standard load 2 µL of stock pGEM DNA marker.
4. Perform electrophoresis as described previously.
5. Visualize the gel under transmitted UV light. The gel may by photographed with Polaroid type 667 film or recorded with an appropriate digital imaging system.

3.6. Computer Analysis of RFLP Patterns

1. Digitize the RFLP patterns with a scanner.
2. Analyze the band patterns using software such as Gel Compar program version 4.0 (Applied Maths, Krotrijk, Belgium) with pGEM markers as the reference standards.
3. Following normalization of the band positions, dendograms are calculated by using the dice coefficient with band settings of minimal profiling of 5%, minimal area of 0.5%, band comparison settings of position tolerance of 2%, increase 0, and minimal area 0.
4. Examples of patterns for *pbp2b* are shown in **Fig. 1**. Susceptible isolates (MIC <0.1 mg/L) invariably demonstrate a single RFLP profile, pattern A. Isolates with an MIC >1 mg/L are defined as having RFLP profiles of pattern K, H, or J. Intermediately resistant strains (MIC of 0.1 to <1 mg/L) are defined as having RFLP profiles of B, C, D, E, F, G, or I. Over time new patterns will emerge and these

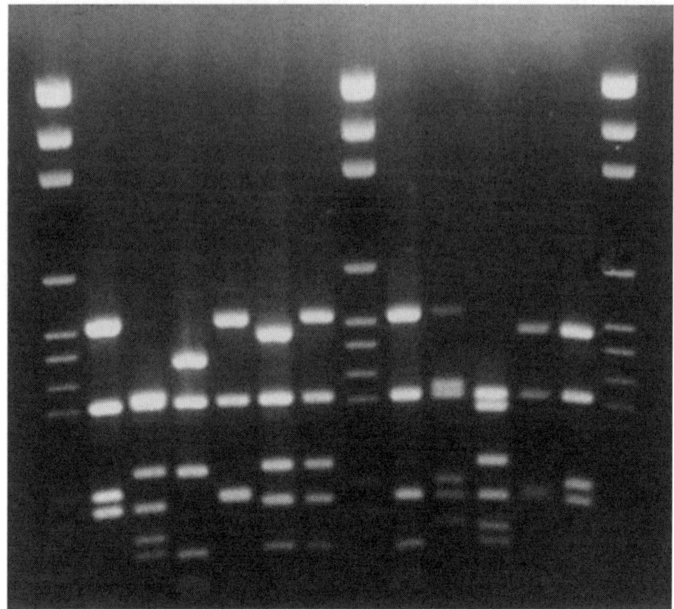

Fig. 1. Examples of all RFLP patterns obtained by *Hin*fI digestion of *S. pneumoniae pbp2b*.

will improve the prediction of intermediate and resistant strains. The performance of this protocol in our laboratory is illustrated in **Table 1**.

4. Notes

1. All pipeting operations should be performed with barrier filter pipet tips in order to contain aerosols and minimize contamination.
2. Ethidium bromide is a powerful mutagen and is moderately toxic. Gloves should be worn when working with solutions that contain this dye.
3. In order to minimize contamination with previously amplified DNA sequences the amplification procedure uses three separate rooms. The PCR mastermix is prepared and aliquoted in the clean room. The individual reactions are transferred to the second (grey) room for addition of DNA to each reaction tube. Finally, analysis of the PCR products is done in the third (dirty) room. Amplified DNA is never taken into the clean or grey rooms. A separate set of supplies and pipets is dedicated for use in each of the three areas. Reagents and supplies for the clean and grey rooms are never taken from the dirty room.
4. It is useful to overestimate the volume of required mastermix by one or two reactions to allow for pipeting inaccuracies and other volume losses during the setup.

5. Positive amplification control: 1 ng *S. pneumoniae* R36A DNA per reaction (one reaction). Negative amplification control: 5 μL of H_2O per reaction instead of sample (one reaction).
6. It is essential to ensure that the DNA is added to the reaction mixture by placing the pipet tip through the mineral oil layer, releasing the 5 μL volume and stirring very gently with the pipet tip.
7. The PCR amplifications described here are established for the Hybaid Omnigene thermocycler and may require modification for other machines.
8. If it is not possible to perform digestion of PCR product soon after completion of the cycle, program the machine to hold at 4°C or place the completed reactions in a refrigerator at 4°C until required.
9. Agarose gel electrophoresis of the PCR reactions is only to control for successful amplification. We routinely proceed from the PCR amplification to the digestion without visualizing the PCR products by electrophoresis.
10. When loading the sample touch the edge of the well with the pipet tip to prevent the oil from rising and dispersing the sample in the gel buffer.
11. It is helpful to run gels under approximately the same conditions to facilitate the comparison of the *Hin*fI RFLP patterns between subsequent gels. Alternatively, equipment that allows digital imaging and computer analysis of RFLP bands from the gel may help interpretation of results once a library of reference patterns is established.

References

1. Baquero, F. (1995) Pneumococcal resistance to β-lactam antibiotics. *Microb. Drug Resist.* **1,** 115–120.
2. Klugman, K. P. and Koornhof, H. J. (1989) Worldwide increase in pneumococcal antibiotic resistance. *Lancet* **ii,** 444.
3. Schutze, G. E., Kaplan, S. L., and Jacobs, R. F. (1994) Resistant pneumococcus: a worldwide problem. *Infect* **22,** 233–237.
4. Hackenbeck, R., Tarpay, M., and Tomasz, A. (1980) Multiple changes of penicillin-binding proteins in penicillin-resistant clinical isolates of *Streptococcus pneumoniae. Antimicrob. Agents Chemother.* **17,** 364–371.
5. Coffey, T. J., Daniels, M., McDougal, L. K., Dowson, C. G., Tenover, F. C., and Spratt, B. G. (1995) Genetic analysis of clinical isolates of *Streptococcus pneumoniae* with high-level resistance to expanded-spectrum cephalosporins. *Antimicrb. Agents Chemother.* **39,** 1306–1313.
6. Munoz, R. C., Dowson, C. G., Daniels, M., Coffey, T. C., Martin, C., Hakenbeck, R., and Spratt, B. G. (1992) Genetics of resistance to third-generation cephalosporins in clinical isolates of *Streptococcus pneumoniae. Mol. Microbiol.* **6,** 2461–2465.
7. Dowson, C. G., Hutchison, A., Brannigan, J. A., George, R. C., Hansman, D., Linares, J., Tomasz, A., Maynard Smith, J., and Spratt, B. G. (1989b) Horizontal transfer of penicillin-binding protein genes in penicillin-resistant clinical isolates of *Streptococcus pneumoniae. Proc. Natl. Acad. Sci. USA* **86,** 8842–8846.

8. Laible, G., Spratt, B. G., and Hackenbeck, R. (1991) Interspecies recombinational events during the evolution of altered PBP 2X genes in penicillin-resistant clinical isolates of *Streptococcus pneumoniae. Mol. Microbiol.* **5,** 1993–2002.
9. Dowson, C. G., Hutchison, A., and Spratt, B. G. (1989) Extensive re-modelling of the transpeptidase domain of penicillin-binding protein 2B of a penicillin-resistant South African isolate of *Streptococcus pneumoniae. Mol. Microbiol.* **3,** 95–102.
10. Smith, A. M. and Klugman, K. P. (1995) Alterations in penicillin-binding protein 2B from penicillin-resistant wild-type strains of *Streptococcus pneumoniae. Antimicrob. Agents Chemother.* **39,** 859–867.
11. du Plessis, M., Smith, A. M., and Klugman, K. P. (1998) Rapid detection of penicillin-resistant *Streptococcus pneumoniae* in cerebrospinal fluid by a seminested-PCR strategy. *J. Clin. Microbiol.* **36,** 453–457.
12. Jalal, H., Organji, S., Reynolds, J., Bennett, D., O'Mason, E., and Millar, M. R. (1997) Determination of penicillin susceptibility of *Streptococcus pneumoniae* using the polymerase chain reaction. *J. Clin. Pathol. Mol. Pathol.* **50,** 45–50.
13. Ubukata, K., Asahi, Y., Yamane, A., and Konno, M. (1996) Combinational detection of autolysin and penicillin-binding protein 2B genes of *Streptococcus pneumoniae* by PCR. *J. Clin. Microbiol.* **34,** 592–596.
14. O'Neill, A. M., Gillespie, S. H., and Whiting, G. C. (1999) Detection of penicillin susceptibility in *Streptococcus pneumoniae* by *pbp2b* PCR-restriction fragment length polymorphism analysis. *J. Clin. Microbiol.* **37,** 157–160.
15. Beall, B., Facklam, R. R., Jackson, D. M., and Starling, H. H. (1998) Rapid screening for penicillin susceptibility of systemic pneumococcal isolates by restriction enzyme profiling of the *pbp2B* gene. *J. Clin. Microbiol.* **36,** 2359–2362.
16. Dowson, C. G., Hutchison, A., and Spratt, B. G. (1989) Nucleotide sequence of the penicillin-binding protein 2B gene of *Streptococcus pneumoniae* strain R6. *Nucleic Acids Res.* **17,** 7518.

9

Detection Methods of Glycopeptide-Resistant *Staphylococcus aureus* I

Susceptibility Testing

Hedeaki Hanaki and Keiichi Hiramatsu

1. Introduction

The breakpoint for resistance to vancomycin for *Staphylococcus aureus* is a minimum inhibitory concentration (MIC) of greater than 8 μg/mL *(1)*. Isolation of the first strain of MRSA resistant to vancomycin (VRSA) Mu50 was made from a Japanese surgical patient with a wound infection who had failed with vancomycin therapy *(2)*. A strain has been described that is heterogeneously resistant to vancomycin (Mu3 strain), and it was found to be susceptible to vancomycin (MIC 2 μg/mL by NCCLS criteria), but there were cells within the Mu3 population that resisted a vancomycin concentration of up to 9 μg/mL) *(1)*. Most of the clinical *S. aureus* strains having reduced susceptibility to glycopeptide antibiotics are heterogeneous in their phenotypic resistance expression. The strains contain small subpopulations of cells that have different levels of glycopeptide resistance. They are designated hetero-resistant strains, and are defined by the population analysis (*see* below). MIC or paper disc susceptibility tests cannot detect hetero-resistant strains. It would appear that heterogeneously resistant VRSA is a preliminary stage that allows development into full resistance upon further exposure to vancomycin. Therefore, it seems reasonable to include VRSA and hetero-VRSA as possible risk factors for vancomycin therapeutic failure in MRSA infection.

From: *Methods in Molecular Medicine, vol. 48: Antibiotic Resistance Methods and Protocols*
Edited by: S. H. Gillespie © Humana Press Inc., Totowa, NJ

Further reports of VRSA associated with vancomycin therapeutic failure have been reported from USA, France, Turkey, and Korea. The resistance level of hetero-VRSA and VRSA is not yet comparable to that of vancomycin-resistant enterococci (VRE).

However, given the limited peak tissue concentration attained by intravenous vancomycin administration (e.g., only 2.46–2.49 μg/mL vancomycin in sputa after a 0.5 g single injection ***(3)*** or 5 μg/mL in an abscess after multiple 2.0 g injection ***(4)***, it is not surprising that pneumonia or wound infections caused by VRSA do not respond to vancomycin therapy. Conventional susceptibility methods are not effective for detecting VRSA, so alternative techniques are required, and these are described in this chapter.

Gradient gel methods are convenient and simple methods to detect resistant strains ***(5,6)***. The minimum inhibitory concentration (MIC) determination, generally used as an evaluation of antibiotic susceptibility of bacteria can only classify the bacteria into discontinuous stepwise levels of resistance. The method that we describe here, is able to detect more subtle differences in the resistance level by using the agar impregnated with continuously increasing concentration of antibiotic. Control strains with a known resistance level should always be used with test strains as a control to monitor batch-to-batch deviation of the gradient gel.

Population analysis is one of the most important methods employed in the study of glycopeptide resistance in *S. aureus* ***(1,7)***. It allows heterogeneous resistance to be detected simply. It is found that vancomycin and β-lactam antibiotics antagonize each other in their action against hetero-VRSA strains in Japan ***(8,9)***. Mu3 agar plate method utilizes this antagonism to detect the hetero-VRSA strains. Our studies have shown that any β-lactam antibiotic so far tested can be used in this method: forty-six commercially available β-lactam antibiotics were examined and all showed the same antagonistic effect ***(8,9)***.

2. Materials

1. Tryptose soy broth (TSB).
2. Brain heart infusion broth (BHIB).
3. Brain heart infusion agar (BHIA).
4. Slope plate 10 × 14 × 1 cm, (Eiken, Tokyo, Japan).
5. Antibiotics: make fresh as required.
6. Vancomycin: stable at 4°C for up to 3 mo or at –20°C for up to 3 mo.
7. Resting medium: 1 m*M* glycine, 1 m*M* glutamic acid, 0.5 m*M*, D-L-alanyl-D-L-alanine, 0.2 m*M* L-lysine, 1 m*M* $MgCl_2$, 0.1 m*M* $MnCl_2$, 0.17 m*M*, uracil, 8.2 μ*M* nicotinamide, 80 m*M* K_2HPO_4, 3 μ*M* thiamine, 28.5 m*M* glucose. Filter with 0.22 μm pore size filter. Stable at 4°C for up to 1 mo.
8. Paper disc: 8 mm diameter thick disc.

9. Paper disc containing β-lactam antibiotics: make fresh as required or use a commercial source.
10. Mu3 agar plates (Becton-Dickinson, Tokyo, Japan).

3. Methods

3.1. Gradient Gel (Fig. 1)

1. Cultivate test and control strains overnight in TSB.
2. Adjust the OD 0.3 at 578 nm (about 10^8 CFU/mL) with fresh TSB (*see* **Note 1**).
3. Prepare a gradient agar plate as follows. Pour 40 mL of BHIA containing appropriate concentration of antibiotic into a slope plate at an angle of about 5 degrees.
4. Keep solidified for 30 min at room temperature. Then set the plate horizontally, and pour 45 mL of fresh BHIA on top of the solidified BHIA. Keep the solidified agar at room temperature for 120 min (*see* **Note 2**).
5. Streak the test and control strains onto the gradient agar plate with a cotton swab. The growth of the bacteria is observed after incubation at 37°C for 48 h.

3.2. Population Analysis (Fig. 2)

1. Culture test and control bacteria overnight in TSB.
2. Adjust the optical density to OD 0.3 at 578 nm (about 10^8 CFU/mL).
3. Make 10-fold serial dilutions from a portion (50 µL) of the cell suspension and spread with sterilized spreader onto the BHIA plates containing varied concentrations of vancomycin, for example, 0, 1, 2, . . .7, 8, 9, 10 µg/mL.
4. Leave the plates for 15 min on a clean bench before use to remove excess moisture on the agar surface (*see* **Note 3**)
5. Count the number of colonies growing on each plate after incubation at 37°C for 48 h.
6. Plot the colony counts on a semi-logarithmic graph with colony counts on the vertical axis and vancomycin concentration on the horizontal axis (*see* **Note 4**).

3.3. Mu3 Agar Method

1. Culture test and control bacteria overnight in TSB.
2. Adjust the optical density of the culture to OD_{578} of 0.3.
3. Inoculate onto the entire surface of a BHI agar plate containing 4 µg/mL of vancomycin and 100% of resting medium ***(10)*** with one stroke of a sterilized cotton wool swab (*see* **Notes 5** and **6**).
4. Place three paper discs (thick, 8 mm in diameter) containing 0.005, 0.05, and 0.5 µg of ceftizoxime, respectively, on the agar plate inoculated with the test organism.
5. Incubate the agar plate at 37°C for 24–48 h.
6. Suspect hetero-resistance if bacterial growth is observed around the discs (*see* **Fig. 3**). Ready-made Mu3 agar plates are commercially available from Becton-Dickinson, Tokyo, Japan.

4. Notes

1. Overnight culture is prepared in TSB to prevent the organism from forming clusters.
2. For the appropriate gradient of antibiotics to be formed in the agar plate, the plate must be kept for 120 min.

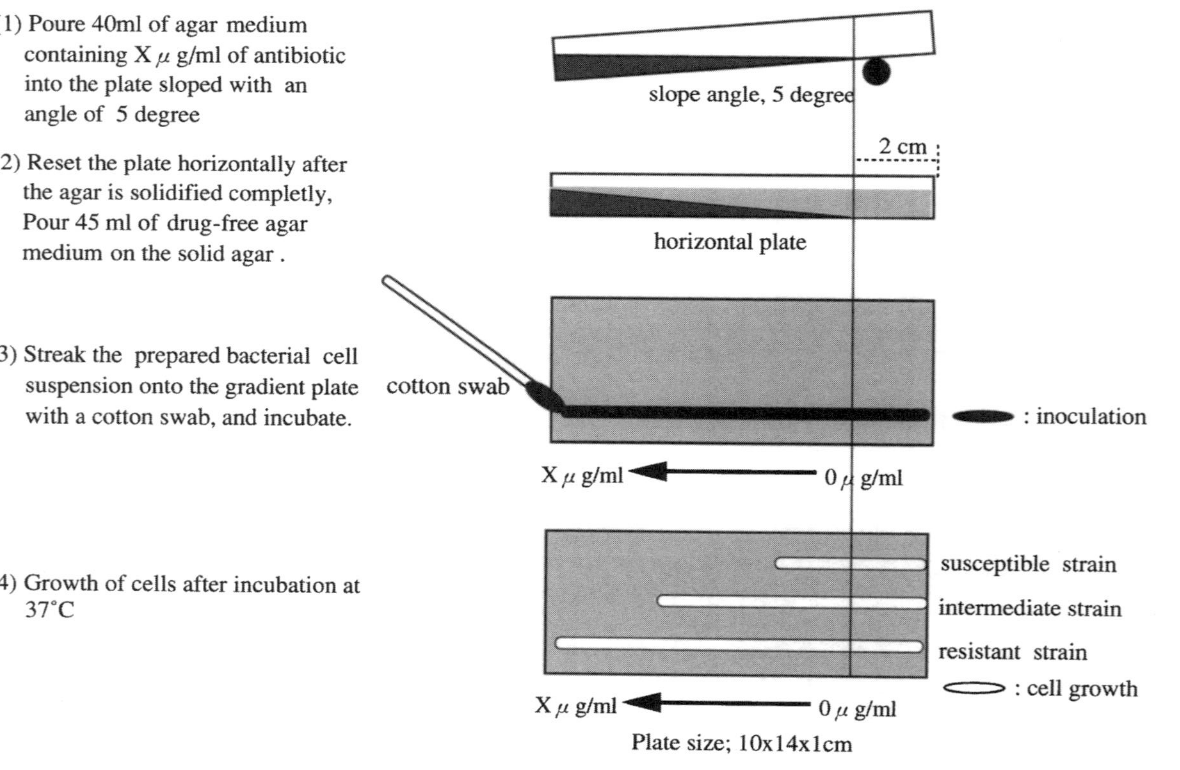

Fig. 1. Process of evaluating vanomycin resistance by gradient gel technology.

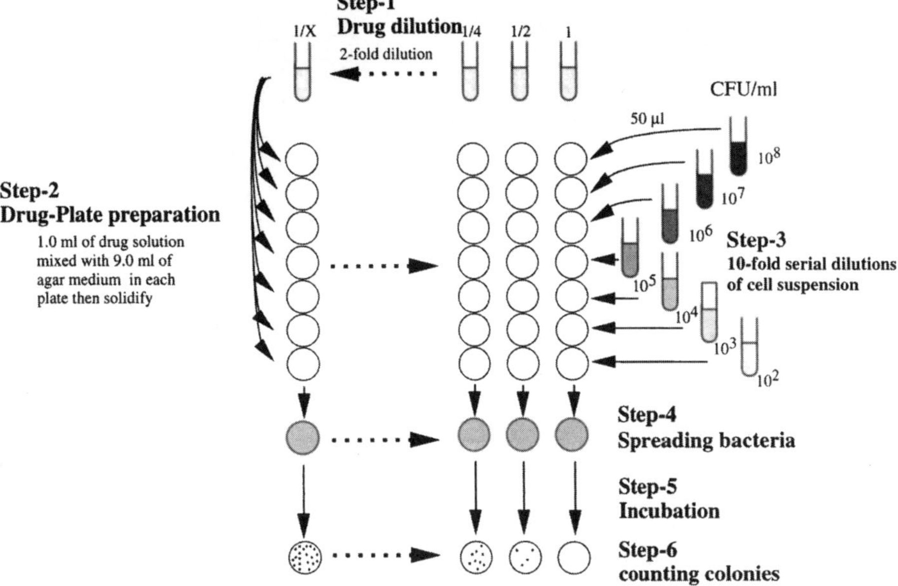

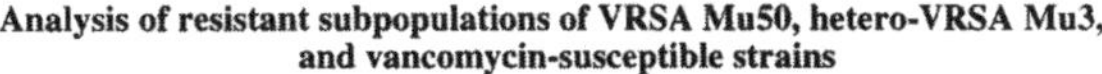

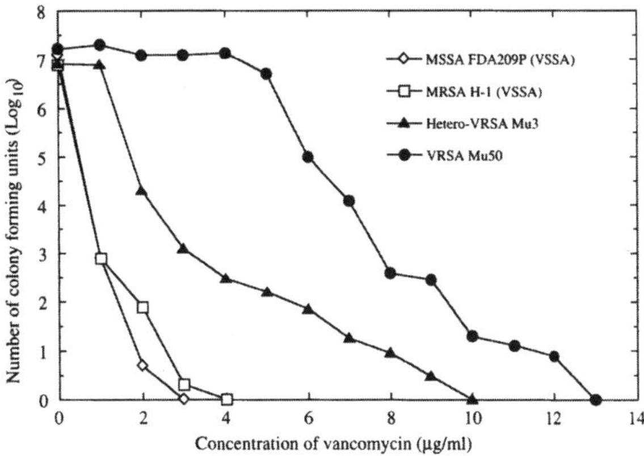

Fig. 2. Population analysis for vancomycin resistant *S. aureus*.

3. The surface of the agar inoculated with bacteria should be dried briefly before incubation, otherwise, patchy growth of "susceptible" cells will appear on the wet surface, which makes the cell count unreliable.
4. The maximum number of cells spread on the agar plate of 9 cm in diameter must be kept less than 10^7 cfu. Otherwise, reliable colony counts cannot be achieved because of some patchy growth of "susceptible" cells on the plate *(1)*.

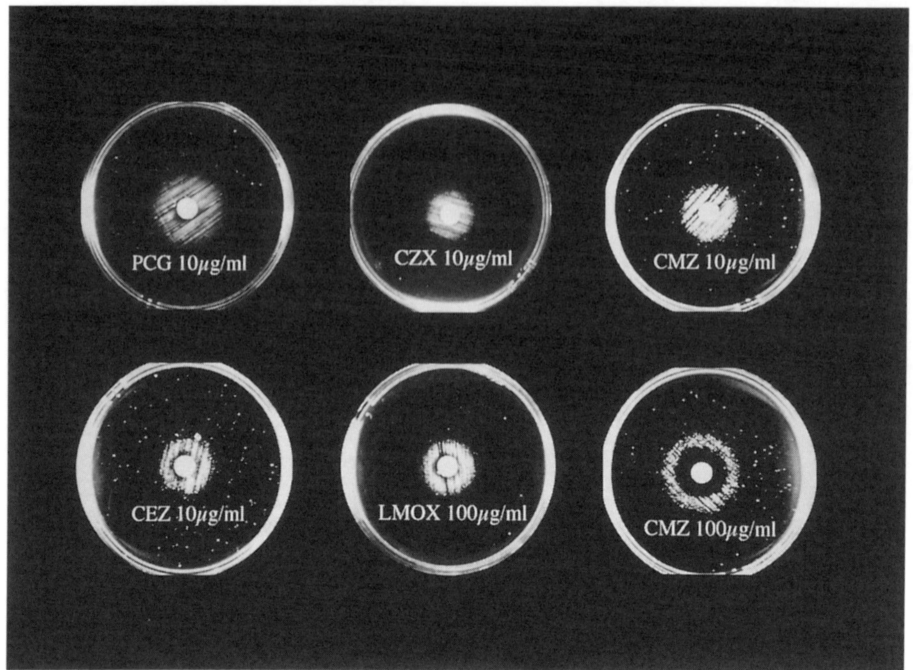

Fig. 3. Example of results using the Mu3 agar method.

5. Multiple inoculation of the cells on the Mu3 agar plate is not recommended. Heavy inoculum makes the result difficult to interpret because of nonspecific growth of the cells all over the plate
6. This method is valid to detect Mu3-type hetero-VRSA prevalent in Japan, but there are some hetero-VRSA (as defined by population analysis) strains in the United States and possibly in other countries which are not detectable by this method.

References

1. Hiramatsu, K., Aritaka, N., Hanaki, H., Kawasaki, S., Hosoda, Y., Hori, S., Fukuchi, F., and Kobayashi, I. (1997) Dissemination in Japanese hospitals of strains of *Staphylococcus aureus* heterogeneously resistant to vancomycin. *Lancet* **350,** 1670–1673.
2. Hiramatsu K., Hanaki, H., Ino, T., Yabuta, K., Oguri, T., and Tenover, F. C. (1997) Methicillin-resistant Staphylococcus aureus clinical strain with reduced vancomycin susceptibility. *J. Antimicrob. Chemother.* **40,** 135–136.
3. Niitsuma, K. and Saito, M. (1996) Vancomycin inhalation therapy a pharmacokinetic and clinical study of vancomycin. *Antibiot. Chemother.* **122,** 123–135.

4. Torres, J. R., Sandres, C. V., and Lewis, A. C. (1979) Vancomycin concentration in human tissues: preliminary report. *J. Antimicrob. Chemother.* **5,** 475–477.
5. Lorian, V. (1966) The gradient plate method, in *Antibiotics and Chemotherapeutic Agents in Clinical and Laboratory Practice* (Thomas, C. C., ed.), Springfield, IL, pp. 102–103.
6. Stranden, A. M., Roos, M., and Berger-Bach, B. (1996) Glutamine synthetase and heteroresistance in methicillin-resistant *Staphylococcus aureus. Microbial. Drug Resistance* **2,** 201–207.
7. Lea, D. and Coulson, C. A. (1949) The distribution of the numbers of mutants in bacterial populations. *J. Genet.* **49,** 264–285.
8. Hanaki H., Inaba, Y., Sasaki, K., and Hiramatsu, K. (1998) A novel method of detecting *Staphylococcus aureus* heterogeneously resistant to vancomycin (Hetero-VRSA). *Jpn. J. Antibiot.* **51,** 521–530.
9. Hanaki H., Ohkawa, S., Inaba, Y., Hashimoto, T., and Hiramatsu, K. (1998) Development of medium (Mu3) for detection of hetero-vancomycin resistant MRSA (hetero-VRSA). Program abstracts of the 38rd Intersci. Confer. Antimicrob. Agents Chemother. abst. C–132.
10. Riley S. and Toennies, G. (1960) Nutritional requirements for bacterial cell wall synthesis. *Nutr. Cell Wall* **84,** 44–50.

10

Detection Methods for Glycopeptide-Resistant *Staphylococcus aureus* II

Cell Wall Analysis

Hedeaki Hanaki and Keiichi Hiramatsu

1. Introduction

1.1. Measuring the Rate of Cell-Wall Synthesis

Vancomycin resistance of Mu50 (VRSA) and Mu3 (hetero-VRSA) is associated with the changes in cell-wall synthesis. Therefore, the analysis of cell-wall synthesis and cell-wall composition study is of cardinal importance for the understanding of this resistance mechanism. The rate of the cell-wall synthesis can be evaluated by measuring the rate of up-take of ^{14}C-N-acetylglucosamine into the cell, since more than 95% of ^{14}C-N-acetylglucosamine is known to be incorporated into the cell wall *(1)*. Murein monomer precursor (UDP-N-acetylmuramyl-pentapeptide) (MMP) is an important intermediate substrate of peptidoglycan synthesis, detection, and quantitation of MMP is useful for the investigation of how the cell-wall synthesis system is altered in *S. aureus* in association with glycopeptide resistance. For example, the cytoplasmic pool size of MMP is several times greater in Mu50 and Mu3 than in vancomycin-susceptible *S. aureus* strains *(2)*.

1.2. Analysis of Cell-Wall Peptidoglycan (Muropeptide)

Peptidoglycan analysis requires a complicated method. However, the degree of cross-linking of the murein (ratio of murein dimer to murein monomer), and the presence of abnormal murein, can be determined by using this method. In VRSA, decreased cross-linking of the peptidoglycan and appearance of nonamidated muropeptide are observed, which explain increased trapping of

From: *Methods in Molecular Medicine, vol. 48: Antibiotic Resistance Methods and Protocols*
Edited by: S. H. Gillespie © Humana Press Inc., Totowa, NJ

vancomycin molecules within the cell wall (affinity trapping mechanism of vancomycin resistance) *(3)*.

2. Materials

1. Resting medium: described in the Mu3 agar plate method Chapter 9.
2. Tryptose Soy Broth (TSB).
3. Spectrophotometer, e.g., U-3200 (Hitachi, Tokyo, Japan).
4. 4C-N-acetylglucosamine: 1.85 MBq in 1.0 mL distilled water (Amersham, Arlington Heights, IL) store at –20°C.
5. N-acetylglucosamine: stable at –20°C for up to 6 mo.
6. SDS.
7. AQUA SOL2 (Packard, Downers Grove, IL).
8. Liquid scintillation counter, e.g., LS3801 (Beckman Instruments, Palo Alto, CA).
9. Brain heart infusion broth (BHIB; Difco Laboratories, Detroit, Michigan).
10. Gyratory shaker Bio-Shaker BR-150L (Taitec, Tokyo, Japan).
11. Ultracentrifuge.
12. Reverse-phase high-pressure liquid chromatography (HPLC) using Galliver HPLC system (consisting of UV970[UV detector], PU-980[pump], LG-980-02 [gradient unit], PG980-50[degasser], and 807-IT[integrator] [Nihonbunko, Tokyo, Japan]).
13. Column: Hypersil ODS, 4.5- by 150-mm Capcell pak (Shiseido, Tokyo, Japan)
14. HPLC development solvent: 0.1% methanol in 50 m*M* sodium phosphate (pH 5.2 containing 0.0005% sodium azide), and 6.0% methanol in 50 m*M* sodium phosphate (pH 5.2, containing 0.0005% sodium azide). Store at room temperature for up to 1 mo.
15. Sodium azide: Highly toxic. Preservative laboratory reagent.
16. Tris-HCl buffer (pH 7.0): Store at 4°C.
17. 0.2 mg/mL trypsin in 1 *M* Tris-HCl buffer (pH 7.0): make fresh as required.
18. 40% (w/v) hydrofluoric acid: Store at 4°C.
19. 0.3 mL sodium citrate buffer (pH 7.0) containing 4 m*M* $MgCl_2$ and 50 µL sodium azide (1 mg/mL): Store at 4°C.
20. Mutanolysin: 0.2 mg/mL from *Streptomyces globisporus* make fresh as required.
21. Phosphoric acid. (Strong acid, irritating.)
22. 1.5 *M* sodium borate buffer (pH 9.0): Store at 4°C.
23. Sodium borohydride (sodium tetrahydroborate): Store at 4°C.
24. HPLC development solvent: 5% methanol in 50 m*M* sodium phosphate (pH 2.5) containing 0.0005% sodium azide, and 30% methanol in 50 m*M* sodium phosphate (pH 2.8) containing 0.0005% sodium azide.
25. Ultrasonic generator, e.g., SONIFIER with 20% duty cycle (cell disruptor 200, Branson, Smithkline).
26. Hydrofluoric acid: 40% (w/v).
27. 4 *N* NaOH.
28. Column: 5-µ*M* Hypersil C18-ODS, 4.5- by 250-nm (Shiseido).
29. HPLC (Nihon-Bunko, JASCO) consisting of a PU-980 pump, an UV-970 detector, and a LG-980-02 gradient unit, an AS-950-10 autosampler, a DG-980-50

degasser. BORWIN chromatography software is used for recording and controlling the system *(4)*.

30. Amino acid analyzer (Biotronic LC5000).

3. Method

3.1. Incorporation of 14C-N-acetylglucosamine (Fig. 1)

1. Cultivate the test organisms at 37°C for 18 h in TSB.
2. Dilute the culture 20-fold with fresh prewarmed TSB, and then cultivate further until an OD_{578} of 0.7 is achieved.
3. Pellet the cells from a 4-mL portion of the culture by centrifugation at 12,000*g* for 10 min.
4. Wash the cell pellet once with resting medium and resuspend in 4 mL of the resting medium.
5. Mix the cell suspension with 8 μL of ^{14}C-N-acetylglucosamine (1.85 MBq/mL) and with 40 μL of cold N-acetylglucosamine to make a final concentration of 6.4 mg/mL.
6. Incubate at 37°C with gentle shaking.
7. After 5, 15, 30, 60, and 120 min of incubation, take a 0.5 mL portion of the cell suspension and transfer into a microfuge tube containing 0.5 mL of 64 μg/mL of cold N-acetylglucosamine and 0.1% sodium dodesylsulfate (SDS).
8. Centrifuge at 12,000*g* for 3 min and discard, the supernatant.
9. Wash the cell pellet once with distilled water and resuspend in 0.5 mL of distilled water (*see* **Note 2**).
10. Mix the cell suspension with 5 mL of AQUA SOL2 (Packard).
11. Determine the radioactivity count using a liquid scintillation counter *(12)*.

3.2. Quantitation of Murein Monomer Precursor (Fig. 2)

1. Cultivate test organisms at 37°C for 18 h in BHIB (*see* **Note 1**).
2. Dilute the culture 20-fold with fresh prewarmed BHIB, and further cultivated until OD_{578} of 0.7 is attained.
3. Add a 25-mL portion of the culture to 225 mL of fresh prewarmed BHIB in a flask, and cultivate further at 37°C until OD_{578} of 0.7 is reached using a gyratory shakerBio-Shaker BR-150L.
4. Harvest the cells by centrifugation at 10,000*g* for 15 min, wash once with distilled water.
5. Resuspend the pellet in 10 mL of distilled water, and add the cell suspension gently into 20 mL of boiling water.
6. Boil the cell suspension continuously for 20 min, and spin down the cell debris by centrifugation at 100,000*g* for 70 min.
7. Take the supernatant and lyophilize it.
8. Dissolve the lyophilized sample in 0.5 mL of distilled water and subject to reverse-phase high-pressure liquid chromatography (HPLC) using Galliver HPLC system (consisting of UV970 [UV detector], PU-980 [pump], LG-980-02

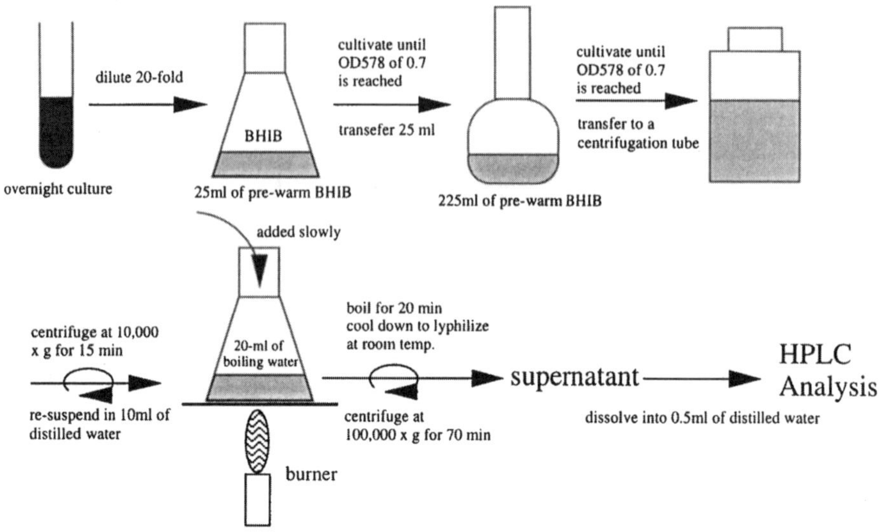

HPLC anlysis of cytoplasmic murein monomer pool.

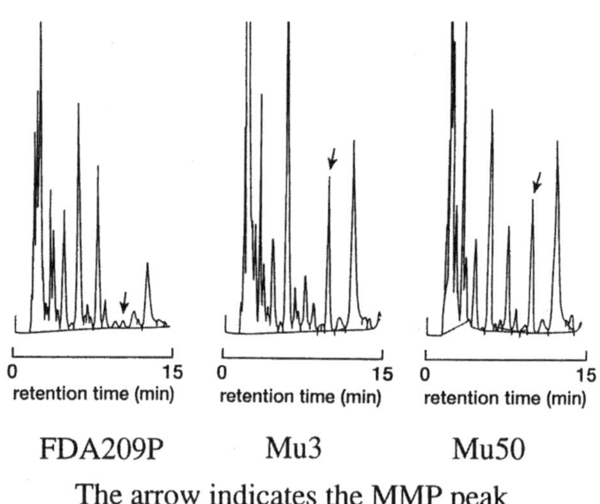

FDA209P Mu3 Mu50

The arrow indicates the MMP peak

Fig. 1. Process for evaluating murein monomer pool and examples of HPLC analysis.

[gradient unit], PG980-50 [degasser], and 807-IT [integrator] [Nihonbunko]). The column 5 μ*M* Hypersil ODS, 4.5- by 150-mm Capcell pak (Shiseido) is eluted at 40°C with a linear gradient from 0.1% methanol in 50 m*M* sodium phosphate (pH 5.2, containing 0.0005% sodium azide) to 6.0% methanol in 50 m*M* sodium

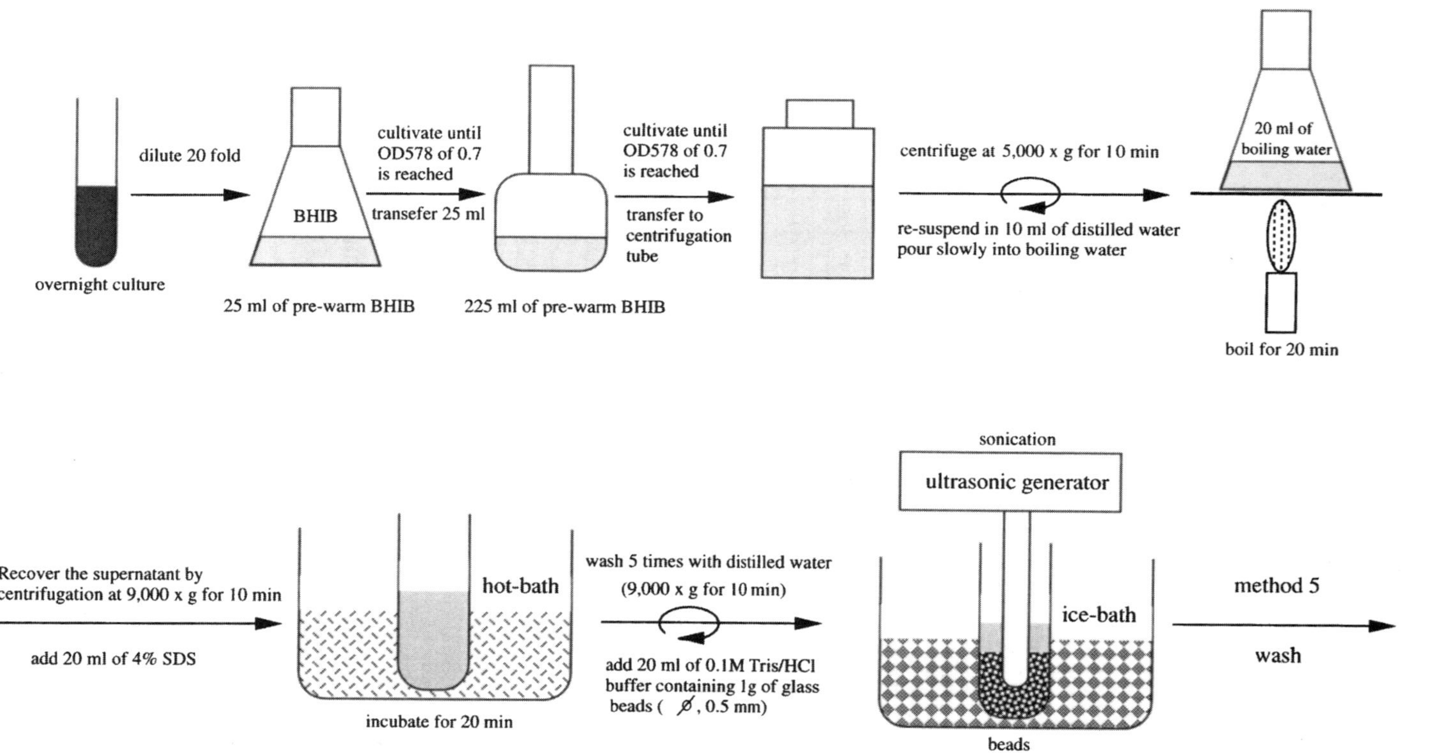

Fig. 2. Process for preparing bacteria for cell wall peptidoglycan analysis.

phosphate (pH 5.2, containing 0.0005% sodium azide) within 15 min. MMP peak is observed at retention time of about 7–10 min by absorption of UV at 265 nm.

3.3. Analysis of Cell Wall Peptidoglycan

Preparation of murein (**Fig. 3A** *[4]*).

1. Inoculate a single colony in 4 mL of brain heart infusion (BHI) broth.
2. Incubate overnight at 37°C.
3. Dilute the overnight culture to 2% in fresh BHI broth, and cultivate at 37°C until OD_{578} value of 0.5 is reached.
4. Pour the culture into 225 mL fresh BHI-broth, and cultivate at 37°C with agitation.
5. Harvest the cells at an OD_{578} of 0.7 by centrifugation (5000*g*) at 4°C for 10 min.
6. Resuspend the pellet in 10 mL of 1 *M* NaCl, and put in boiling water for 20 min.
7. Harvest the pellet at OD_{578} of 0.7 by centrifugation (5000*g*) at 4°C for 10 min.
8. Add the pellet to 20 mL of 4% SDS in H_2O, and boil for another 20 min to remove noncovalently bound materials.
9. Cool to room temperature.
10. Harvest the crude cell wall [CCW] by centrifugation at 5000*g* for 10 min, and resuspend in 20 mL of water.
11. Wash the CCW five times with 20 mL of water to remove SDS and resuspend in 20 mL of 0.1 *M* Tris-HCl buffer (pH 7.0).
12. Break the CCW mechanically in 20 mL of 0.1 *M* Tris-HCl buffer (pH 7.0) with glass beads (diameter 0.5 mm) and an ultrasonic generator SONIFIER with 20% duty cycle (cell disruptor 200, Branson, Smithkline) for 10 min at 4°C, or with glass beads (diameter 0.1 mm) using a cell grinder for 5 min at 4°C *(5)*.
13. Harvest the CCW suspension by decanting.
14. Wash the glass beads twice with 2 mL of 4% SDS, and add recovered CCW to the CCW suspension.
15. Centrifuge the CCW suspension (5000*g*) for 10 min, and wash the CCW pellet with 20 mL of 1 *M* Tris-HCl buffer (pH 7.0).
16. Resuspend the CCW pellet in 20 mL of 0.2 mg/mL trypsin in 1 *M* Tris-HCl buffer (pH 7.0) and incubate at 37°C for 24 h with agitation to eliminate cell-wall proteins.
17. Wash the CCW pellet with 20 mL of 1 *M* NaCl in 1 *M* Tris-HCl buffer (pH 7.0) by centrifugation (13,000*g*), and then with 20 mL of 1 *M* Tris-HCl buffer (pH 7.0), and finally three times with water.
18. Resuspend the CCW in 1 mL of 40% (w/v) hydrofluoric acid and incubate at 4°C for 18 h to eliminate teichoic acids.
19. Harvest the purified murein by centrifugation (13,000*g*) at 4°C for 10 min.
20. Wash four times with 1 mL of water, and lyophilize *(1)* (*see* **Note 3**).

3.3.1. Preparation and Reduction of Muropeptides (*Fig. 3B*).

1. Degrade the lyophilized murein in 0.3 mL sodium citrate buffer (pH 7.0) containing 4 m*M* $MgCl_2$ and 50 µL sodium azide (1 mg/mL) with 50 µL mutanolysin (0.2 mg/mL) from *Streptomyces globisporus* by incubating at 37°C overnight with agitation.

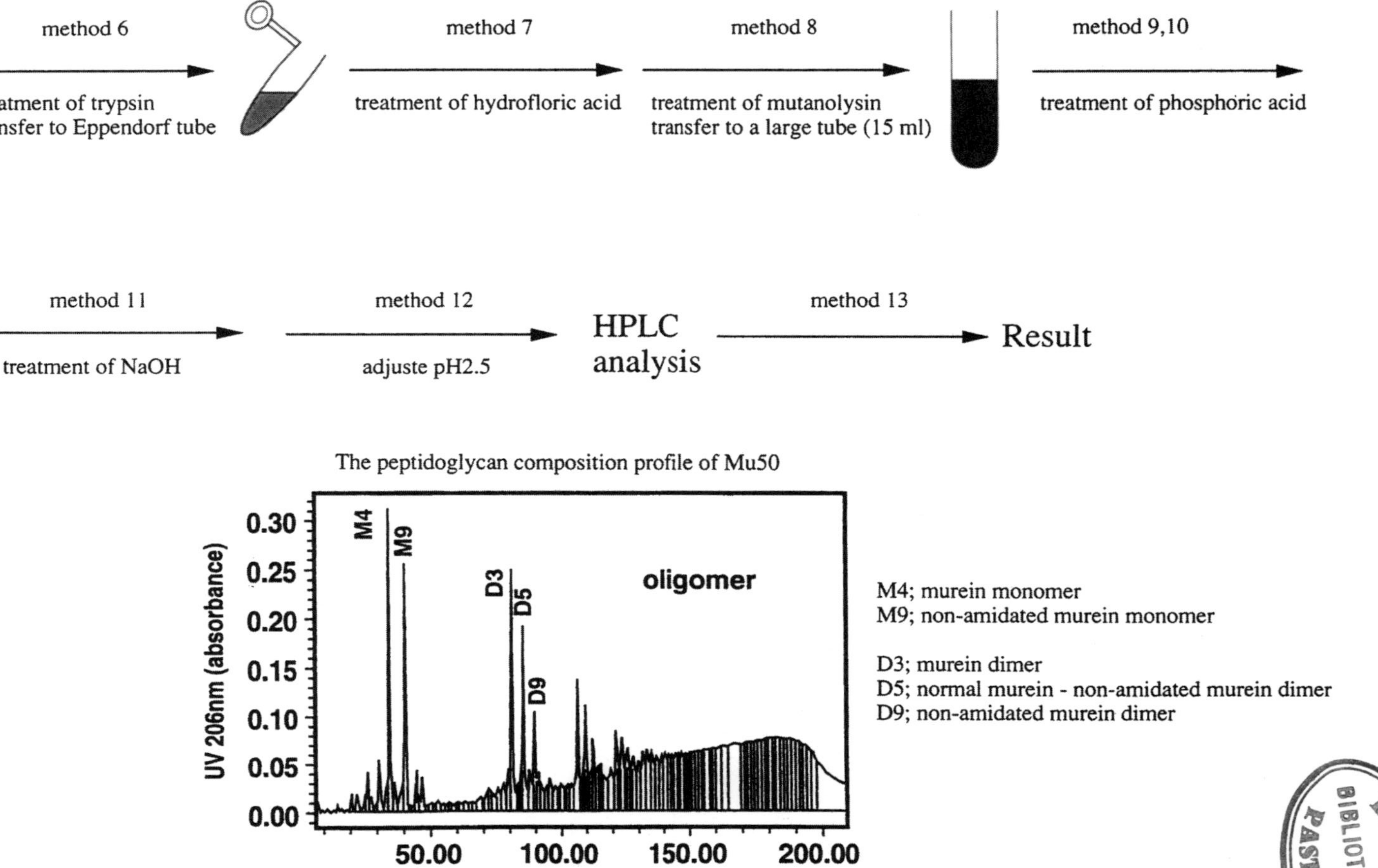

Fig. 3. Process of cell wall analysis and example of HPLC trace.

2. Adjust the samples to pH 4.0 with 20% phosphoric acid, and incubate at 100°C for 5 min to inactivate the enzyme.
3. Add 175 mL of 1.5 *M* sodium borate buffer (pH 9.0), then add 10 mg solid sodium borohydride.
4. Incubate at room temperature for 15 min to reduce the muropeptides. Excess borohydride is destroyed by the addition of 20% H_3PO_4 until no bubbling is observed.
5. Adjust the samples to pH 11.5–12.5 with about 120 µL of 4 *N* NaOH and incubate at 37°C for 1.5 h to hydrolyze remaining O-acetyl groups present at the muramic acid residues.
6. Adjust the muropeptide solution to pH 2.5 with 4 *N* HCl prior to centrifugation (13,000*g*; 10 min) and filtration (0.22 µ*M* pore size) to remove insoluble material *(1)*.

3.3.2. Fractionation of Muropeptides by HPLC

Separate muropeptides by reversed-phase high performance liquid chromatography (HPLC). The column (5-µ*M* Hypersil C18-ODS, 4.5- by 250-nm, Shiseido) is eluted with a linear gradient from 5% methanol in 50 m*M* sodium phosphate (pH 2.5) containing 0.0005% sodium azide to 30% methanol in 50 m*M* sodium phosphate (pH 2.8) within 210 min. The flow rate is 0.75 mL/min. Normally injection volume is 100–200 µL. Muropeptide peaks are detected by absorption at 206 nm.

3.3.3. Amino acid composition analysis

Muropeptide peaks are fractionated, lyophilized, and then hydrolyzed in 6 *N* HCl at 166°C for 1 h. Samples are analyzed by an amino acid analyzer (Biotronic LC5000) (*see* **Note 4**).

4. Notes

1. Test organism should be grown to OD578 of 0.7 (log-phase) before harvesting.
2. The washing of cell pellet should be done carefully to remove as much of the adherent ^{14}C-N-acetylglucosamine from the cell surface as possible.
3. Check the pH of the sample before treatment with mutanolysin.
4. The amino acid components of the suspected murein monomer precursor can be confirmed by amino-analyzer, which, if normal, should be two molecules of alanine, one glutamic acid or glutamine, and one lysine *(2)*.

References

1. Wong W., Young, F. E., and Chatterjee, A. N. (1974) Regulation of bacterial cell walls: turnover of cell wall in *Staphylococcus aureus*. *J. Bacteriol.* **120,** 837–843.
2. Hanaki H., Kuwahara-Arai, K., Boyle-Vavra, S., Daum, R. S., Labischinski, H., and Hiramatsu, K. (1998) Activated cell-wall synthesis is associated with vanco-

mycin resistance in methicillin-resistant *Staphylococcus aureus* clinical strains Mu3 and Mu50. *J. Antimicrob. Chemother.* **42,** 199–209.

3. Hiramatsu, K. and Hanaki, H. (1998) Glycopeptide resistance in staphylococci. *Curr. Opinion Infect. Dis.* **11,** 653–658.
4. Hanaki H., Labischinski, H., Murakami, H., and Hiramatsu, K. (1998) Increase in glutamine-non-amidated muropeptides in the peptidoglycan of vancomycin-resistant *S. aureus* (VRSA) strain Mu50. *J. Antimicrob. Chemother.* **42,** 315–320.
5. Stranden A. M., Ehlert, K., Labischinski, H., and Berger-Bachi, B. (1997) Cell wall monoglycine cross-bridges and methicillin hypersuscepribility in a *fem*AB null mutant of methicillin-resistant *Staphylococcus aureus*. *J. Bacteriol.* **179,** 9–16.

11

Multiplex PCR for the Rapid Simultaneous Speciation and Detection of Methicillin-Resistance and Genes Encoding Toxin Production in *Staphylococcus aureus*

Mark E. Jones, Karl Köhrer, and Franz-Josef Schmitz

1. Introduction

The use of polymerase chain reaction (PCR) to rapidly amplify target DNA molecules has evolved a place within diagnostic microbiology allowing the sensitive and specific identification of microorganisms concurrent with the detection of specific genes involved in resistance or virulence. This is particularly helpful when dealing with problem pathogens such as *Staphylococcus aureus*, where the rapid diagnosis and detection of methicillin-resistance can assist in the fast implementation of appropriate treatment and infection control measures ***(1–4)***. In addition, the rapid assessment of toxin production can ascertain whether toxin-related symptoms need to be considered ***(5)***. The protocol described here enables the simultaneous differentiation between *S. aureus* (and coagulase negative staphylococci) from other eubacterial organisms. Concomitant with species identification this protocol allows for the detection of specific staphylococcal resistance genes, such as *mecA*, encoding methicillin resistance, or staphylococcal virulence genes, such as *seb*, *sec1* and *tst*, encoding enterotoxin B, enterotoxin C, and toxic shock syndrome toxin-1, respectively. In *S. aureus* the detection of methicillin-resistance using agar diffusion or broth micro-dilution techniques, or toxin production using immunodiffusion, agglutination, or ELISA is often difficult. This is because the *mecA* gene and the genes involved in toxin production may be poorly expressed and influenced significantly by culture conditions ***(5–10)***. Other methods, in particular various hybridization techniques have been used as diagnostic tools. However,

From: *Methods in Molecular Medicine, vol. 48: Antibiotic Resistance Methods and Protocols*
Edited by: S. H. Gillespie © Humana Press Inc., Totowa, NJ

these have several disadvantages over PCR techniques in that a relatively large number of bacterial cells is initially required, a DNA extraction step is often necessary, and the procedure is more complicated requiring the construction of labeled probe molecules. PCR avoids some of these problems in that DNA preparation is simpler and the whole process can be completed in one working day ***(4,5)***. Numerous studies have used the PCR technique to detect methicillin resistance in staphylococci ***(1,2,11–13)***. In most, extracted DNA was incubated with restriction enzymes before the start of the assay. However, more recently several methods have been described that pick bacterial colonies directly from agar plates for use in subsequent PCR methodologies which have advantages for routine use in diagnostic laboratories ***(4,5,14)***.

The method described in this chapter is a multiplex-PCR using target DNA derived directly from bacterial colonies picked from fresh overnight agar plates without any preceding DNA preparation. Within four hours from start a molecular fingerprint derived using routine agarose gel electrophoresis, can be produced facilitating the identification of *S. aureus* and the presence or absence of genes conferring methicillin resistance and toxin production. The basic method described can be adjusted in a number of ways. For example organisms can be detected directly from cerebrospinal or peritoneal fluids (*see* **Note 1**). Furthermore primer sets can be excluded, included, or exchanged depending on the interests of the user or developments in our understanding of the pathogenesis of *S. aureus* infection (*see* **Note 2**). In particular other resistance genes can be detected in addition to *mecA*, such as genes encoding aminoglycoside modifying enzymes or mupiricin resistance, by the use of alternative oligonucleotide primer sets ***(15,16)***. The PCR method described here can either be used as a basic screen for *S. aureus* or can be incorporated into the arsenal of methods available for use in the rapid diagnosis and targeted treatment of staphylococcal infections.

2. Materials

Unless described below all materials should be stored according to the manufacturers' instructions.

2.1. Bacterial Isolates

Fresh cultures of each of the bacterial isolates to be tested should be available. In addition appropriate control strains are necessary to correctly interpret results.

1. *S. epidermidis* strain ATCC 27626 as a positive control for the *mecA* gene and negative control for the *coa* gene.
2. *S. aureus* ATCC 29213 for the positive control of the *coa* gene and negative control of the *mecA* gene (*see* **Note 3**).

2.2. PCR Reaction

2.2.1. Oligonucleotide Primers

Based on published DNA sequences of relevant bacterial genes the following oligonucleotide primers should be available (*see* **Note 2**). High purity primers dissolved in sterile water should be ordered in advance from your local supplier. From the oligonucleotide stock solutions a 100 µ*M* dilution for use on subsequent PCR reactions should be made in sterile water. Primer stock solutions and dilutions must be stored at –20°C at all times.

1. Primer set 1*:* *mecA* gene for the detection of methicillin resistance ***(17)***;
   5'-primer: [5']-GTTGTAGTTGTCGGGTTTGG-[3'],
   3'-primer: -[5']-CGGACGTTCAGTCATTTCTAC-[3'],
   (Amplification product length, 161 nucleotides)
2. Primer set 2: *coa* gene for the detection of coagulase encoding gene ***(18)***;
   5'-primer: [5']-GCTTCTCAATATGGTCCGAG-[3'],
   3'-primer: [5']-CTTGTTGAATCTTGGTCTCGC-[3'],
   (Amplification product length, 131 nucleotides)
3. Primer set 3: 16S eubacteria rRNA gene for the detection of eubacteria ***(19)***;
   5'-primer: [5']-AACTGGAGGAAGGTGGGGAT-[3'],
   3'-primer: [5']-AGGAGGTGATCCAACCGCA-[3'],
   (Amplification product length, 371 nucleotides)
4. Primer set 4: 16S rRNA gene for the detection of staphylococci ***(19)***;
   5'-primer: [5']-GCCGGTGGAGTAACCTTTTAGGAGC-[3'],
   3'-primer: [5']-AGGAGGTGATCCAACCGCA-[3']
   (Amplification product length, 106 nucleotides)
5. Primer set 5: *seb* gene for the detection of the enterotoxin B encoding gene ***(5,20)***;
   5'-Primer: [5']-GTATAAGAGATTATTTATTTCACATG-[3'],
   3'-Primer: [5']-TATATTAAGTCAAAGTATAGAAATTG-[3'],
   (Amplification product length 231 nucleotides)
6. Primer set 6: *sec-1* gene for the detection of the enterotoxin C-1 encoding gene ***(5,21,22)***;
   5'-Primer: [5']-CCACTTTGATAATGGGAACTTAC-[3'],
   3'-Primer: [5']-GATTGGTCAAACTTATCGCCTGG-[3'],
   (Amplification product length 270 nucleotides)
7. Primer set 7: *tst* gene for the detection of the TSST-1 encoding gene ***(5,23)***;
   5'-Primer: [5']-AAGCCCTTTGTTGCTTGCGAC-[3'],
   3'-Primer: [5']-AGCAGGGCTATAATAAGGACTC-[3'],
   (Amplification product length 250 nucleotides)

2.2.2. PCR Reagents.

1. A high quality *Taq* DNA polymerase (e.g., Ampli-*Taq* DNA polymerase®, Perkin-Elmer Biosystems, Weiterstadt, Germany).

2. 10X PCR reaction buffer: 100 m*M* Tris-HCl pH 8.3, 500 m*M* KCl, 25 m*M* $MgCl_2$. This is normally supplied with *Taq* DNA polymerase (e.g., GeneAmp 10X PCR buffer® Perkin Elmer Biosystems).
3. 5X dNTP nucleotide mix (500 µ*M*) containing equal concentrations of dATP, dCTP, dGTP and dTTP (e.g., GeneAmp dNTPs® mixes, Perkin Elmer Biosystems).
4. Sterile water. Store at room temperature.
5. PCR thermocycler.

2.3. Agarose Gel Electrophoresis

1. 10X stock agarose gel sample buffer: 50% glycerine, 0.1% BPB, 0.1 *M* EDTA pH 7.8. Stored at room temperature indefinitely.
2. High quality normal-melting temperature agarose (e.g., Metaphor® agarose Biozym Diagnostik).
3. Ethidium bromide (10 mg/mL stock solution). Stored at 4°C in darkness. Can be stored indefinitely. Take care as EtBr is a carcinogen and all skin contact should be avoided.
4. 10X TBE buffer: 890 m*M* Tris-HCl, 890 m*M* boric acid, 2 m*M* EDTA, pH 8.0. This can be stored sterile at room temperature for up to 3 mo.
5. 1 kb DNA size marker. Store at –20°C or keep on ice when in use.
6. Submarine gel electrophoresis rig.
7. Suitable power pack.

3. Methods

3.1. Bacterial isolates

1. Culture each bacterial isolate to be tested overnight (*see* **Note 4**).
2. Culture control strains in parallel with test isolates. For *S. aureus* best results can be obtained by inoculating isolates on Mueller-Hinton 5% blood agar plates and incubating overnight at 35°C.

3.2. PCR Reaction

1. Prepare a PCR amplification mixture with an end volume of 50 µL containing 5 µL of 10X PCR reaction buffer, 10 µL of 5X dNTP mixture, and 2.0 µL of each of the primers from the 7 primer sets (*see* **Note 2**).
2. Add 20 µL of water bringing the volume up to 49 µL.
3. Add 1 µL (5 Units) of *Taq* DNA polymerase after an initial denaturation step described later, bringing the final reaction volume to 50 µL (*see* **Note 5**). The final concentration of the PCR reaction mix components is 10 m*M* Tris-HCL (pH 8.3), 50 m*M* KCl, 2.5 m*M* $MgCl_2$, 100 µ*M* of dNTPS (25 µ*M* of each dNTP) and 0.4 µ*M* of each of the respective primers (*see* **Note 6**). This reaction mix should be stored on ice at all times.
4. Using a sterile toothpick take approximately one-tenth of a single overnight bacterial colony and gently mix into the PCR amplification mixture (*see* **Note 7**). Cultures can be used directly from the incubator.

5. Mix each sample thoroughly for a few seconds using a bench vortex mixer followed by a few seconds spin in a bench centrifuge to ensure the PCR reaction mixture is coalesced at the bottom of the tube.
6. Include at least two PCR control samples in parallel with test samples. The first should contain no bacterial culture, and the second should contain no oligonucleotide primers. Other PCR control reaction mixes can be made as appropriate. Sterile water should be used to make each control tube to a final volume of 50 µL (*see* **Note 5**).
7. Overlay the PCR reaction mixture with 2 drops of sterile paraffin oil. N.B. certain PCR thermal cycler apparatus are designed for use with no overlaying paraffin oil. Please refer to the appropriate manufacturers' instructions.
8. Program the PCR thermal cycler to achieve two separate conditions. The first is a denaturation program in which sample mixes and control tubes are heated to 94°C for 10 min. The second is an amplification program which enables amplification of target DNA molecules to take place by achieving the following parameters: an initial denaturation of 5 min at 94°C, followed by 25 cycles of the following parameters, 94°C 20 s (denaturation), 55°C 20 s (annealing) and 72°C 50 s (final elongation), followed immediately by a final elongation step of 72°C for 5 min.
9. From ice place each sample (containing no *Taq* DNA polymerase) into the PCR apparatus and run the first denaturation PCR program. This "hot-start" step is designed to achieve a temperature at which all bacterial template DNA and oligonucleotide primers are fully denatured, abolishing any nonspecific annealing (and subsequent amplification) that has occurred (*see* **Note 8**).
10. Once the denaturation program is complete, remove samples from the PCR apparatus and place on ice.
11. Add 1 µL of *Taq* DNA polymerase to each reaction mix below the paraffin oil.
12. Mix the reaction mix gently with the end of the pipet tip. A small-volume pipet should be used to facilitate the accurate dispensation of the *Taq* DNA polymerase.
13. From ice place each test sample including control tubes in the PCR thermal cycler and run samples using the second amplification PCR program.
14. After the PCR reaction is complete remove samples for immediate use or store at 4ºC for up to 12 h or freeze indefinitely for future use (*see* **Note 9**).

3.3. Agarose Gel Electrophoresis

1. Remove 15 µL of the amplified sample, avoiding as much as possible the paraffin oil.
2. Mix gently with 1.5 µL of 10X stock agarose sample buffer.
3. Load all samples, including control samples, onto a premade 4% agarose gel (*see* **Note 10**) in 0.5X TBE buffer containing a final concentration of 0.5 µg/mL EtBr (*see* **Note 11**). Each gel must contain amplified DNA from control organisms and from the control PCR reactions.
4. Load a 1 kb DNA size marker into the outside lane to allow proper sizing of resolved amplified DNA fragments (*see* **Note 12**).

5. Use fresh 0.5X TBE buffer containing no EtBr as a running buffer (*see* **Note 11**).
6. Run the gel at a constant 80 volts for 45 min or until the sample buffer dye front has reached 2/3rd of the distance through the gel.
7. Visualize amplified DNA fragments using an ultraviolet trans-illuminator and a computerized or Polaroid image taken, depending on apparatus available in your lab.
8. Calculate the sizes of amplified bands from each sample by comparison to the size markers on either side of the gel (*see* **Note 12**). By this and by comparison to the amplified gene products derived from samples containing control organisms the presence or absence of genes can be deduced. Special attention should be paid to PCR control lanes running samples containing no template DNA or no oligonucleotide primers prior to drawing firm experimental conclusions. Any amplified fragments detected in these samples would suggest that nonspecific DNA amplification has occurred and results should be interpreted with caution or repeated after taking appropriate precautionary steps (*see* **Note 13**).

4. Notes

1. Multiplex-PCR for the detection of *S. aureus* can be used directly from peritoneal and cerebrospinal fluids, replacing the need to first culture organisms. In the case of infections with staphylococci, and especially methicillin-resistant organisms this enables the early introduction of proper therapeutic management, something that classical techniques take 48 h to achieve. The clinical sensitivity and specificity of this method has been demonstrated to be at least as good as conventional methods and able to detect $\geq 10^2$ colony forming units/mL ***(24)***. To detect organisms directly from cerebrospinal or peritoneal fluids, 100 µL of fresh sterile fluid should be centrifuged at 5000*g* for 10 min at room temperature and the sediment resuspended in 10 µL of sterile water. Use 5 µL as a DNA template in a subsequent PCR reaction. When performing PCR on liquid samples such as this, the amount of sample must be incorporated into the calculated end volume of the PCR reaction, which is not necessary when using a small fraction of bacterial colonies ***(24)***.
2. The types and combinations of oligonucleotide primers described in this protocol can be adjusted according to the wishes of the experimenter. For example a simpler technique would be to screen only for *S. aureus*, coagulase negative staphylococcus and other eubacterial species, simultaneously screening for methicillin resistance should staphylococcal species be present. For this one needs to include only primer sets 1–4, omitting those primer sets specific for staphylococcal toxin genes ***(4)***. The volume of sterile water added to bring the reaction mix to a final volume of 50 µL should be adjusted accordingly. However, caution should be taken when adding new or novel primer sets. Oligonucleotides included in this study do not form primer-dimers with each other, have similar annealing temperatures within target DNA sequences, and amplify gene products with different low molecular weight sizes. New or novel primers must first be tested with appropriate controls prior to use.
3. Since specific *S. aureus* isolates strains are not routinely available as controls for toxin-type production, it is recommended to perform one of a number of com-

mercially available biochemical tests able to identify specific toxin producing strains from your own collection that can be subsequently stored for use as control organisms.

4. Fresh overnight bacterial colonies always work best. Older cultures contain higher amounts of cell debris and possible PCR inhibitors.
5. The final volume of the reaction mix can be adjusted as appropriate but should always be kept to a minimum, 50 μL usually being a maximal volume. In changing the final volume of the reaction mix, make sure to adjust the corresponding volumes of 10X PCR reaction buffer, nucleotides and *Taq* DNA polymerase used, so that appropriate end concentrations are maintained. Whatever adjustments are made, sterile water should be used to make the reaction mix to the desired final volume. If you are using multiple primer sets, different stock concentrations of nucleotides, or samples other than bacterial colonies, e.g., cerebrospinal fluids (*see* **Note 1**) it is a good idea to make a quick calculation to ensure that all reagents, buffers, and samples can be incorporated without exceeding the calculated final volume amount.
6. To save time, in addition to ensuring better inter-experimental standardization of this technique, stocks of reaction mixes can be made in bulk and stored at –20°C for up to 6 mo. Such stock mixes should not contain *Taq* DNA polymerase or template DNA, which can be added immediately after thawing stock. *Taq* DNA polymerase should be added before aliquoting stock PCR mix into separate reaction tubes.
7. Do not be tempted to take larger quantities of bacterial colony for sample tubes. PCR is an exquisitely sensitive technique and larger amounts of template DNA can reduce the performance of the PCR.
8. During sample preparation nonspecific annealing can occur between oligonucleotide primers and template DNA. The addition of *Taq* DNA polymerase prior to complete denaturation of these complexes may lead to amplification of nontarget DNA reducing the performance of the technique and clarity of results. The addition of the first denaturation PCR program prevents this. An alternative "hot-start" method can be used that involves prior denaturation of the bacterial samples. This is the preferred method when studying coagulase negative staphylococci as prior removal of the capsule by heating can improve amplification results. For this, reaction mixes can be prepared to a total volume of 49 μL, including addition of the *Taq* DNA polymerase. Concomitant with this, a single bacterial colony from each isolates is resuspended in 10 μL of sterile water and denatured using the first denaturation PCR program described previously. When complete sample tubes are immediately removed, placed on ice and 1 μL of each denatured bacterial colony added to the prepared reaction mixes. The same amplification conditions are then used to amplify target DNA sequences. In addition a number of commercially available "hot-start" PCR kits are available.
9. After the PCR program is complete sample tubes can be left in the PCR machine at room temperature for 1–2 h until further use, although best results are ensured

by immediate removal of samples for storage at 4°C (short-term storage) or direct freezing at –20°C (long-term storage). It is often optimal to keep the PCR thermal cycler at 4°C, meaning that samples can be left overnight without removing samples from the PCR apparatus. For long-term storage appropriate volumes of 10X stock agarose gel sample buffer can be added directly to the sample tube prior to freezing. Samples can be taken from the freezer, thawed and loaded directly onto agarose gels.

10. Each of the oligonucleotide primer sets described here amplify DNA fragments ranging in size from 106 bp (16S staphylococcal rRNA gene) to 371 bp (16S eubacterial rRNA gene), thus agarose gel conditions used needs to able to satisfactorily resolve fragment sizes encountered. 4% agarose gels are considerably denser than the 1% agarose gels used in routine molecular techniques and allow for better resolution of smaller fragments.
11. Appropriate precautionary steps must be taken when using or disposing of ethidium bromide, and any substances containing even trace amounts of ethidium bromide, especially agarose gels and running buffers. Standard operating procedures controlling the use of ethidium bromide within a laboratory vary from laboratory to laboratory. It should make no difference to the end result, whether ethidium bromide is added directly to the agarose gel prior to resolving PCR amplified fragment or whether gels are stained after use.
12. Any DNA size marker can be used as long as it allows for the accurate sizing of DNA fragments in the range of 100–500 bp. Space permitting size markers should be run in the middle and on one side of the gel allowing compensation for "smiling" in lanes toward the edge of the gel.
13. As with any other PCR technique appropriate attention to control wells provide a necessary level of confidence in interpreting test results. The amplification of DNA in negative control wells casts doubt on the validity of results from any of the samples. The contaminating substance can be identified by setting up control samples sequentially omitting individual reagent from the sample mix and checking for nonspecific amplification.

References

1. Ubukata, K., Nakagami, S., Nitta, A., Yamane, A., Kawakami, S., Sugiura, M., and Konno, M. (1992) Rapid identification of the *mecA* gene in methicillin-resistant staphylococci by enzymatic detection of polymerase chain reaction products. *J. Clin. Microbiol.* **30,** 1728–1733.
2. Tokue, Y., Shoji, S., Satoh, K., Watanabe, A., and Motomiya, M. (1992) Comparison of a polymerase chain reaction assay and a conventional microbiologic method for detection of methicillin-resistant *Staphylococcus aureus. Antimicrob. Agents Chemother.* **36,** 6–9.
3. Geha, D. J., Uhl, J. R., Gustaferro, C. A., and Persing, D. H. (1994) Multiplex PCR for identification of methicillin-resistant staphylococci in the clinical laboratory. *J. Clin. Microbiol.* **32,** 1768–1772.
4. Schmitz, F.-J., MacKenzie, C. R., Hofmann, B., Verhoef, J., Finken-Eigen, M., Heinz, H.-P., and Köhrer, K. (1998) Specific information concerning taxonomy,

pathogenicity and methicillin resistance of staphylococci obtained by a multiplex PCR. *J. Med. Microbiol.* **46,** 773–778.

5. Schmitz, F.-J., Steiert, M., Hofmann, B., Verhoef, J., Hadding, U., Heinz, H.-P., and Köhrer, K. (1998) Development of a multiplex-PCR for the direct detection of the genes for enterotoxin B and C, and toxic shock syndrome toxin-1 in *Staphylococcus aureus* isolates. *J. Med. Microbiol.* **47,** 335–340.
6. Hartman, B. J. and Tomasz, A. (1986) Expression of methicillin resistance in heterogeneous strains of *Staphylococcus aureus. Antimicrob. Agents Chemother.* **29,** 85–92.
7. Madiraju, M. V. V. S., Brunner, D. P., and Wilkinson, B. J. (1987) Effects of temperature, NaCl, and methicillin on penicillin-binding proteins, growth, peptidoglycan synthesis, and autolysis in methicillin-resistant *Staphylococcus aureus. Antimicrob. Agents Chemother.* **31,** 1727–1733.
8. Watanakunakorn, C. (1985) Effect of inoculum size on in-vitro susceptibility of methicillin-resistant *Staphylococcus aureus* to 18 antimicrobial agents. *Eur. J. Clin. Microbiol.* **4,** 68–70.
9. Wong, A. C. L. and Bergdoll, M. S. (1990) Effect of environmental conditions on production of toxic shock syndrome toxin-1 by *Staphylococcus aureus. Infect. Immun.* **58,** 1026–1029.
10. Mills, J. T., Parsonnet, J., Tsai, Y. C., Kendrick, M., Hickman, R. K., and Kass, E. H. (1985) Control of production of toxic shock syndrome toxin-1 (TSST-1) by magnesium ion. *J. Infect. Dis.* **151,** 1158–1161.
11. Murakami, K., Minamide, W., Wada, K., Nakamura, E., Teraoka, H., and Watanabe, S. (1991) Identification of methicillin-resistant strains of staphylococci by polymerase chain reaction. *J. Clin. Microbiol.* **29,** 2240–2244.
12. Predari, S. C., Ligozzi, M., and Fontana, R. (1991) Genotypic identification of methicillin-resistant coagulase-negative staphylococci by polymerase chain reaction. *Antimicrob. Agents Chemother.* **35,** 2568–2573.
13. Ünal, S., Hoskins, J., Flokowitsch, E., Wu, C. Y. E., Preston, D. A., and Skarud, P. L. (1992) Detection of methicillin-resistant staphylococci by using the polymerase chain reaction. *J. Clin. Microbiol.* **30,** 1685–1691.
14. Hedin, G. and Löfdahl, S. (1993) Detecting methicillin-resistant *Staphylococcus epidermidis:* disc diffusion, broth breakpoint or polymerase chain reaction. *APMIS* **101,** 311–318.
15. Schmitz, F.-J., Lindenlauf, E., Hofmann, B., Fluit, A. C., Verhoef, J., Heinz, H.-P. and Jones, M. E. (1998) The prevalence of low and high-level mupirocin-resistance in staphylococcal clinical isolates from 19 European hospitals. *J. Antimicrob. Chemother.* **42,** 489–495.
16. Schmitz, F.-J., Gondolf, M., Fluit, A. C., Hofmann, B., Verhoef, J., Heinz, H.-P. and Jones, M. E. (1999) The prevalence of aminoglycoside-resistance and corresponding resistance genes in staphylococcal clinical isolates from 19 European hospitals. *J. Antimicrob. Chemother.* **43,** 253–259.
17. Ryffel, C., Tesch, W., Birch-Machin, I., Reynolds, E., Barberis-Maino, L., Kayser, F. H., and Berger-Bächi, B. (1990) Sequence comparison of *mecA* genes isolated

from methicillin-resistant *Staphylococcus aureus* and *Staphylococcus epidermidis. Gene* **94,** 137–138.

18. Phonimdaeng, P., O'Reilly, M., Nowlan, P., Bramley, A. J., and Foster, T. J. (1990) The coagulase of *Staphylococcus aureus* 8325–4. Sequence analysis and virulence of site-specific coagulase-deficient mutants. *Mol. Microbiol.* **4,** 393–404.
19. Greisen, K., Loeffelholz, M., Purohit, A., and Leong, D. (1994) PCR-primers and probes for the 16S rRNA gene of most species of pathogenic bacteria, including bacteria found in cerebrospinal fluid. *J. Clin. Microbiol.* **32,** 335–351.
20. Ranelli, D. M., Jones, C. L., Johns, M. B., Mussey, G. J., and Khan, S. A. (1985) Molecular cloning of staphylococcal enterotoxin B gene in *Escherichia coli* and *Staphylococcus aureus. Proc. Natl. Acad. Sci. USA* **82,** 5850–5854.
21. Bohach, G. A. and Schlievert, P. M. (1987) Nucleotide sequence of the staphylococcal enterotoxin C1 gene relatedness to other pyrogenic toxins. *Mol. Gen. Genet.* **209,** 15–20.
22. Lee, P. K. and Schlievert, P. M. (1991) Molecular genetics of pyrogenic exotoxin 'superantigens' of group A streptococci and *Staphylococcus aureus. Curr. Top. Microbiol. Immunol.* **174,** 1–19.
23. Blamster-Hautamaa, D. A., Kreiswirth, B. N., Kornblum, J. S., Novick, R. P., and Schlievert, P. M. (1986) The nucleotide and partial amino acid sequence of toxic shock syndrome toxin-1. *J. Biol. Chem.* **261,** 15783–15786.
24. Schmitz, F.-J., Steiert, M., Hofmann, B., Fluit, A. C., Verhoef J., Heinz, H.-P. and Jones, M. E. (1998) Detection of staphylococcal genes directly from cerebrospinal and peritoneal fluid samples using a multiplex polymerase chain reaction. *Eur. J. Clin. Microbiol. Infect. Dis.* **17,** 272–274.

12

Chromogenic Detection of Aminoglycoside Phosphotransferases

Ana M. Amoroso and Gabriel O. Gutkind

1. Introduction

Acquired resistance to aminoglycosides is most frequently due to the presence of the so-called aminoglycoside modifying enzymes (AGME) *(1)* able to catalyze one or more of three general reactions: N-acetylation, O-nucleotidylation and O-phosphorylation *(2)*. Although resistance phenotype (to different (substrate or not for enzymatic modification) may serve as an approach for identifying actual enzymes present in a given isolate *(3)*, results can be obscured or confusing, particularly when several different enzymes *(4)* (even, isoenzymes with different affinities) are superimposing their action in a single microorganism with potential "permeability" or target alterations. Thus, identification of the AGME content of a given strain also requires screening at the DNA level using probes specific to all the known AGME *(5)*. However, the complete set of probes is available only to a few laboratories around the world, making surveillance for the appearance of novel enzymes, or the unlikely evolution of those already known, a relatively nonfeasible goal, as search for new enzymes may begin only after failing to hybridize to all known probes.

We developed a chromogenic *(6–8)* system that can be used for qualitative, semiquantitative assay or for detecting different aminoglycoside phosphotransferase activities in resistant cell extracts after separating the enzymes by analytical isoelectrofocusing. The method can prove helpful for the analysis of clinical multiresistant isolates where the phenotypic resistance may not be caused by a single enzyme or isozyme. It can also be used as a rapid method for comparative studies on enzymatic activity expression in strains with similar genotype but different phenotypes. Surveillance for enzymes with pIs different from those already described may be used for presumption of novel enzymes.

From: *Methods in Molecular Medicine, vol. 48: Antibiotic Resistance Methods and Protocols*
Edited by: S. H. Gillespie © Humana Press Inc., Totowa, NJ

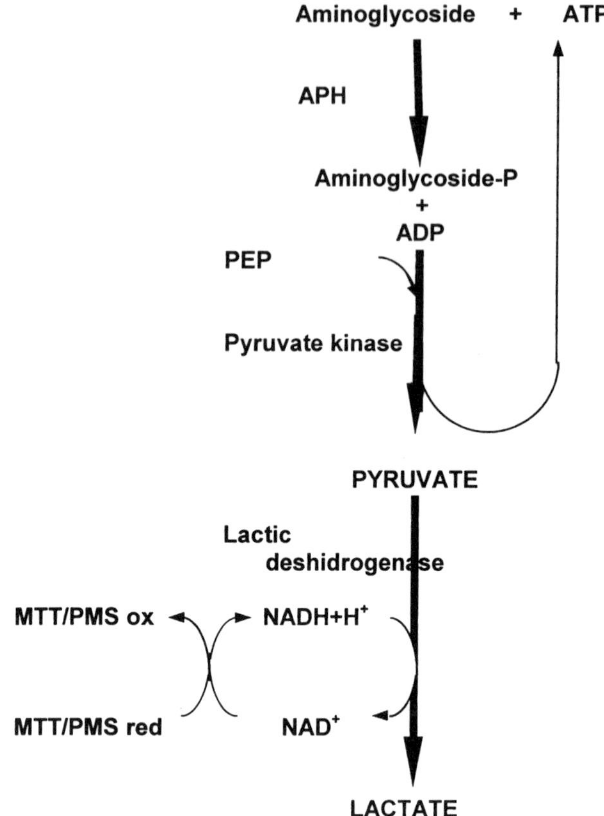

Fig. 1. Enzymatic reaction used for APH activity detection.

Clarified bacterial extracts activity is detected (after analytical isoelectrofocusing [IEF]) by coupling pyruvate production by pyruvate kinase (from phosphoenolpyruvate) in the presence of the ADP obtained by phosphorylation of selected aminoglycosides. Pyruvate can be easily reduced to lactate (by lactate dehydrogenase) in the presence of NADH, which can, in due time, be regenerated by oxidation of phenazine methosulphate and thiazolyl blue to a colored formazan. The enzymatic reaction is outlined in **Fig. 1**.

2. Materials

1. Culture media: Brain Heart Infusion (sterile, use within one week of prepared).
2. Coupled colorimetric reaction for detection of phosphotranferase activity. Buffer A; 10 m*M* tris chloride, 10 m*M* magnesium acetate, 25 m*M* ammonium chloride pH 7.8.

3. Concentrated Agarized buffer A; 20 m*M* tris chloride, 20 m*M* magnesium acetate, 50 m*M* ammonium chloride, 1.5% Agar pH 7.8 (melt and heat and hold at 42°C).
4. Solution a: 160 m*M* NADH, 10X (make fresh as required).
5. Solution b: 1200 UI/mL pyruvate kinase (approx 15.8X) 635 µL (make fresh as required).
6. Solution c: 320 m*M* phosphoenolpyruvate, 10X (make fresh as required).
7. Solution d: 80 m*M* ATP, 10X (make fresh as required).
8. Solution e: Commercial lactate deshidrogenase (Sigma L-1378), 20X.
9. Solution f: 23 m*M* kanamycin sulphate (Armstrong, Argentina), 10X (stable at 4°C for at least two months).
10. Solution g: 10 m*M* MTT (thiazolyl blue)/L m*M* PMS (phenazine methosulphate, Sigma (P-9625) solution (stable for weeks at 4°C, light sensitive, toxic).
11. Sonicator.
12. Ultrafiltration system (Amicon 10 membranes).
13. Pharmacia precast gel Immobiline Dry Plates, pH 4.0–7.0.

3. Methods

3.1. Bacterial Extracts

1. Grow cells to late logarithmic phase in Brain Heart Infusion at 37°C in the presence of 50 mg/l kanamycin (our selective antibiotic, may be replaced by other aminoglycosides) (*see* **Note 1**).
2. Harvest by low speed refrigerated centrifugation (6000*g*, 10 min, 4°C).
3. Wash bacteria in cold buffer A.
4. Resuspend in the same buffer.
5. Cool the bacterial suspension on an ice-water bath, and disrupt by sonication (other methods may be used for different bacterial amounts) (six 30-s bursts in a Vibracell VC 500 sonicator, one minute cooling between bursts should be satisfactory) (*see* **Note 2**).
6. Clarify cell extracts by centifugation (15,000*g*, 10 min, at 4°C). Supernatants can be tested for enzymatic activity by monitoring loss of antibiotic activity with a small amount of kanamycin and ATP by a standard disk method (*see* **Notes 3** and **4**).
7. Concentrate extracts by ultrafiltration using Amicon 10 membrane (*see* **Note 5**).

3.2. Analytical Isoelectrofoccusing (IEF)

This process can be carried out using different ampholytes, depending on the expected pIs of the enzymes. In our case, after confirming in broad range gels (3–10 lab-made gels) presence and position of active bands, Pharmacia precast gel Immobiline Dry Plates T.M., pH 4.0–7.0 were used for monitoring more precisely apparent relative pIs. Runs are performed following general techniques as suggested by supplier's instructions.

3.3. Developing the Reaction

1. After completing IEF, remove paper electrode strips, and wash hels briefly in buffer A.

2. Prepare reaction mixture as follows: add one mL of solutions a, c, d, and f, 635 µL of solution b and 500 µL of solution e to melted and agarized concentrated buffer A.
3. Pour the mixture onto the gel, incubate for an hour in the dark at 37°C; then pour onto a in solution g until appearance of blue color.
4. Record position of decolorized bands and compare to position of reference pI standards (*see* **Note 6**).

4. Notes

1. Different aminoglycosides can be used both as selective agents and/or as enzymatic substrates. We have experienced with neomycin, gentamicin, and kanamycin, in the range of 0.5 to 2.3 m*M* (final concentration).
2. Different (cold) bacterial disruption systems can be used (depending on the amount of bacterial cells to be extracted) ***(9)***. An Aminco French Press (using a concentrated bacterial paste) is a good alternative for bacteria in the range of 2–40 g (wet weight); other alternatives to be considered should include a X-Press (frozen bacterial paste).
3. Be sure to test different antibiotic batches for absence of reducing agents (some pharmaceutical preparations may contain low amounts of sulfites (or other reducing agents), which may interact producing spontaneous reaction with the reagents.
4. Recheck different reactive batches with those already in use. Some of the enzymes and reagents are temperature sensitive, and (at least in our hands) noncontrolled storage conditions during transportation and clearance from customs proves to affect their suitability.
5. Extraction procedures need to be developed for each particular enzyme and bacteria, as enzymatic activity is easily lost during purification.
6. Qualitative and/or semiquantitative enzymatic detection can be performed placing small (10 µL) bacterial extracts (or serial dilutions) drops onto the agarized reaction solution.

References

1. Foster, T. J. (1983) Plasmid determined resistance to antimicrobial drugs and toxic ions in bacteria. *Microbiol. Rev.* **47,** 361–409.
2. Davies, J. E. (1991) Aminoglycoside aminocyclitol antibiotics and their modifying enzymes, in *Antibiotics in Laboratory Medicine* (Lorian, V., ed.), Williams and Wilkins, Baltimore, MD, pp. 691–713.
3. Miller, G. H., Sabatelli, F. J. Hare, R. S. and Waitz, J. A. (1980) Survey of aminoglycoside resistant patterns. *Dev. Ind. Microbiol.* **21,** 91–104.
4. Rossi, M. A., Gutkind, G. O., Quinteros, M., Marino, M., Couto, E., Tokumoto, M., Woloj, M., Miller, G., and Medeiros, A. (1991) A *Proteus mirabilis* with a novel extended spectrum β-lactamase and six different aminoglycoside resistant genes. 31th. ICAAC abst #939.

5. Shaw, K. J., Rather, P. N., Hare, R. S., and Miller, G. H. (1993) Molecular genetics of aminoglycoside resistance genes and familial relationships of the aminoglycoside modifying enzymes. *Microb. Rev.* **57,** 138–163.
6. Amoroso, A. and Gutkind, G. (1998) Chromogenic detection of aminoglycoside phospho transferases. *Antimicrob. Agents Chemother.* **42,** 228–330.
7. Shaw, C. R. and Prasad, R. (1970) Starch gel electrophoresis of enzymes. A compilation of enzymes. *Biochem. Genet.* 4, 297–320
8. Goldman, P. and Northrop, D. (1976) Purification and sprectrophotometric assay of neomycin phosphotransferase II. *Biochem. Biophys. Res. Commun.* **69,** 230–236.
9. Hughes, D. E, Wimpenny, J. W. T., and Lloyd, D. (1971) The disintegration of micro-organisms in *Methods in Microbiology*, vol. 5b (Norris, J. R. and Ribbons, D. W., eds.), Academic, London and New York, pp. 1–54.

II

Monitoring Response to Treatment

13

Quantification of *M. tuberculosis* DNA in Sputum During the Treatment of Pulmonary Tuberculosis

Lucy E. DesJardin and Gery L. Hehman

1. Introduction

The most common laboratory measures of response to therapy for patients with pulmonary tuberculosis are conversion of acid-fast bacilli (AFB) sputum smear to negative, or culture positive sputum to negative. AFB enumeration lacks sensitivity and specificity and the culture of *M. tuberculosis* (MTB) bacteria can take weeks. Quantitative estimates of MTB DNA in sputum have been shown to correlate with numbers of viable bacilli before the onset of chemotherapy ***(1–3)***. Once effective treatment has been initiated, DNA levels remain high in comparison to viable MTB counts in a majority of smear-positive patients and thus do not serve as a marker for the bactericidal response observed in sputa.

Although not an entirely reliable prognostic indicator, the quantification of MTB DNA in sputum is potentially useful in certain cases. First, a DNA level obtained during the first week of treatment will give an approximate estimate of the number of bacilli present before the start of treatment. This may be used to gauge the infectious potential of a pulmonary tuberculosis patient. Second, an estimate of bacillary load may be determined for a patient treated at a remote location where quantitative culture data could not be obtained. Such an estimate might be of particular value in locations that lack facilities to perform quantitative culture. In that event, a small amount of frozen specimen can be processed for DNA quantification at a later time. Third, polymerase chain reaction (PCR) quantification of DNA may be more sensitive in detecting a relapse case by sputum converting to PCR positive before culture positive ***(4–6)***. Finally, a recent study showed that 6 of 19 smear positive patients exhibited a

From: *Methods in Molecular Medicine, vol. 48: Antibiotic Resistance Methods and Protocols*
Edited by: S. H. Gillespie © Humana Press Inc., Totowa, NJ

≥10,000-fold reduction in levels of sputum MTB over the first two months of treatment, correlating with conversion of cultures to negative *(2)*. For those subjects, the quantitative decline in MTB DNA did appear to reflect treatment efficacy. Although the studies on relative DNA and CFU levels after the initiation of chemotherapy were conducted on smear-positive subjects, it is likely that quantitative DNA levels might prove more useful to monitor therapy in the smear-negative population. A note of caution to the above studies is that quantitative PCR, as compared to qualitative PCR, is necessary since MTB DNA can persist for months to years by qualitative analysis. A study by Hellyer et al. showed that the qualitative assessment of MTB DNA in sputum does not correspond to the stage or severity of disease in patients receiving a standard chemotherapeutic regimen *(7)*.

Competitive PCR is a standard method used for quantification of DNA and has been applied successfully in a number of studies *(8,9)*. However, this technique is labor-intensive and requires analysis of multiple reactions for each specimen. Furthermore, analysis of PCR products postamplification increases the chance of laboratory contamination leading to inaccurate estimations of bacillary load including false positive reactions. Recently, the ABI Prism 7700 (*Taq*Man) (Applied BioSystems/Perkin-Elmer (ABI/PE), Foster City, CA) has been shown to be a rapid and sensitive instrument for quantification of PCR and reverse transcriptase-polymerase chain reaction (RT-PCR) products *(2,3,10,11)*. The system uses a dually-labeled fluorogenic probe that hybridizes to sequences internal to the flanking PCR primers. When the two fluorophores are in close proximity, as is the case with an intact oligonucleotide probe, the quencher dye (TAMRA) absorbs the emission of the reporter dye (FAM). During the course of PCR, the 5' exonuclease activity of *Taq* Polymerase degrades the internally hybridizing oligonucleotide probe *(12)*. Degradation of the probe leads to separation of the two dyes in solution, with a subsequent increase in the level of fluorescence in the reaction when excited by a laser. The level of fluorescence measured in a sample is proportional to the amount of specific PCR product generated. The amount of target DNA in a sample is interpolated from a standard curve run simultaneously with the unknown samples. Quantification of PCR products occurs in "real-time" during each amplification step, thus samples are quantified during the exponential phase of amplification, the phase considered to produce the most accurate results, and not just at the conclusion of the last PCR cycle. This also increases the dynamic range of the assay; for example, we have achieved linearity over six logs of input DNA *(3)*. Since measurements are made during the amplification process there are no postamplification steps, which eliminates potential sources of carryover contamination and allows for greater throughput.

Sputum contains a complex mixture of DNA from human and assorted microbial sources. It is important that the PCR primers and reaction conditions are specific for detection of the MTB DNA only. For this assay we chose the insertion element IS*6110* as the DNA target ***(13,14)***. The advantage of this sequence is that it is specific for organisms of the MTB complex ***(15)***. The disadvantage is that the element is found in a variable number of copies per genome and thus could potentially lead to an overestimation of the number of MTB bacilli present. However, in practical terms, variation observed with multiple sputum specimens from the same subject appear to effect enumeration as much or more than the relatively small differences in the copy number of the IS*6110* element ***(3)***. Additionally, enumeration of MTB DNA within a single patient over time of treatment would not be affected by IS*6110* copy number. Other MTB DNA sequences could be used for enumeration provided those sequences were specific for the MTB complex.

2. Materials

2.1. Collection and Homogenization of Sputum

1. 50 mL sterile graduated polypropylene centrifuge tube or other sterile specimen collection container.
2. N-acetyl-L-cysteine (NALC) powder combined with 2.9% sodium citrate (NaCitrate) to achieve a final concentration of 50 mg/mL.
3. 2% NaOH/1.45% NaCitrate (NaOH/NaCitrate).
4. 68 m*M* phosphate buffer, pH 6.7
5. 4 mm glass beads.
6. Graduated transfer pipets.
7. Disposable serological pipets (1 mL, 5 mL).
8. pH indicator strips.
9. Aerosol resistant barrier tips P20, P200, P1000.
10. Disposable gloves.

2.2. Isolation of DNA from Sputum Specimens

1. Gene Clean III Kit (NaI, glass milk, New Wash) (BIO 101, Carlsbad, CA).
2. 100% Ethanol.
3. 1 *M* Tris-HCl, pH 7.2.
4. Nuclease-free H_2O (Amresco, Solon, OH).
5. 2 mL sterile polypropylene screw cap tubes.
6. 50 mL polypropylene screw cap tubes.
7. Aerosol resistant barrier tips (ART) P20, P200, P1000.
8. Disposable gloves.

2.3. PCR Quantification of MTB DNA

1. Plasmid DNA for standard curve. Plasmid pIS*6110,* containing the entire IS*6110* sequence, was isolated from recombinant DH5α cells (Gibco-BRL Life Technologies) by the PERFECTprep DNA isolation kit (5 Prime→3 Prime, Boulder, CO).

2. Oligonucleotide primers. Forward PCR primer (IS6) corresponds to the region of IS*6110* from base 807 to base 824, sequence 5'GGCTGTGGGTAGCAGACC-3'. The reverse primer (IS7) corresponds to the region from base 952 to base 969, sequence 5'-CGGGTCCAGATGGCTTGC-3'. Bases numbered as in GenBank accession #X52471. For primer preparations, each primer (IS6 and IS7) is diluted in sterile water to 10 µ*M* solutions (10 pmol/µL). Aliquots are stored in 100 µL vol in 0.5 mL polypropylene microcentrifuge tubes at –20°C.
3. TaqMan Probe. The internal oligonucleotide (TaqMan) probe is labeled with the fluorescent dyes 5-carboxyfluoroscein (FAM) on the 5' end and N,N,N',N'-tetramethyl-6-carboxyrhodamine (TAMRA) on the 3' end. The internal probe hybridizes within the 163-bp region amplified by the PCR primers and has the sequence 5-(FAM)-TGTCGACCTGGGCAGGGTTCG-(TAMRA)-3'.
4. *Taq* Polymerase (5 U/µL) (Biolase, ISC BioExpress).
5. 10X PCR Buffer (100 m*M* Tris-HCl, pH 8.3; 500 m*M* KCl).
6. $MgCl_2$ (50 m*M*). Generally supplied with *Taq* Polymerase.
7. Bovine Serum Albumin (BSA) (DNase-Free) stock solution. BSA can be purchased as a nonacetylated, DNase-free, 10 mg/mL solution (Pharmacia). Until needed the solution is stored as supplied at –20°C. A 1 mg/mL working stock solution is prepared by mixing 100 mL of the 10 mg/mL BSA with 900 mL nuclease-free H_2O. Aliquots of the BSA working stock are stored at –20°C in 1.5-mL microcentrifuge tubes.
8. Deoxynucleotide stock solutions. Solutions of dATP, dCTP, and dGTP can be purchased individually as 100 m*M* solutions (Pharmacia). Until needed they are stored as supplied at –20°C. A working stock of dNTP (a solution containing 10 m*M* dATP, 10 m*M* dCTP, and 10 m*M* dGTP) is prepared by mixing 100 µL of each of the 100 m*M* dNTPs with 700 µL nuclease-free H_2O. Aliquots of the dNTP working stock are stored at –20°C in 1.5 mL microcentrifuge tubes.
9. dUTP can be purchased as a 100 m*M* solution (Pharmacia). Until needed the solution is stored as supplied at –20°C. A 10 m*M* working stock of dUTP is prepared by mixing 100 µL of 100 m*M* dUTP with 900 µL nuclease-free H_2O. Aliquots of the dUTP working stock are stored at –20°C in 1.5 mL microcentrifuge tubes.
10. Yeast RNA 5 µg/µL (Ambion).
11. Uracil DNA glycosylase (UDG, 1 U/µL) (New England BioLabs).
12. Nuclease-free H_2O (Amresco).
13. 96-well optical reaction plate (Perkin-Elmer).
14. Optical caps (Perkin-Elmer).
15. Aerosol resistant barrier tips P20, P200, P1000.
16. Disposable gloves.

3. Methods

3.1. Collection and Homogenization of Sputum (see Notes 1 and 2)

1. Samples should be collected and stored using sterile materials and aseptic technique. Record sample volume. Sterile polypropylene screw cap tubes are

preferred for sample storage (*see* **Note 3**). Maintain the sample at 4°C until homogenized.

2. Using a serologic pipet add to the specimen collection container an amount of freshly prepared NALC/NaCitrate equal to 10% of the volume of the sample. Recap the container, swirl slightly to loosen adherent specimen, and decant into a 50 mL centrifuge tube. If specimen is collected in a centrifuge tube, the 1/10 vol of NALC/NaCitrate may be added directly to that tube.
3. Add ten 4 mm glass beads, close tube and vortex 20 s.
4. Incubate the mixture for 5 min at room temperature and vortex again for 20 s.
5. Add a volume of NaOH/NaCitrate equal to the specimen volume.
6. Vortex the mixture for 20 s and incubate at room temperature for 15 min. Bring the volume to 50 mL with phosphate buffer. Mix suspension by vortex.
7. Centrifuge the tubes at 4000*g* at 8–10°C for 15 min.
8. Decant the supernatant (and discard) into a splash-proof container.
9. Resuspend the pellet in 1 to 3 mL phosphate buffer and record volume used. It is essential to record the volume of sputum initially processed and the buffer volume used for pellet resuspension in order to calculate the initial concentration of MTB DNA per mL sputum.
10. Check pH of the sample with indicator strips and, if necessary, adjust to pH 7.2 to 7.5 using 1 *M* Tris buffer.

3.2. Isolation of DNA from Sputum Specimens

3.2.1. GeneClean III New Wash Preparation (16)

1. In a PCR cabinet located in a DNA-free area, add 280 mL of nuclease-free H_2O to a 1-Liter bottle dedicated for mixing New Wash.
2. To the bottle add the contents of 1 tube of New Wash Concentrate (14 mL) and swirl to mix.
3. Add 310 mL of 100% ethanol and swirl to mix.
4. Divide diluted New Wash into 40–45 mL aliquots by dispensing into 50 mL polypropylene screw cap tubes. Store tubes at –20°C.

3.2.2. Isolation of DNA Using Gene Clean III Protocol

1. Work should be performed in a Biosafety exhaust protective hood, equipped with UV light. Clean the Biosafety hood with 10% bleach. Turn the UV light on for 20 min before using the cabinet (*see* **Note 2**).
2. Prepare a boiling water bath and a water bath set at 55°C.
3. Label one 2 mL sterile polypropylene screw cap tube for each specimen. Include positive controls containing known numbers of MTB cells and negative control samples containing water and reagents only.
4. Add 100 µL of 1 *M* Tris-HCl, pH 7.2 to each tube.
5. Add 400 µL of nuclease-free H_2O to each negative control tube.
6. Transfer 400 µL of each sample to the appropriate tube.
7. Addpositive control cells to the appropriate tubes and bring the final volume to 400 µL with H_2O.

8. Transfer the tubes to a floating tube rack and place them in the boiling water bath for 10 min. Allow tubes to cool for 5 min then pulse centrifuge for 20 s.
9. Add 3 vol (1500 µL) Gene Clean NaI to each tube. Vortex Gene Clean III glass milk stock until well suspended and add 10 µL to each tube.
10. Vortex tubes briefly to mix and agitate by rocking the tubes for 30 min on a platform rocker.
11. Centrifuge for 1 minute at 10,000*g*. Aspirate the supernatant and discard.
12. Wash the pellet by adding 500 µL of Gene Clean III New Wash. Vortex until glass milk is resuspended and pellet the glass milk by centrifugation.
13. Repeat above step for a total of 3 washes, aspirate off and discard the supernatant, and allow the tube to air dry for 30 min.
14. Elute the DNA by adding 50 µL nuclease-free H_2O to the pellet and mix by vortex. Heat at 55°C for 10 min. Centrifuge samples for 1 min to pellet the glass milk away from the aqueous phase containing the DNA.

3.3. PCR Quantification of MTB DNA

3.3.1. Preparation of DNA for Standard Curve

To accurately quantify the number of MTB target DNA molecules present, a stock of ultra-pure DNA must be prepared for use as a standard. The source of the DNA can be MTB or *M. bovis* genomic DNA purified from cultured cells, or, if the target sequence of interest has been cloned onto a plasmid, the purified plasmid can be used. In this protocol, the recombinant plasmid, pIS6110 was used for a standard curve. The PERFECT prep plasmid isolation kit (Ambion) was used to purify plasmid DNA from DH5α cells following manufacturer's instructions. The concentration and purity of DNA is determined spectrophotometrically, and requires an A260/280 ratio of at least 1.9. If necessary the plasmid DNA can be further purified by phenol:$CHCl_3$ extraction followed with repeated washing using a Centricon filter (*see* **Note 3**).

3.3.2. PCR Amplification

The PCR master mix is assembled in a designated clean room or area (i.e., DNA-free room that is not used for culture or sample preparation) in a UV equipped PCR cabinet. The master mix contains all the components necessary for PCR except control and sample DNA. Control and sample DNA are added in a designated template room or area in a UV equipped PCR cabinet.

1. Prepare the PCR master mix by combining the following reagents (per 50 µL PCR reaction):
   5 µL of 10X PCR Buffer (final 1X);
   5 µL of 50 m*M* $MgCl_2$ (final 5 m*M*);
   0.5 µL of 1 mg/mL BSA (final 10 ng/µL);
   0.1 µL of 5 mg/mL Yeast RNA (final 10 ng/µL);

2 µL of 10 m*M* dUTP working stock (final 400 µ*M*);
1 µL of 10 m*M* ea dNTP working stock (final 200 µ*M* ea);
1 µL of 10 µ*M* IS6 oligo (final 0.2 µ*M*);
1 µL of 10 µ*M* IS7 oligo (final 0.2 µ*M*);
0.5 µL of 10 µ*M* IS*6110* *Taq*Man probe (final 100 n*M*);
1 µL of 1 U/µL UDG (final 1 U);
0.2 µL of 5 U/µL *Taq* Polymerase (final 1 U); and
32.7 µL of Nuclease-free H_2O.

2. Dispense 45 µL of PCR master mix per well to a 96-well optical reaction plate (Perkin-Elmer). Fill enough wells to assay test samples in duplicate, control DNA in duplicate, and no-template control wells.
3. Add 5 µL of sample or standard DNA to individual wells of the 96-well plate. Seal wells with optical caps (Perkin-Elmer).
4. Place the plate in the ABI 7700 and set amplification profile. The amplification profile consists of 1 cycle at 50°C, 2 min to allow for uracil DNA glycosylase ([UDG] decontamination); 1 cycle at 95°C, 5 min; and 40 cycles of 94°C, 30 s, and 68°C, 1 min.
5. Following the conclusion of the run, do not remove the caps from the plate. Because the PCR products have been quantified by the ABI 7700 during the PCR run, no further manipulation of the PCR reaction mix is required. The plate can be discarded without ever exposing the surrounding environment to post-amplification PCR products (*see* **Note 4**).

3.3.3. Quantification Using the ABI Prism 7700

Amplification and detection is performed with the ABI 7700 using SDS software and following the manufacturer's instructions ***(17)***. The TAMRA signal is used to standardize the reaction. The threshold is set at 10 times the standard deviation of the mean base-line emission calculated for PCR cycles 3 to 15. The fractional cycle number reflecting a positive PCR is called the cycle threshold (Ct). The Ct for standard amounts of pIS*6110* plasmid DNA and test samples are usually in the range of 18 and 32 cycles of amplification ***(18)***. The amount of product in a particular reaction is measured by interpolating from a standard curve of Ct values generated from known starting concentrations of DNA, consisting of 10-fold increments of 5 to 500,000 molecules per reaction. The coefficient of variation should be less than 1% between replicate standards and an average of ~10% for samples ***(1–3,10,11)*** (*see* **Note 5**).

4. Notes

1. Sputum is viscous and requires homogenization to obtain a representative level of MTB DNA present throughout the sample. Any standard laboratory protocol for sputum digestion and decontamination can most likely be used provided it results in a homogenous solution and will not degrade DNA. The traditional method of pretreatment involves decontamination and digestion of sputum with

NALC and NaOH (19). The result of this treatment is a specimen with a much-reduced viscosity; however, pretreatment often results in an acidic or basic pH. It is essential that the sample pH be adjusted to 7.2 to 7.5 for adequate recovery of DNA.

2. *M. tuberculosis* is a biohazard group 3 organism and all processes up to the stage in which nucleic acid is precipitated are carried out in a Bio Safety Level III laboratory.
3. PCR is an extremely sensitive and powerful technique with the potential to amplify a single molecule of input target, resulting in a positive reaction. For this reason precautions must be taken to avoid contamination during each phase of specimen collection and processing. Protocols for the proper collection and handling of specimens must be generated and followed with frequent checks for false-positive reactions. The preparation of specimen DNA should be done in a biological safety cabinet that is not used for routine culture work. Avoid specimen contact with any potential source of MTB bacteria (alive or dead) or DNA, such as BACTEC bottles, LJ slants, and other processed or unprocessed samples. The use of sterile disposable plastics, tubes, disposable gloves and gowns, and Aerosol-Resistant (ART) sterile pipet tips is recommended. Assemble PCR reactions in a dedicated UV-equipped, dead-space, cabinet. If at all possible, maintain separate areas for sample preparation, PCR master mix preparation, and template addition to PCR reactions. Decontaminate all surfaces and racks with 10% bleach. Since every PCR reaction can generate up to 1 billion copies of the target molecule, the UDG decontamination system is highly recommended to help control amplicon contamination from previous reactions. UDG removes uracil residues from uracil-containing DNA, leading to a degradation of DNA. With this system, the nucleotide dUTP is substituted for dTTP in all PCR reactions. By adding UDE enzyme and initally incubating PCR reactions at 50°C, contaminating products from previous PCR reactions are degraded and prevented from serving as a target or template in the reaction. The UDG is then inactivated during the 95°C step.
4. The exact quantification of DNA for use in the standard curve can be challenging. To improve accuracy it is useful to isolate DNA three times from the same source independently to compare results between preparations. With the availability of commercial plasmid purification kits on the market it is easier to isolate highly purified plasmid DNA containing target DNA than it is to isolate genomic DNA. This also obviates the need to grow and harvest your own mycobacterial cultures. We prepared standard curves using DNA from *M. bovis* 410 (containing one copy of IS*6110*) and the plasmid pIS*6110* in parallel. Both curves were linear over 6 orders of magnitude with the R^2 of the lines greater than 0.99 in each case *(3)*. The slopes of the curves were similar, with no appreciable differences between genomic and plasmid DNA. These data suggest that amplification efficiency was similar for mycobacterial genomic DNA and plasmid DNA and either could be used as a standard.
5. Biological specimens have been noted to contain inhibitors to the PCR reaction in certain cases. Using the protocol described, no inhibition of the PCR reaction

was found in either sputum or cerebralspinal fluid (CSF) samples, however, bone marrow and pleural fluids were, on occasion, found to contain inhibitors. The usual method to determine whether inhibitors are present is to coamplify an exogenously introduced internal control DNA template with the sample in the same PCR reaction. Postamplification products from the internal control are distinguished from the endogenous template by product size ***(14)***. With the ABI Prism 7700 system, size differentiation of products is not possible unless one were to subject the products of the PCR reactions to gel electrophoresis postamplification, requiring that PCR tubes are opened after target amplification therefore defeating one of the major advantages of the system. However, it is still possible to detect inhibitors of PCR using a couple of different strategies. First, a known amount of purified MTB DNA can be added with the test sample to a separate sample PCR reaction well. The quantity of MTB molecules in this well should be equal to the sum of the endogenous template plus the added MTB DNA. An amount of product less than expected is an indication of inhibition. A second strategy is to modify the internal control sequence by adding a sequence of DNA base pairs foreign to the region under analysis. This same approach is used to prepare a competitive PCR template ***(3)***. The altered DNA is added to the test sample and PCR performed. A second TaqMan detector probe can be designed to detect the foreign sequence. This second probe can either be labeled with a dye other than FAM for simultaneous detection, or the samples can be assayed in parallel for side by side detection.

6. Although not many laboratories presently have access to a "real-time" PCR instrument such as the ABI Prism 7700, several methods for the quantification of PCR products postamplification exist. The most common method is competitive PCR, where the test sample and various known amounts of internal control DNA are amplified simultaneously but detected independently using gel electrophoresis ***(8,9)***. Comparisons are made between the signals from the test sample PCR product and the internal control. Reactions in which the signal of the test sample PCR product is equivalent to that of the internal control indicate an equivalent amount of starting target DNA. A second method of quantitative PCR utilizes limiting dilution ***(20)***. Although less accurate, limiting dilution PCR can provide a rough estimate by measurement of the titer, or the greatest dilution at which a PCR product is observed. This system is advantageous in that internal control DNA or recombinant plasmid constructs are not required. However, since the titer is determined through the presence of a band observed on a gel, this system may lead to an overestimation due to the presence of contaminating DNA. Since it has been noted that some samples may contain agents that completely or partially inhibit PCR, this system may also lead to underestimation.

Acknowledgments

We are grateful to Dr. Kathleen Eisenach and members of the laboratory at the University of Arkansas for Medical Sciences for their support and scientific input. We thank Tobin Hellyer for his scientific insight into these studies and Tobin Hellyer and Larry Schlesinger for critical reading of the manuscript. This work was supported by The Tuberculosis Research Unit (NIH contract #NO-AI-45244).

References

1. Hellyer, T. J., DesJardin, L. E., Teixeira, L., Perkins, M. D., Cave, M. D., and Eisenach, K. D. (1999) Detection of viable *Mycobacterium tuberculosis* by reverse transcriptase-strand displacement amplification of mRNA. *J. Clin. Microbiol.* **37,** 518–523.
2. DesJardin, L. E., Perkins, M. D., Wolski, K., Haun, S., Teixeira, L., Chen, Y., Johnson, J. L., Ellner, J. J., Dietze, R., Bates, J., Cave, M. D., and Eisenach, K. D. (1999) Measurement of sputum *Mycobacterium tuberculosis* mRNA as a surrogate for response to chemotherapy. *Am. J. Resp. Crit. Care Med.* **160,** 203–210.
3. DesJardin, L. E., Chen, Y., Perkins, M. D., Teixeira, L., Cave, M. D., and Eisenach, K. D. (1998) Comparison of the ABI 7700 system (TaqMan) and competitive PCR for quantification of *IS6110* DNA in sputum during treatment of tuberculosis. *J. Clin. Microbiol.* **36,** 1964–1968.
4. Kennedy, N., Gillespie, S. H., Saruni, A. O. S., Kisyombe, G., McNerney, R., Ngowi, F. I., and Wilson, S. (1994) Polymerase chain reaction for assessing treatment response in patients with pulmonary tuberculosis. *J Infect Dis* **170,** 713–716.
5. Levée, G., Glaziou, P., Gicquel, B., and Chanteau, S. (1994) Follow-up of tuberculosis patients undergoing standard anti-tuberculosis chemotherapy by using a polymerase chain reaction. *Res Microbiol* **145,** 5–8.
6. Yuen, K.-Y., Chan, K.-S., Chan, C.-M., Ho, P.-L., and Ng, M.-H. (1997) Monitoring the therapy of pulmonary tuberculosis by nested polymerase chain reaction assay. *J Infect* **34,** 29–33.
7. Hellyer, T. J., Fletcher, T. W., Bates, J. H., Stead, W. W., Templeton, G. L., Cave, M. D., and Eisenach, K. D. (1996) Strand displacement amplification and the polymerase chain reaction for monitoring response to treatment in patients with pulmonary tuberculosis. *J. Infect. Dis.* **173,** 934–941.
8. Piatak, M. Jr., Luk, K. C., Williams, B., and Lifson, J. D. (1993) Quantitative competitive polymerase chain reaction for accurate quantitation of HIV DNA and RNA species. *BioTechniques* **14,** 70–77.
9. Zimmermann, K. and Mannhalter, J. W. (1996) Technical aspects of quantitative competitive PCR. *BioTechniques* **21,** 268–279.
10. Gibson, U. E. M., Heid, C. A., and Williams, P. M. (1996) A novel method for real time quantitative RT-PCR. *Genome Res* **6,** 995–1001.
11. Heid, C. A., Stevens, J., Livak, K. J., and Williams, P. M. (1996) Real time quantitative PCR. *Genome Res.* **6,** 986–994.
12. Holland, P. M., Abramson, R. D., Watson, R., and Gelfand, D. H. (1991) Detection of specific polymerase chain reaction product by utilizing the 5'→ 3' exonuclease activity of *Thermus aquaticus* DNA polymerase. *Proc. Natl. Acad. Sci. USA* **88,** 7276–7280.

13. Thierry, D., Cave, M. D., Eisenach, K. D., Crawford, J. T., Bates, J. H., Gicquel, B., and Guesdon, J. L. (1990) IS611**0,** an IS-like element of *Mycobacterium tuberculosis* complex. *Nucleic Acids Res.* **18,** 188.
14. Eisenach, K. D., Sifford, M. D., Cave, M. D., Bates, J. H., and Crawford, J. T. (1991) Detection of *Mycobacterium tuberculosis* in sputum samples using a polymerase chain reaction. *Am. Rev. Resp. Dis.* **144,** 1160–1163.
15. Hellyer, T. J., DesJardin, L. E., Assaf, M. K., Bates, J. H., Cave, M. D., and Eisenach, K. D. (1996) Specificity of IS*6110*-based amplification assays for *Mycobacterium tuberculosis* complex. *J. Clin. Microbiol.* **34,** 2843–2846.
16. BIO 101. '97/'98 Protocols, Procedures & References Gene Clean. Technical Manual.
17. ABI Prism 7700 Sequence Detection System, User's Manual, P-E Applied BioSystems, copyright 1998.
18. Hellyer, T. J., DesJardin, L. E., Hehman, G. L., Cave, M. D. and Eisenach, K. D. (1999) Quantitative analysis of mRNA as a marker for viability of *Mycobacterium tuberculosis. J. Clin. Microbiol.* **37,** 290–295.
19. Kent, P. T. and Kubica, G. P. (1985) Isolation procedures, in *Public Health Mycobacteriology: A Guide for the Level III Laboratory*, Centers for Disease Control and Prevention, Atlanta, pp. 31–70.
20. Ferre, F. (1992) Quantitative or semi-quantitative PCR: reality versus myth. *PCR Methods Appl.* **2,** 1–9.

14

Isolation of *M. tuberculosis* RNA from Sputum

Lucy E. DesJardin

1. Introduction

Analysis of RNA has many applications and has become increasingly important both in basic research and clinical application. The type and number of particular mRNA transcripts expressed in *M. tuberculosis* (MTB) bacilli under various conditions can provide insight into models of pathogenesis. MTB mRNA has also been demonstrated to correspond to viability in drug-treated MTB culture systems *(1)*, thus providing an alternative to the lengthy and often difficult bacterial viability assays used in determining drug susceptibility.

Isolation of MTB RNA has an immediate application in evaluation of treatment efficacy in patients. Recent studies on smear-positive pulmonary tuberculosis patients undergoing treatment with an optimal chemotherapeutic regimen show that quantitative estimates of MTB 85B mRNA in sputum taken before and after initiation of chemotherapy correlate with numbers of viable bacilli *(2–4)*. This methodology has potential advantages over conventional microbiological methods of assessing chemotherapeutic efficacy. The most common indicators used to monitor the response to therapy of patients with pulmonary tuberculosis are conversion of an acid fast bacilli (AFB)-positive sputum smear and positive sputum culture to negative *(5–8)*. AFB enumeration lacks sensitivity and specificity whereas culture for MTB bacilli requires a minimum of two weeks before results are available *(5,9,10)*. Specificity and sensitivity of MTB mRNA as a surrogate for viability is achieved by targeting a message unique to the tubercle bacilli in an RT-PCR analysis, allowing for amplification, and thus detection, of low numbers of MTB specific target molecules. RNA analysis as a measure of bactericidal effect could benefit the design of clinical trials for the evaluation of new treatment regimens or drugs, by allowing for trials of shorter duration. With the increasing prevalence of

From: *Methods in Molecular Medicine, vol. 48: Antibiotic Resistance Methods and Protocols*
Edited by: S. H. Gillespie © Humana Press Inc., Totowa, NJ

MTB strains resistant to the first line drugs rifampin and isoniazid, analysis of MTB mRNA levels may provide an earlier indication of therapeutic efficacy than is possible through conventional culture methods.

Recovery of RNA presents certain challenges, particularly with biological materials that contain limited numbers of tubercle bacilli in a complex milieu. RNA, particularly mRNA, has a rapid turnover and is degraded in nonliving cells by release of endogenous RNases unless precautions are taken to prevent this. The normal methods of collecting and processing sputum, and other MTB-containing biological specimens may reduce the viability and permit of degradation of the RNA making it unreliable for study. The focus of this protocol is on a method that is sufficiently efficient to enable an adequate amount of MTB RNA to be obtained from a small volume of sputum containing limited numbers of bacilli. This protocol can also be adapted to other biological materials and pure cultures of MTB. Although the amount of RNA obtained is relatively small it is possible to detect 10 to 1000 CFU/mL for an mRNA target (depending upon the particular message) and less than one CFU/mL if using a 16S rRNA target with a well designed RT-PCR assay (*see* **Note 1**).

2. Materials

2.1. Sputum Collection and Homogenization

N-acetyl-l-cysteine (NALC) powder combined with 1.3% sodium citrate (NaCitrate) to a final concentration of 50 mg/mL. Make fresh before use (*see* **Note 2**).

2.2. RNA Isolation

1. 5 *M* ammonium acetate (NH_4OAc).
2. Diethyl pyrocarbonate (DEPC) treated dH_2O (Ambion #9915G).
3. Glycogen.
4. 0.2 *M* Tris-HCl, pH 7.5.
5. 0.5 *M* KCl.
6. DNase I (Ambion #2224).
7. 10X DNase I Buffer: 0.2 *M* Tris-HCl, pH 7.5, 0.5 *M* KCl.
8. TRIzol-LS (Gibco-BRL #10296-010).
9. Fast RNA tubes-Blue (BIO 101, #6020-601).
10. Cleanascite (CPG #LGC1050).
11. 25 *mM* Manganese acetate ($Mn(OAc)_2$) (Perkin-Elmer #N808-0177).
12. Prime RNase Inhibitor (5 Prime→3 [Prime #9-903250]).
13. Isopropyl alcohol.
14. 95% ethanol.
15. 75% ethanol.
16. Chloroform:isoamyl alcohol ($CHCl_3$:IAA, 24:1).
17. Chloroform.

18. 1.5 mL screw cap tube.
19. Aerosol resistant (ART) barrier tips P20, P200, P1000.

3. Methods

3.1. Collection and Homogenization of Sputum for RNA Isolation

1. Samples should be collected and stored using sterile materials and aseptic technique. Sterile polypropylene screw cap tubes are preferred for sample storage. Maintain the sample at 4°C until homogenized. Process samples within 24 h of collection (*see* **Note 3**).
2. Using a serologic pipet add to the specimen collection container freshly prepared NALC/NaCitrate (50 mg/mL) equal to 10% of the volume of the sample. Recap the container, swirl to loosen the adherent specimen, and decant into a 50 mL centrifuge tube. If the specimen is collected in a centrifuge tube, the 1/10 volume of NALC/NaCitrate may be added directly to that tube.
3. Add ten 4 mm glass beads, close the tube and vortex for 20 s.
4. Incubate the tube for 5 min at room temperature and vortex again for 20 s.
5. Transfer 500 µL of the liquefied sputum to screw-cap polypropylene tubes and store frozen at –70°C until it is to be processed for RNA isolation.

3.2. Isolation of RNA

1. Using an ART P1000 barrier tip, add 1000 µL TRIzol-LS to the sputum sample tube (containing 500 µL homogenized sputum) and mix with the pipet to resuspend. Transfer the contents of the tube to a FastRNA glass matrix tube. If the samples are difficult to resuspend, pour the contents of the sample tube into the FastRNA glass matrix tube.
2. Process in a FastPrep FP120 cell disrupter (BIO101) using a setting of 6.5 for 45 s. Do not remove the tube. After 2 min, repeat processing using the above settings. Allow the sample tubes to cool 5 min before removing (*see* **Note 4**).
3. Add 200 µL chloroform directly to the processed sample and vortex for 2 min.
4. Centrifuge the tubes gently (800*g*) for 5 min to pellet glass matrix. Transfer the tube's liquid contents (aqueous and organic layer) to a fresh 1.5 mL polypropylene tube leaving the glass matrix behind (*see* **Note 5**). Centrifuge for 15 min at room temperature (14,000*g*). The sample should now be separated into a clear aqueous phase and a red organic phase. Remove the aqueous phase (usually ~700 µL) and place it in a fresh 1.5 mL polypropylene tube taking care not to disturb the interface where the DNA is located (*see* **Note 6**).
5. Add 100 µL Cleanascite (CPG) to aqueous layer. Gently mix samples for 10 min on rocker table. Centrifuge for 1 min at maximum speed (14,000*g*). Remove supernatant carefully without disturbing the CPG pellet and place in a fresh 1.5 mL tube.
6. Add 500 µL $CHCl_3$:IAA (24:1) to the aqueous phase. Vortex for 2 min. Centrifuge 5 min (14,000*g*) at room temperature. Remove the aqueous phase and place in a fresh 1.5-mL polypropylene tube—take care not to disturb the interface.

7. Add 4 µL glycogen coprecipitant (Ambion) and 1/10 vol 5 *M* NH_4OAc to the aqueous phase. Precipitate RNA with an equal volume of isopropanol at –20°C for at least 3 h. Centrifuge (14,000*g*) for 30 min at 4°C. Wash pellet twice with 75% EtOH. Air-dry for 10 to 20 min (*see* **Note 7**).
8. Resuspend RNA pellet in 79 µL DEPC dH2O (Ambion) by allowing it to stand at room temperature for 10 min followed by vortex mixing for 2 min. Add 10 µL 10X DNase I Buffer (0.2 *M* Tris-HCl, pH 7.5; 0.5 *M* KCl), 4 µL 25 *mM* MnOAc (Perkin-Elmer), 2 µL Prime RNase Inhibitor (5 Prime→3 Prime), 5 µL DNase I (2 U/µL, Ambion). Pulse-spin the sample to the bottom of the tube and incubate at 37°C for 30 min.
9. Centrifuge tubes for 1 min (14,000*g*) to remove any condensation on lid and sides. Place in 75°C water bath for 10 min to inactivate the DNase I. Remove from bath and place samples on ice for 2 min. Centrifuge tubes for 1 min (14,000*g*) to remove condensation on lid and sides of tube.
10. RNA is now ready for RT-PCR (*see* **Note 8**). Keep RNA samples on ice during handling or stored frozen at –70°C (*see* **Note 9**).

4. Notes

1. To increase the validity of MTB RNA isolation and subsequent analysis, RNA extraction controls should be processed at the same time as the clinical specimens using the same reagents. Cultures of MTB that have been quantified by both CFU and measurement of log phase A580 are good controls for RNA isolation. Aliquots of 5×10^5 and 5×10^3 cells per isolation should be analyzed and the amount of message per cell determined. Previous studies have shown 1 to 25 molecules of 85B mRNA per cell ***(1,3)***. Lower amounts may indicate that the extraction efficiency was less than optimal.
2. RNA, particularly mRNA, is extremely labile, and care must be taken to avoid degradation. All reagents used in the isolation of RNA should be dedicated to RNA work only. Gloves must be worn at all times because skin contains RNase. All glassware, tubes and disposable items such as pipet tips, should be sterile and RNase-free. A separate work-space should be used if possible.
3. Sputum is viscous and requires homogenization to obtain a representative level of MTB RNA throughout the sample. The traditional method of pretreatment involves decontamination and digestion of sputum with NALC and NaOH ***(11)***. However, this treatment results in a substantial reduction of RNA in sputum ***(12)***. Therefore, alkaline reagents should not be used in the homogenization process. Additionally, use of NALC at concentrations exceeding those recommended will result in the loss of mRNA. Samples not maintained at 4°C after collection and not processed and frozen within 24 to 48 h are also subject to degradation.
4. Heat is generated in sample tubes during processing in the FP120, resulting in an increase in pressure and occasional leakage. Use caution when handling and opening tubes. Allowing them to cool in the instrument reduces the risk of pressurized release of the contents.

5. As a safety precaution, it is advisable to transfer the sample to a fresh tube at this step since we have, in some cases, noted a failure of tubes during high speed centrifugation after processing in the FP 120. The reason for tube failure is not clear but may be due to weakening of the tube during the vigorous agitation with the glass matrix.
6. To avoid DNA contamination of the RNA containing fraction, it is important to avoid mixing the aqueous fraction with the interface. Pipette slowly starting from the top of the aqueous phase and moving down. The DNA fractions can be stored –20°C if DNA isolation is desired (*see* **ref. *3*** for complete DNA isolation protocol and Chapter 13).
7. If there is a pause in the preparation of mRNA, this safely can occur at this step by precipitating the RNA overnight in isopropanol. However, after pelleting the RNA by centrifugation and washing with 75% ethanol, do not let the RNA pellet dry completely or it will be resistant to dissolving in aqueous solution.
8. Biological materials contain complex mixtures of RNA from both the host and other microbial sources. This RNA can present a confounding factor in the analysis of specific MTB mRNA targets. Particular care must be taken to prevent cross-reaction with other molecules that may not be apparent when using RNA from cultured MTB. We have employed several techniques to ensure the specificity of our RT-PCR assays.

   To quantify a particular MTB mRNA in RNA isolated from sputum samples, the RNA is initially reverse transcribed to cDNA using a primer specific for the target gene ***(1,3,12)***. The use of a specific reverse transcription (RT) primer results in greater yield of a particular product. The majority of RNA isolated from a biological specimen is likely to be RNA from host cells and other microbes present in the specimen. Additionally, the majority of total RNA is comprised of ribosomal RNA. If random primers are used for the RT reaction, there is competition between different priming events for the limited amount of reverse transcriptase enzyme present, whereas a specific primer will target the enzyme to the specific message.

   Sensitivity and specificity are enhanced by use of conditions that favor formation of cDNA from the target message. In some instances, the use of a short RT primer located 50 to 200 bases 3' to the region amplified during subsequent PCR is necessary (unpublished observations). This shorter primer is constructed to have a lower melting temperature that allowed for added targeting during the RT reaction. A second set of primers that amplify a region 5' to the RT primer are then used in subsequent PCR of the cDNA. The PCR primers are designed to have a higher melting temperature (TM) than the shorter RT primer. The RT primer will, therefore, not form PCR products at the annealing temperature used during PCR.

   The choice of enzyme used for reverse transcription will also effect the yield. We employed RT from the avium myeloblastosis virus (AMV). This enzyme is not as processive as that from Moloney murine leukemia virus (M-MLV), however, the more frequent initiation of RT allows for greater sensitivity of detection.

For accurate quantification of a specific target, a source of purified RNA is necessary to measure the efficiency of the RT reaction. For this control, a gene corresponding to the mRNA of interest is cloned into a plasmid vector containing an RNA polymerase promoter flanking the cloned sequence. In vitro transcripts can then be prepared using commercially available kits such as the MegaScript Transcription Kit (Ambion). Known amounts of in vitro RNA are used in RT reactions and the cDNA quantified. The difference between the observed and expected amount of target cDNA is a measure of the efficiency of the RT reaction. In addition to correcting for the efficiency of RT, dilution factors involved in the RT reaction and PCR amplification, as well as the dilution factor for the original processing of sputum must all be taken into account when calculating the levels of any particular transcript.

To monitor for DNA contamination of the RNA extract, reactions must also be performed which contain all RT reagents except the AMV RT enzyme. Perform RT reactions and mock RT reactions on samples, MTB control RNA, and in vitro transcript RNAs simultaneously.

As with any nucleic acid amplification reaction, precautions must be taken to avoid false-positive results in addition to those precautions used for handling RNA. PCR is an extremely sensitive and powerful technique, with the potential to amplify a single molecule of input target, resulting in a positive reaction. For this reason precautions must be taken to avoid contamination during each phase of specimen collection and processing. Protocols for the proper collection and handling of specimens must be generated and followed with frequent checks for false-positive reactions. The preparation of specimen RNA should be done in a biological safety cabinet that is not used for routine culture work. Avoid specimen contact with any potential source of MTB bacteria, such as BACTEC bottles, LJ slants, and other processed or unprocessed samples. The use of sterile disposable plastics, tubes, disposable gloves and gowns, and aerosol resistant (ART) barrier pipet tips is recommended. Assemble PCR reactions in a dedicated UV-equipped, dead-space, cabinet. If at all possible maintain separate areas for sample preparation, PCR master mix preparation, and template addition to PCR reactions. Decontaminate all surfaces and racks with 10% bleach. Since every PCR reaction can generate up to 1 billion copies of the target molecule, the UDG decontamination system may also help to control amplicon contamination from previous reactions.

9. To avoid repeated freezing and thawing of an RNA sample, freeze the sample in small aliquots.

Acknowledgments

I am grateful to Dr. Kathleen Eisenach and members of the laboratory at the University of Arkansas for Medical Sciences, in particular Shirley Haun, Maria Winters, Ying Chen, and Marjorie Beggs for their support and scientific input. I thank Gery Hehman, Tobin Hellyer, and Larry Schlesinger for critical reading of the chapter and numerous suggestions and insights. This work was supported by The Tuberculosis Research Unit (NIH contract #NO-AI-45244).

References

1. Hellyer, T. J., DesJardin, L. E., Hehman, G. L., Cave, M. D., and Eisenach, K. D. (1999) Quantitative analysis of mRNA as a marker for viability of *Mycobacterium tuberculosis. J. Clin. Microbi*ol. **37,** 290–295.
2. Hellyer, T. J., DesJardin, L. E., Teixeira, L., Perkins, M. D., Cave, M. D., and Eisenach, K. D. (1999) Detection of viable *Mycobacterium tuberculosis* by reverse transcriptase-strand displacement amplification of mRNA. *J. Clin. Microbi*ol. **37,** 518–523.
3. DesJardin, L. E., Perkins, M. D., Wolski, K., Haun, S., Teixeira, L., Chen, Y., Johnson, J. L., Ellner, J. J., Dietze, R., Bates, J., Cave, M. D., and Eisenach, K. D. (1999) Measurement of sputum *Mycobacterium tuberculosis* mRNA as a surrogate for response to chemotherapy. *Am. J. Respir. Crit. Care Med.* **160,** 203–210.
4. DesJardin, L. E., Chen, Y., Perkins, M. D., Teixeira, L., Cave, M. D., and Eisenach, K. D. (1998) Comparison of the ABI 7700 system (TaqMan) and competitive PCR for quantification of *IS6110* DNA in sputum during treatment of tuberculosis. *J. Clin. Microbi*ol. **36,** 1964–1968.
5. Gangadharam, P. R. (1981) The role of the laboratory in the management of tuberculosis patients. *Sem. Respir. Med.* **2,** 182–195.
6. Kim, T. C., Blackman, R. S., Heatwole, K. M., Kim, T., and Rochester, D. F. (1984) Acid-Fast bacilli in sputum smears of patients with pulmonary tuberculosis. *Am. Rev. Respir. Dis.* **129,** 264–268.
7. Hobby, G. L., Holman, A. P., Iseman, M. D., and Jones, J. M. (1973) Enumeration of tubercle bacilli in sputum of patients with pulmonary tuberculosis. *Antimicrob. A. Chemother.* **4,** 94–104.
8. Yeager, H., Jr., Lacy, J., Smith, L. R., and LeMaistre, C. A. (1967) Quantitative studies of mycobacterial populations in sputum and saliva. *Am. Rev. Respir. Dis.* **95,** 998–1004.
9. Suzuki, K., Kimoto, T., Tsuyuguchi, K., Matsumoto, H., Niimi, A., Tanaka, E., Murayama, T., and Amitani, R. (1998) Modification of results of drug susceptibility tests by coexistence of *Mycobacterium avium* complex with *Mycobacterium tuberculosis* in a sputum sample: case report and experimental considerations. *J. Clin. Microbi*ol. **36,** 2745–2747.
10. Wright, P. W., Wallace, R. J., Jr., Wright, N. W., Brown, B. A., and Griffith, D. E. (1998) Sensitivity of fluorochrome microscopy for detection of *Mycobacterium tuberculosis* versus nontuberculous mycobacteria. *J. Clin. Microbi*ol. **36,** 1046–1049.
11. Kent, P. T. and Kubica, G. P. (1985) Isolation procedures, in *Public Health Mycobacteriology: A Guide for the Level III Laboratory*, Centers for Disease Control and Prevention, Atlanta, pp. 31–70.
12. DesJardin, L. E., Perkins, M. D., Teixeira, L., Cave, M. D., and Eisenach, K. D. (1996) Alkaline decontamination of sputum specimens adversely affects stability of mycobacterial mRNA. *J. Clin. Microbi*ol. **34,** 2435–2439.

15

Detection of Viable *Mycobacterium tuberculosis* by Reverse Transcriptase-Strand Displacement Amplification of mRNA

Tobin J. Hellyer

1. Introduction

The continued dominance of tuberculosis as a cause of morbidity and mortality *(1)* has fueled the search for more rapid and reliable means of diagnosis. Numerous systems have now been described for the amplification and detection of DNA or rRNA sequences that are specific for the *Mycobacterium tuberculosis* complex *(2–7)*. While useful in reducing the amount of time required for definitive diagnosis, these techniques have not proved suitable for monitoring therapeutic efficacy, owing to the persistence of amplifiable nucleic acids for long periods beyond the point of smear and culture conversion *(8–14)*. This presumably reflects both the shedding of dead or dormant bacilli from pulmonary lesions as well as the inherent stability of bacterial DNA and rRNA. In contrast with these nucleic acid targets, bacterial mRNA is typically short-lived with a half-life of only a few minutes *(15,16)*. Consequently, an mRNA-based assay is likely to detect only living organisms and thus be a good indicator of bacterial viability and therefore therapeutic response *(9,12,13)*.

This chapter describes a method for Reverse Transcriptase-Strand Displacement Amplification (RT-SDA) of mRNA that encodes for the *M. tuberculosis* complex α-antigen (85B protein), one of the most highly expressed proteins of *M. tuberculosis* in both broth culture and human phagocytic cells *(17–19)*. SDA is an isothermal process that achieves amplification of a DNA target sequence through the coordinated activity of two enzymes: a restriction enzyme and an exonuclease-deficient DNA polymerase *(7,20–24)*. In the RT-SDA system described here, the RNA target sequence is first reverse transcribed into cDNA using avian myeloblastosis virus (AMV) reverse transcriptase and the buffer

From: *Methods in Molecular Medicine, vol. 48: Antibiotic Resistance Methods and Protocols*
Edited by: S. H. Gillespie © Humana Press Inc., Totowa, NJ

conditions are then adjusted to those suitable for SDA. The products of amplification are detected by DNA polymerase extension of ^{32}P-labeled probes, although alternative nonradioactive means of detection can also be employed.

We have recently described the application of the α-antigen RT-SDA assay to sequential sputum specimens from patients receiving treatment for pulmonary tuberculosis ***(13)***. During the first week of chemotherapy, levels of α-antigen mRNA declined rapidly, reflecting a drop in the number of viable organisms present in each sputum sample. In contrast, levels of α-antigen DNA did not appear to diminish significantly over the same period. Analysis of bacterial mRNA may, therefore, provide a more rapid means of assessing chemotherapeutic efficacy than is possible using conventional microbiological methods of patient follow-up ***(9)***. Given the protracted nature of antituberculous therapy, such assays have an important practical application in the development of novel antituberculous drug regimen and in rapid susceptibility testing of mycobacterial isolates, both of which have become increasingly important with the rise in drug resistant tuberculosis ***(1,25,26)***.

2. Materials

All reagents should be of molecular biology grade and stored at –20°C unless otherwise indicated.

2.1. RT-SDA

1. 0.5 mL Safe-Lock microcentrifuge tubes.
2. Dry baths for 0.5 mL tubes: 95°C, 45°C, and 52.5°C.
3. Sterile, RNase-free water (store at room temperature or 4°C).
4. HPLC- or gel-purified primers (**Table 1**) (*see* **Notes 1** and **2**).
5. 500 m*M* potassium phosphate buffer (K_iPO_4), pH 7.6 (*see* **Note 3**) ***(28)***.
6. Dimethyl sulfoxide (DMSO) (store at room temperature).
7. 55% v/v glycerol.
8. 250 ng/µL human placental DNA (ultra-pure) (Sigma).
9. 5 µg/µL acetylated bovine serum albumin (Gibco-BRL).
10. Nucleotide mixture: 40 m*M* 2'-deoxycytosine 5'-O-(1-thiotriphosphate) (dCTPαS), 10 m*M* dATP, 10 m*M* dGTP and 10 m*M* dUTP (all Amersham-Pharmacia).
11. 100 m*M* and 650 m*M* magnesium acetate.
12. Enzyme diluent: 50% v/v glycerol, 50 m*M* K_iPO_4, pH 7.6, 0.1 m*M* EDTA.
13. 30 U/µL PRIME RNase inhibitor (Eppendorf Scientific).
14. 25 U/µL AMV reverse transcriptase (Roche Molecular Biochemicals).
15. 20 U/µL exonuclease-deficient (exo^-) *Bst* polymerase (New England Biolabs).
16. DNA polymerase diluent: 50% v/v glycerol, 50 m*M* K_iPO_4, pH7.6, 0.1 m*M* EDTA, 1 m*M* dithiothreitol (DTT).
17. 160 U/µL *Bso*BI restriction enzyme (NEB).

Table 1
Primer Sequences for RT-SDA of *M. tuberculosis* Complex α-Antigen mRNA

Primer Name	5'-3' Sequence	Position[a]
SDA Primers		
S1	CGA TTC CGC TCC AGA CTT CTC GGG TTT GTC CGC CAA CAG G	445–459
S2	ACC GCA TCG AGT ACA TGT CTC GGG TTT GAC AAG CCG ATT GCA G	497–482
Bumper Primers[b]		
B1	ACC TTC CTG ACC AGC GAG	415–432
B2	AGA TCA TTG CCG ACG AGC	523–506
B3	GCT GGG GGT GGT AGG C	544–529
B4	CCG ACA GCG AGC CG	571–558
Detector Primer		
D1	CGG TGG GCT TCA CGG	475–461

[a]Position within α-antigen sequence of *M. tuberculosis* strain Erdman ***(27)***.

[b]*Bso*BI recognition sequences are in bold face. SDA primer target binding regions are underlined.

2.2. Probe Labeling

1. 37°C water or dry bath.
2. Boiling water bath.
3. Microcentrifuge for 2.0 mL tubes.
4. 10 μ*M* detector probe (**Table 1**).
5. 10X polynucleotide kinase buffer: 700 m*M* Tris-HCl, pH 7.6, 100 m*M* $MgCl_2$, 50 m*M* DTT (NEB).
6. 15 U/μL polynucleotide kinase (NEB).
7. 0.01 mCi/μL $^{32}P\gamma$-ATP (New England Nuclear).
8. G25 Sephadex TE Midi-SELECT-D spin columns (Eppendorf Scientific) (store at room temperature or 4°C).

2.3. Primer Extension

1. 37°C dry bath for 0.5 mL tubes.
2. Boiling water bath.
3. Nucleotide mixture: 5 m*M* dCTPαS, 2 m*M* dATP, 2 m*M* dGTP, 2 m*M* dUTP.
4. 10X REACT 1 buffer: 500 m*M* Tris-HCl, pH 8.0, 10 m*M* $MgCl_2$ (Gibco-BRL).
5. 5 U/μL exonuclease-deficient (exo^-) Klenow polymerase (NEB).
6. Formamide stop buffer: 95% v/v deionized formamide, 20 m*M* EDTA, pH 8.0, 0.02% w/v bromophenol blue, 0.02% w/v xylene cyanol.

2.4. Gel Electrophoresis

1. Sequencing apparatus with 0.4 mm spacers and analytical comb.
2. Power supply for DNA sequencing (up to 4000 V).
3. Siliconizing agent, e.g., Sigmacote® (Sigma) or Acryl-Glide® (Amresco) (store at room temperature).
4. Whatman paper No. 3 (14" × 17" or larger).
5. PVC plastic wrap.
6. X-ray film (e.g., Fuji RX, 14" × 17") and suitable cassettes with intensifying screens.
7. 50 mL syringe fitted with 22-gage needle.
8. 8% w/v denaturing polyacrylamide sequencing gel mix (Gibco-BRL) (store at 4°C).
9. 10% w/v ammonium persulfate, fresh solution.
10. 10X Tris-borate EDTA (TBE) buffer: 1 *M* Tris, 0.9 *M* boric acid, 0.01 *M* EDTA, pH 8.4 (store at room temperature).

3. Methods

3.1. RT-SDA

The following protocol is designed specifically for RT-SDA of *M. tuberculosis* α-antigen mRNA using the primers described in Table 1 (*see* **Notes 1**, **2**, and **4**). Amplification of alternative mRNA target sequences may require reoptimization of the conditions for reverse transcription and/or SDA (*see* **Note 5**).

1. Prepare the following buffer and enzyme mixtures in advance in a clean, amplicon-free environment (*see* **Notes 6** and **7**) and maintain on ice until use. The volumes given below are per reaction and can be scaled up accordingly.

   Reverse Transcriptase Buffer (*see* **Notes 8–11**): 2.4 µL sterile distilled water, 1.2 µL 500 m*M* K_iPO_4, 2.4 µL DMSO, 1.2 µL 250 ng/µL human placental DNA, 1 µL 5 µg/µL acetylated BSA, 0.4 µL nucleotide mix (40/10/10/10 m*M*), 1 µL primer mix (25 µ*M* S2, 2.5 µ*M* B2, 0.25 µ*M* B3, and 0.025 µ*M* B4), 1 µL enzyme diluent, 1 µL 30 U/µL RNase inhibitor and 0.4 µL 100 m*M* magnesium acetate. Aliquot into 0.5 µL microcentrifuge tubes in 12 µL vol.

   Reverse Trancriptase Enzyme Mix: 2.9 µL enzyme diluent and 0.1 µL 25 U/µL AMV reverse transcriptase.

   Supplemental SDA Buffer: 16.95 µL sterile distilled water, 3.6 µL DMSO, 4.05 µL 500 µ*M* K_iPO_4, 0.8 µL 250 ng/mL human DNA, 0.6 µL nucleotide mix (40/10/10/10 m*M*), and 1 µL primer mix (25 µ*M* S1, 2.5 µ*M* B1).

   SDA Enzyme Mix: 0.25 µL 160 U/µL *Bso*BI, 0.75 µL 20 U/µL exo$^-$ *Bst* polymerase, 0.48 µL 650 m*M* magnesium acetate, and 1.52 µL DNA polymerase diluent.
2. To each 12 µL vol of reverse transcriptase buffer, add 5 mL mRNA target (*see* **Notes 12–14**) and maintain the mixtures on ice until ready to begin amplification.
3. Equilibrate the tubes containing the reverse transcriptase buffer and mRNA target at 45°C for 3 min. At the same time, allow the reverse transcriptase enzyme mix to equilibrate to room temperature.
4. To each tube, add 3 µL reverse transcriptase enzyme mix, vortex briefly and continue to incubate at 45°C for 15 min.
5. Transfer the tubes to a second dry bath at 52.5°C and equilibrate for 3 min. Meanwhile, equilibrate the supplemental SDA buffer to the same temperature and allow the SDA enzyme mix to come to room temperature.
6. To each tube, add 27 µL supplemental SDA buffer and vortex briefly to mix.
7. Add 3 µL SDA enzyme mix per reaction (*see* **Note 15**), vortex briefly to mix and incubate the tubes at 52.5°C for 45 min. Stop the reactions by heating at 95°C for 3 min. Store the completed reactions at –20°C.

3.2. Probe Labeling

The following protocol provides sufficient labeled oligonucleotide for the detection of approx 80–100 RT-SDA reactions, depending on the volume of probe recovered from the Sephadex spin column. Removal of unincorporated nucleotides from the reaction mixture is optional but reduces the amount of liquid radioactive waste produced during electrophoresis of the primer extension products. All manipulations involving radioactive substrates should be performed in a designated work area according to established safety guidelines.

1. Mix the following in order: 23.5 µL sterile distilled water, 5 µL 10X polynucleotide kinase buffer, 5 µL 10 µ*M* D1 detector primer, 15 µL 0.01 mCi/µL $^{32}P\gamma$-ATP, and 1.5 µL 15 U/mL T4 polynucleotide kinase.

2. Incubate the mixture for 30 min at 37°C and stop the reaction by heating at 95°C for 2 min in a boiling water bath.
3. Prepare a G25 Sephadex spin column for use by removing the top and bottom seals and placing in a 2 mL microcentrifuge tube. Centrifuge for ~1 min at maximum speed (10,000*g*) (*see* **Note 16**).
4. Transfer the spin column to a clean microcentrifuge tube and carefully load the probe labeling mixture onto the middle of the angled bed of Sephadex. Allow to stand for 2–3 min then centrifuge at maximum speed for 2 min. The labeled probe passes through the column whereas unincorporated nucleotides are retained and can be discarded with the solid radioactive waste.
5. Store the labeled primer at –20°C and use within 10–14 d.

3.3. Primer Extension

Primer extension with the D1 detector probe generates products of 37 and 56 bases corresponding to the full-length and nicked SDA products (**Fig. 1**) *(13)*. These are separated by denaturing electrophoresis and visualized by autoradiography.

1. Prepare the extension buffer and extension enzyme mix in advance and keep on ice until use. The volumes given are per reaction and can be scaled up accordingly.
   Extension Buffer: 3.5 µL sterile distilled water, 0.5 µL 500 m*M* K_iPO_4, 0.5 µL nucleotide mix (5/2/2/2 m*M*) and 0.5 µL ^{32}P-labeled detector probe.
   Extension Enzyme Mix: 0.7 µL sterile distilled water, 0.1 µL 10X REACT 1 buffer and 0.2 µL 5 U/µL exo$^-$ Klenow polymerase.
2. Transfer 5 µL amplified sample to a clean 0.5 µL Safe-Lock microcentrifuge tube and add 5 mL extension buffer.
3. Heat the tubes for 2 min at 95°C in a boiling water bath, centrifuge briefly to remove condensation and equilibrate in a dry bath at 37°C for 1 min.
4. Add 1 mL extension enzyme mix to each sample and incubate for 10 min at 37°C (*see* **Note 17**).
5. Add 10 µL formamide stop buffer and store at –20°C until ready for electrophoresis.

3.4. Gel Electrophoresis

The following protocol assumes the use of a commercially available denaturing polyacrylamide sequencing gel mix and a standard sequencing apparatus. Procedures for setting up gel electrophoresis equipment vary between manufacturers and the reader should refer to the appropriate users manual for details.

1. Clean the glass plates thoroughly with detergent and ethanol. Coat either or both plates with a siliconizing agent to prevent the gel from sticking to the surface and rewash thoroughly before assembling the apparatus using 0.4 mm spacers.
2. Add the required volume of ammonium persulfate to the sequencing gel mix and swirl gently (*see* **Note 18**). Pour the gel using an analytical comb and allow to set for 30–40 min before proceeding.

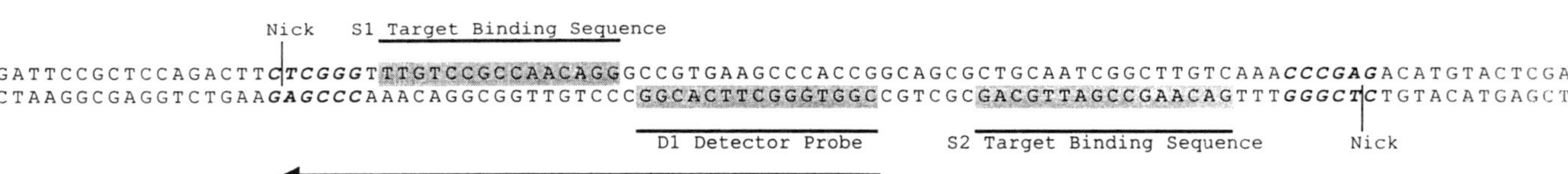

Fig. 1. Sequence of the double-stranded SDA amplicon showing extension products of detector probe D1. The target binding sequences of primers S1, S2, and D1 are indicated. DNA polymerase extension from the 3'-end of D1 leads to generation of products of 37 and 56 bases, corresponding to the nicked and full-length SDA products.

3. Run the gel using 0.5X TBE buffer. For best results, prerun the gel for 30–40 min at ~55 W or until the glass plates are warm to the touch (~50°C). This ensures that the denatured extension products remain single stranded and do not form any secondary structures that could influence their migration through the gel.
4. Using a syringe, thoroughly flush the wells with running buffer to remove any urea that accumulates during the prerun.
5. Denature the samples by heating for 2 min in a boiling water bath. Centrifuge briefly to remove condensation and load 5 µL per well (*see* **Note 19**).
6. Electrophorese at constant power until the lower dye front (bromophenol blue) is ~3–4" from the bottom of the gel.
7. Carefully pry apart the plates and transfer the gel to 3 MM Whatman paper by smoothing the paper over the gel. Seal the gel in Saran wrap and place in an autoradiography cassette.
8. Expose the gel to X-ray film for 1–12 h before developing (**Fig. 1**) (*see* **Notes 20** and **21**).

4. Notes

1. SDA primers and bumpers should be HPLC- or gel-purified. Use of less stringent means of purification may have a detrimental effect on RT-SDA performance. We have observed lot-to-lot variation in performance between primers purified in the same manner by the same company as well as differences in performance between manufacturers. Where possible, all reactions within a given set of experiments should be conducted with the same lot of primers. Functional testing of new primer lots should be conducted using existing primer mixtures for comparison.
2. We have had success using SDA primers with a T_m of 42–50°C. The specificity of SDA derives from the amplification and detector primers, rather than the bumpers. As a consequence, the T_m of the bumper primers is less critical but where possible it should be matched to the T_m of the SDA primers. The efficiency of SDA decreases as the distance between the SDA primers increases. An intervening region of 25–30 nucleotides is considered ideal. When designing SDA primers for a new target sequence, it is generally advisable to use the tail sequences from primers that are known to function well, modified as necessary in order to avoid primer interactions. It is particularly important to avoid interactions at the 3' ends of the SDA primers that may lead to exponential amplification of nonspecific products.
3. 500 m*M* K_iPO_4 should be prepared using fresh anhydrous stocks of KH_2PO_4 and K_2HPO_4. Prepare 500 m*M* solutions of each of the two salts using sterile distilled water. Transfer 87 mL K_2HPO_4 to a sterile flask and bring the pH to 7.6 by adding approx 13 mL KH_2PO_4. Store in the final solution in 1 mL vol at –20°C.
4. The RT-SDA protocol given here is extremely sensitive and is capable of detecting less than 10 purified in vitro transcripts of the *M. tuberculosis* α-antigen gene *(13)*. The ability to detect mRNA extracted from cultured organisms or clinical samples is largely dependent on the efficiency of the RNA extraction procedure

and the purity of the recovered nucleic acid. This is particularly a problem for mycobacteria that possess a tough, resilient cell wall that must be breached in order to release the enclosed nucleic acids. Many manufacturers provide kits for the isolation of mRNA from eukaryotic cells using oligo(dT) capture probes. These are not suitable for isolation of mRNA from prokayotes and alternative protocols using silica-based chromatographic resins are costly and often provide variable yields, particularly with clinical samples. The procedure described by DesJardin (***29*** and Chapter 14) permits efficient recovery of high quality RNA and DNA from clinical samples containing as few as 1000 cells of *M. tuberculosis*.

5. In our hands, the reverse transcription reaction is robust to changes in salt and cosolvent concentrations. However, these parameters together with magnesium ion and enzyme concentration may have a profound effect on the efficiency of SDA. For example, the optimum concentration of K_iPO_4 can vary between 25 and 55 m*M* and optimum DMSO concentration ranges from 3–12% v/v. Optimization of SDA conditions involves titration of all these components in a matrix that permits recognition of interactions between different parameters. The optimum temperature for SDA is typically between 50 and 54°C, although successful amplification can be achieved as high as 60°C ***(22,30)***. Manipulation of temperature can, therefore, play an important part in assay optimization.
6. Precautions must be taken in handling samples containing RNA owing to the ubiquitous presence of RNases. Wear gloves at all times and use dedicated pipettes with certified RNase-free tips, tubes and reagents. It is often helpful to provide a designated RNase-free area in the laboratory in which no target DNA is handled and no other work is conducted.
7. Care must be exercised in order to minimize the potential for contamination of reactions with amplicons from previous amplifications. Adopt a unidirectional workflow including separate areas and dedicated equipment for reagent preparation, target manipulation, amplification, and detection. Use barrier pipette tips and, where possible, aliquot reagents in single-use volumes. Discard tips and tubes that are contaminated with target nucleic acid or amplicons in sealed plastic bags and regularly decontaminate work areas with 10% v/v bleach.
8. The final reverse transcription reaction contains the following concentrations of reagents in a 20 µL vol: 30 m*M* K_iPO_4 pH 7.6, 12% v/v DMSO, 12.5% v/v glycerol, 1250 n*M* primer S2, 125 n*M* primer B2, 12.5 n*M* primer B3, 1.25 n*M* primer B4, 300 ng human placental DNA, 5 µg acetylated BSA, 0.8 m*M* dCTPαS, 0.2 m*M* dATP, 0.2 m*M* dGTP, 0.2 m*M* dUTP, 2 m*M* magnesium acetate, 30 U RNase inhibitor, and 2.5 U AMV reverse transcriptase.
9. Use of three bumper primers in the reverse transcriptase reaction is designed to take advantage of the strand displacement activity of AMV reverse transcriptase ***(31)*** and facilitate synthesis of multiple copies of cDNA from a single mRNA target molecule. Together with the inherent RNase H activity of AMV reverse transcriptase, this means that no denaturation step is necessary to dissociate the cDNA from the mRNA template. SDA can, therefore, be initiated directly

following the reverse transcription reaction and appropriate adjustment of buffer conditions.

10. The protocol outlined in this chapter can readily be modified to incorporate decontamination of the reverse transcription reaction with uracil DNA glycosylase (UDG) (Gibco-BRL), as a further precaution toward amplicon control. UDG hydrolyses uracil-glycosidic bonds in dU-containing single- and double-stranded DNA, releasing uracil and creating alkali-sensitive apyridiminic sites ***(32)***. UDG is included in the reverse transcriptase buffer at a concentration of 1 U/reaction and the volume of enzyme diluent is adjusted accordingly. Following addition of target RNA to the reverse transcriptase buffer, tubes are incubated at 45°C for 15 min to facilitate decontamination of the reaction mixtures. Subsequent cleavage by the UDG of newly synthesized cDNA molecules is prevented by the inclusion of 2–4 U UDG inhibitor (Gibco-BRL) in the reverse transcriptase enzyme mix.
11. We have found that the best tubes in which to perform SDA reactions are clear 0.5 mL Safe-Lock microcentrifuge tubes. These are easy to manipulate and the lids do not open when the tubes are boiled. Use of colored tubes for SDA should be avoided as the dye may have a deleterious effect on amplification efficiency ***(33)***.
12. The presence of contaminating α-antigen DNA in the RNA samples may give rise to false-positive results. For this reason, it is important to include appropriate controls comprising parallel reactions conducted without the addition of reverse transcriptase. In these reactions, the volume of diluent in the reverse transcriptase enzyme mix is increased to account for the absence of the enzyme and maintain the overall glycerol concentration in the reaction. DNA contamination is most likely to occur with clinical samples containing large numbers of bacteria ($\geq 10^6$) but can often be overcome by appropriate dilution of the RNA extracts ***(13)***.
13. As a control for the sensitivity of the RT-SDA, at least one positive control should be included in each run. This may comprise α-antigen mRNA recovered from a known number of cultured cells or, preferably, in vitro transcripts of the α-antigen gene. The latter have the advantage that they can be quantified spectophotometrically and accurately diluted to the desired level. In vitro transcripts can be prepared by cloning the target sequence into an *Escherichia coli* plasmid vector that possesses an RNA polymerase promoter, such as pBlueScript (Stratagene) or pGEM (Promega) ***(13)***.
14. Target RNA should be diluted in 10 ng/µL yeast carrier RNA to prevent loss through nonspecific binding to plastic tips and tubes.
15. The final SDA reaction contains the following concentrations of reagents in a 50 µL vol: 52.5 m*M* K_iPO_4 pH7.6, 12% v/v DMSO, 7.7% v/v glycerol, 500 n*M* primers S1 and S2, 50 n*M* primers B1 and B2, 5 n*M* primer B3, 0.5 n*M* primer B4, 500 ng human placental DNA, 5 µg acetylated BSA, 0.8 m*M* dCTPαS, 0.2 m*M* dATP, 0.2 m*M* dGTP, 0.2 m*M* dUTP, 7 m*M* magnesium acetate, 40 U *Bso*BI and 15 U exo$^-$ *Bst* polymerase. Some additional components, such as RNase inhibitor and reverse transcriptase enzyme, are carried over from the reverse transcription reaction but do not participate in the SDA.

16. The spin columns for removal of unincorporated radioactive label should be used according to the manufacturer's instructions since there is lot-to-lot variation in the centrifugation conditions necessary for efficient recovery of oligonucleotide DNA.
17. Primer extension reactions can be performed at 50–55°C using exo$^-$ *Bst* polymerase instead of exo$^-$ Klenow polymerase. Owing to the high T_m of the D1 probe (52°C) it is not necessary to modify of the detector primer to function at the higher temperature. Although not usually a problem with the α-antigen assay, use of the higher temperature for primer extension can reduce the appearance of nonspecific background products.
18. For the Gibco-BRL sequencing gel mixes, 0.6 mL 10% v/v ammonium persulfate is used per 100 mL gel. Gels can be prepared several days in advance as long as precautions are taken to prevent dehydration of the acrylamide around the comb.
19. An appropriate radiolabeled size marker should be included on the gel to facilitate orientation of the primer extension products. Alternatively, use a positive sample from a previous experiment as a positive control for the primer extension reaction and to orientate the gel.
20. A negative RT-SDA result can be due either to the absence of amplifiable RNA or to inhibition of the reverse transcription and/or SDA by contaminants in the target sample. A control mRNA sequence may therefore be included in the RT-SDA reaction that coamplifies with the α-antigen target but which can be discriminated on detection with ^{32}P-labeled probes or other means. For this purpose, we have used in vitro transcripts of the *M. tuberculosis* α-antigen gene that possess a 6 base mutation in the region intervening S1 and S2 and corresponding to the 3' end of the D1 detector probe. As a further development of this concept, Nycz et al. ***(34)*** have described a quantitative RT-SDA assay for HIV which is based upon competitive amplification of the target sequence and an internal control.
21. In addition to ^{32}P-based detection of the products of RT-SDA, we have developed both chemiluminescent and fluorescence-based detection formats. The chemiluminescent microtiter assay provides much higher throughput of samples than is possible with radioactive primer extension. This technique employs a biotinylated capture probe (5'-GCTTCACGGCCCT-(Biotin)$_3$) which hybridizes to the SDA amplicon in the intervening region between primers S1 and S2 ***(35)***. The amplicon-capture probe hybrid is in turn captured to the surface of a streptavidin-coated microtiter plate. Captured target is detected through hybridization of an alkaline phosphatase-conjugated detector probe (5'-CGCTGCCGGTGG-(AP)). After the wells are washed to remove unhybridized probes, a chemiluminescent substrate (Lumiphos 530, Lumigen) is added and light emitted from the breakdown of the substrate by the phosphatase enzyme is detected using a luminometer.

    The fluorescence polarization assay relies upon the difference in tumbling rates between a single-stranded oligonucleotide and its double-stranded counterpart ***(30,36–38)***. A fluorescein-labeled oligonucleotide (5'-FAM-CGCTGCCGGTGGGCTTCACG) is included in the SDA buffer at a concentration of 5 n*M*. Extension of the oligonucleotide and conversion to a double-stranded form during the course of amplification results in slower tumbling of the dye and a corresponding increase in fluorescence polarization value of the sample.

A further refinement of fluorescence detection has been the development of an energy transfer-based system. Included in the reaction mixture is an oligonucleotide that is labeled with donor and acceptor fluorophores, separated by a *Bso*BI restriction site. The 3' end of the detector probe hybridizes to the target sequence between SDA primers S1 and S2. In this state, the proximity of the acceptor and donor fluors quenches flourescence but extension and amplification of the detector probe results in formation of a double-stranded restriction site that is cleaved by the *Bso*BI enzyme. The resulting spatial separation of the two fluors leads to a target-specific increase in fluorescence intensity that can be monitored in "real-time" during the course of amplification. By conducting amplification and detection in an enclosed vessel, such real-time assays eliminate many of the problems associated with amplicon contamination. This format is the basis of the BDProbeTec® ET diagnostic SDA assays marketed by Becton Dickinson and Company ***(39)***.

Acknowledgments

This work was supported by a research agreement between Becton Dickinson and Company and the University of Arkansas.

References

1. Raviglione, M. C., Snider, D. E., and Kochi, A. (1995) Global epidemiology of tuberculosis: morbidity and mortality of a worldwide epidemic. *JAMA* **273**, 220–226.
2. Eisenach, K. D., Sifford, M. D., Cave, M. D., Bates, J. H., and Crawford, J. T. (1991) Detection of *Mycobacterium tuberculosis* in sputum samples using a polymerase chain reaction. *Am. Rev. Respir. Dis.* **144**, 1160–1163.
3. Iovannisci, D. M. and Winn-Deen, E. S. (1993) Ligation amplification and fluorescence detection of *Mycobacterium tuberculosis* DNA. *Mol. Cell. Probes* **7**, 35–43.
4. Jonas, V., Alden, M. J., Curry, J. I., Kamisango, K., Knott, C. A., Lankford, R., Wolfe, J. M., and Moore, D. F. (1993) Detection and identification of *Mycobacterium tuberculosis* directly from sputum sediments by amplification of rRNA. *J. Clin. Microbiol.* **31**, 2410–2416.
5. Shah, J. S., Liu, J., Buxton, D., Hendricks, A., Robinson, L., Radcliffe, G., King, W., Lane, D., Olive, D. M., and Klinger, J. D. (1995) Q-beta replicase-amplified assay for detection of *Mycobacterium tuberculosis* directly from clinical specimens. *J. Clin. Microbiol.* **33**, 1435–1441.
6. Van der Vliet, G. M. E., Schukkink, R. A. F., van Gemen, B., Schepers, P., and Klatser, P. R. (1993) Nucleic acid sequence-based amplification (NASBA) for the identification of mycobacteria. *J. Gen. Microbiol.* **139**, 2423–2429.
7. Walker, G. T., Little, M. C., Nadeau, J. G., and Shank, D. D. (1992) Isothermal *in vitro* amplification of DNA by a restriction enzyme/DNA polymerase system. *Proc. Natl. Acad. Sci USA* **89**, 392–396.

8. DesJardin, L. E., Chen, Y., Perkins, M. D., Teixeira, L., Cave, M. D., and Eisenach, K. D. (1998) Comparison of the ABI 7700 System (TaqMan) and competitive PCR for quantification of IS*6110* DNA in sputum during treatment of tuberculosis. *J. Clin. Microbiol.* **36**, 1964–1968.
9. DesJardin, L. E., Perkins, M. D., Wolski, K., Haun, S., Teixeira, L., Chen, Y., Johnson, J. L., Ellner, J. J., Dietze, R., Bates, J., Cave, M. D., and Eisenach, K. D. (1999) Measurement of sputum *Mycobacterium tuberculosis* mRNA as a surrogate for response to chemotherapy. *Am. J. Respir. Crit. Care Med.* **160**, 203–210.
10. Gamboa, F., Manterola, J. M., Vinado, B., Matas, L., Gimenez, M., Lonca, J., Manzano, J. R., Rodrigo, C., Cardona, P. J., Padilla, E., Dominguez, J., and Ausina, V. (1997) Direct detection of *Mycobacterium tuberculosis* complex in nonrespiratory specimens by Gen-Probe Amplified Mycobacterium tuberculosis Direct Test. *J. Clin. Microbiol.* **35**, 307–310.
11. Hellyer, T. J., Fletcher, T. W., Bates, J. H., Stead, W. W., Templeton, G. L., Cave, M. D., and Eisenach, K. D. (1996) Strand displacement amplification and the polymerase chain reaction for monitoring response to treatment in patients with pulmonary tuberculosis. *J. Infect. Dis.* **173**, 934–941.
12. Hellyer, T. J., DesJardin, L. E., Hehman, G. L., Cave, M. D., and Eisenach, K. D. (1999) Quantitative analysis of mRNA as a marker for viability of *Mycobacterium tuberculosis. J. Clin. Microbiol.* **37**, 290–295.
13. Hellyer, T. J., DesJardin, L. E., Teixeira, L., Perkins, M. D., Cave, M. D., and Eisenach, K. D. (1999) Detection of viable *Mycobacterium tuberculosis* by reverse transcriptase-Strand Displacement Amplification of mRNA. *J. Clin. Microbiol.* **37**, 518–523.
14. Moore, D. F., Curry, J. I., Knott, C. A., and Jonas, V. (1996) Amplification of rRNA for assessment of treatment response of pulmonary tuberculosis patients during antimicrobial therapy. *J. Clin. Microbiol.* **34**, 1745–1749.
15. Belasco, J. G., Nilsson, G., von Gabain, A., and Cohen, S. N. (1986) The stability of *E. coli* gene transcripts is dependent on determinants localized to specific mRNA segments. *Cell.* **46**, 245–251.
16. Von Gabain, A., Belasco, J. G., Schottel, J. L., Chang, A. C. Y., and Cohen, S. N. (1983) Decay of mRNA in *Escherichia coli*: investigation of the fate of specific segments of transcripts. *Proc. Natl. Acad. Sci. USA.* **80**, 653–657.
17. Harth, G., Lee, B.-Y., Wang, J., Clemens, D. L., and Horwitz, M. A. (1996) Novel insights into the genetics, biochemistry, and immunocytochemistry of the 30-kilodalton major extracellular protein of *Mycobacterium tuberculosis. Infect. Immun.* **64**, 3038–3047.
18. Lee, B.-Y. and Horwitz, M. A. (1995) Identification of macrophage and stress-induced proteins of *Mycobacterium tuberculosis. J. Clin. Invest.* **96**, 245–249.
19. Wiker, H. G. and Harboe, M. (1992) The antigen 85 complex: a major secretion product of *Mycobacterium tuberculosis. Microbiol. Rev.* **56**, 648–661.
20. Hellyer, T. J., DesJardin L. E., Assaf, M. K., Bates, J. H., Cave, M. D., and Eisenach, K. D. (1996) Specificity of IS*6110*-based amplification assays for *Mycobacterium tuberculosis* complex. *J. Clin. Microbiol.* **34**, 2843–2846.

21. Milla, M. A., Spears, P. A., Pearson, R. E., and Walker, G. T. (1998) Use of the restriction enzyme *Ava*I and exo⁻ *Bst* polymerase in strand displacement amplification. *Biotechniques* **24**, 392–396.
22. Spargo, C. A., Fraiser, M. S., Van Cleve, M., Wright, D. J., Nycz, C. M., Spears, P. A., and Walker, G. T. (1996) Detection of *M. tuberculosis* DNA using thermophilic strand displacement amplification. *Mol. Cellular Probes* **10**, 247–256.
23. Walker, G. T., Fraiser, M. S., Schram, J. L., Little, M. C., Nadeau, J. G., and Malinowski, D. P. (1992) Strand displacement amplification- an isothermal, *in vitro* DNA amplification technique. *Nucleic Acids Res.* **20**, 1691–1696.
24. Walker, G. T. (1993) Empirical aspects of strand displacement amplification. *PCR Methods and Applications* **3**, 1–6.
25. Ellner, J. J., Hinman, A. R., Dooley, S. W., Fischl, M. A., Sepkowitz, K. A., Goldberger, M. J., Shinnick, T. M., Iseman, M. D., and Jacobs, W. R. (1993) Tuberculosis symposium: emerging problems and promise. *J. Infect. Dis.* **168**, 537–551.
26. Shinnick, T. M. and Good, R. C. (1995) Diagnostic mycobacteriology laboratory practices. *Clin. Infect. Dis.* **21**, 291–299.
27. De Wit, L., Palou, M., and Content, J. (1994) Nucleotide sequence of the 85B-protein gene of *Mycobacterium bovis* BCG and *Mycobacterium tuberculosis*. *DNA Seq.* **4**, 267–270.
28. Sambrook, J., Fritsch, E. F, and Maniatis, T., eds. (1998) *Molecular Cloning: A Laboratory Manual*, 2nd ed. Appendix B p21. Cold Spring Harbor Laboratory, Cold Spring Harbor, NY.
29. DesJardin L. E., Perkins, M. D., Teixiera, L., Cave, M. D., and Eisenach, K. D. (1996) Alkaline decontamination of sputum specimens adversely affects stability of mycobacterial mRNA. *J. Clin. Microbiol.* **34**, 2435–2439.
30. Walker, G. T. and Linn, C. P. (1996) Detection of *Mycobacterium tuberculosis* DNA with thermophilic strand displacement amplification and fluorescence polarization. *Clin. Chem.* **42**, 1604–1608.
31. Collett, M. S., Leis, J. P., Smith, M. S., and Faras, A. J. (1978) Unwinding-like activity associated with avian retrovirus RNA-directed DNA polymerase. *J. Virol.* **26**, 498–509.
32. Longo, M. C., Berninger M. S., and Hartley, J. L. (1990) Use of uracil DNA glycosylase to control carry-over contamination in polymerase chain reactions. *Gene* **93**, 125–128.
33. Keating, W., Donahue, C., Nycz, C., Schram, J., Weng, J., Haaland, P., Jurgensen, S., Nadeau, J., and Little, M. (1993) Enhanced performance of a sensitive, rapid method for the detection of *Mycobacterium tuberculosis* using strand displacement DNA amplification (SDA). 93rd Annual General Meeting of the American Society for Microbiology, Abstract U40.
34. Nycz, C. M., Dean, C. H., Haaland, P. D., Spargo, C. A., and Walker, G. T. (1998) Quantitative reverse transcription strand displacement amplification: quantification of nucleic acids using an isothermal amplification technique. *Anal. Biochem.* **259**, 226–234.

35. Spargo, C. A., Haaland, P. D., Jurgensen, S. R., Shank, D. D., and Walker, G. T. (1993) Chemiluminescent detection of strand displacement amplified DNA from species comprising the *Mycobacterium tuberculosis* complex. *Mol. Cellular Probes* **7**, 395–404.
36. Spears, P. A., Linn, C. P., Woodard, D. L., and Walker, G. T. (1997) Simultaneous strand displacement amplification and fluorescence polarization detection of *Chlamydia trachomatis* DNA. *Anal. Biochem.* **247**, 130–137.
37. Walker, G. T., Linn, C. P., and Nadeau, J. G. (1996) DNA detection by strand displacement amplification and fluorescence polarization with signal enhancement using a DNA binding protein. *Nucleic Acids Res.* **24**, 348–353.
38. Walker, G. T., Nadeau, J. G., Linn, C. P., Devlin R. F., and Dandliker, W. B. (1996) Strand displacement amplification (SDA) and transient-state fluorescence polarization detection of *Mycobacterium tuberculosis* DNA. *Clin. Chem.* **42**, 9–13.
39. Little, M. C., Andrews, J., Moore, R., Bustos, S., Jones, L., Embres, C., Durmowicz, G., Harris, J., Berger, D., Yanson, K., Rostkowski, C., Yursis, D., Price, J., Fort, T., Walters, A., Collis, M., Llorin, O., Wood, J., Failing, F., O'Keefe, C., Scrivens, B., Pope, B., Hansen, T., Marino, K., Williams, K., and Boenisch, M. (1999) Strand displacement amplification and homogeneous real-time detection incorporated in a second-generation DNA probe system, BDProbeTecET. *Clin. Chem.* **45**, 777–784.

III

Molecular Epidemiology

16

BOX PCR Fingerprinting for Molecular Typing of *Streptococcus pneumoniae*

Alex van Belkum and Peter W. M. Hermans

1. Introduction

A highly conserved repeated DNA element has been identified in the chromosome of *Streptococcus pneumoniae* (pneumococcus) and given the name of the BOX repetitive element *(1)*. This was the first demonstration of the presence of such a repetitive DNA moiety in a Gram positive bacterial species. Approximately 25 of these elements are found in noncoding regions dispersed throughout the entire pneumococcal genome. The BOX repeat is found to consist of three discriminate regions: *box*A, *box*B, and *box*C, which are 59, 45, and 50 basepairs in length, respectively. Various different combinations of these three elements are found to be present in different BOX loci and limited sequence heterogeneity is encountered among different elements from the same strain or elements sequenced from different strains. The first publication on the BOX repetitive elements also described its intricate secondary structure, supported by compensating basepairing in different loci where the repeat is encountered (*see* **Fig. 1**). Moreover, their location in the vicinity of genes involved in the regulation of various aspects of bacterial competence, genetic transformation and virulence suggest that the elements might well be involved in coordination of the control of gene expression. More recently, Saluja and Weiser *(2)* demonstrated that the presence of a BOX element is associated with variation in colony opacity of the pneumococcus. The frequency with which the colonies switched from transparent to opaque clearly depended on the presence of *box*A and *box*C elements. It has also been shown that BOX elements form targets for site-specific recombination events *(3)*, which provides another possibility for involvement in regulation of gene expression and genome evolution.

From: *Methods in Molecular Medicine, vol. 48: Antibiotic Resistance Methods and Protocols*
Edited by: S. H. Gillespie

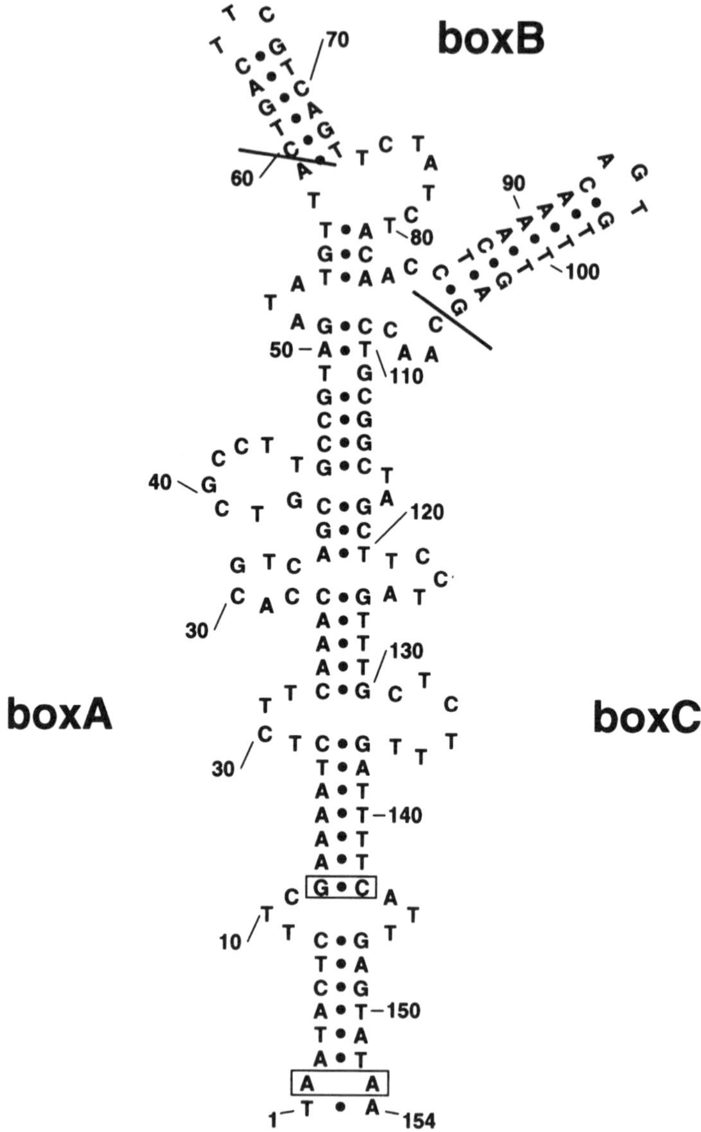

Fig. 1. Predicted secondary structure of the consensus BOX sequence containing one copy of boxB. The figure is adapted from reference *(1)*. Boxed basepairs indicate interactions that have been supported by phylogenetic comparisons, the basepairs themselves are highlighted by dots. The border between boxA and boxB is at nucleotide position 60, whereas boxB borders boxC at nucleotide 104. The PCR primer locations and the corresponding primer codes can be found in **Table 1**.

Table 1
Survey of the DNA Sequence for the Different Primers Used in Various Studies on BOX PCR for Typing of *Streptococcus pneumoniae*

Primer Code	Sequence 5' → 3'	Position in **Fig. 1**	Literature reference
boxA1	CGTCAGCGTCGCCTTGCCGTAG	30-51	*(5)*
boxA1R	CTACGGCAAGGCGACGCTGACG	51-30	*(5,8,9)*
boxA2R	ACGTGGTTTGAAGAGATTTTCG	32-11	*(5)*
boxA	ATACTCTTCGAAAATCTCTTCAAAC	3-27	*(6,10)*
boxB1	TTCGTCAGTTCTATCTACAACC	65-86	*(5)*
boxB2	AACCTCAAAACAGTGTTTTGAG	83-104	*(5)*
boxC1	TGCGGCTAGCTTCCTAGTTTGC	110-131	*(5)*
boxC1R	AGCAAACTAGGAAGCTAGCCGC	132-111	*(5)*
boxC2	TTGCTCTTTGATTTTCATTGAG	128-149	*(5)*

Note: The primers boxA1R and boxA have been employed most successfully for molecular typing of pneumococci. Although both primers derive from the boxA region there is no overlap in primary structure. Primers boxA1 and boxA1R are each others precise complement, as are primers boxC and boxC1R. *See* **Fig. 1** for a precise localisation of some of the primers in the entire BOX element.

It has been recognized that multicopy BOX elements might provide targets that might be useful for molecular discrimination among pneumococcal strains. Initially, a hybridization assay was developed that employed either the *box*B element alone or a full copy of a 154 basepairs long BOX element as a molecular probe *(4)*. Through a Southern hybridization protocol, DNA fingerprints could indeed be generated. A striking degree of polymorphism was encountered among nonrelated isolates of *S. pneumoniae*, whereas multiple isolates obtained from the blood and the cerebrospinal fluid of the same patients were identical. The data thus produced were amenable to straightforward computer analysis and interpretation. Moreover, some of the BOX probes used did not cross-hybridize to genomic DNA from a large variety of other bacterial species, thereby establishing a species-specific typing test. The species specificity for the *box*B and *box*C sequences has been confirmed by another study, which showed in addition that *box*A sequences did cross-hybridize to genomic digests from other bacterial species *(5)*. The same authors during the same study demonstrated the feasibility of polymerase chain reaction (PCR) mediated amplification using BOX motif primers for molecular typing of *S. pneumoniae*. It has been shown that *box*A sequences are appropriate typing targets not only for the pneumococcus but also for other bacterial species. Similar conclusions are drawn from an independent, contemporary study, where, again, the *box*A sequence motif appeared to provide an adequate means of detecting genetic polymorphism among various pneumococcal strains *(6)*. Interestingly, by using other types of thermostable polymerases during the PCR process the specificity of the reaction could be, modified for typing staphylococci and other bacterial species as well *(6)*.

The value of the BOX PCRs for clinical epidemiological studies has been demonstrated on various occasions *(7)*. The evaluation of pharyngeal colonization of individuals infected by the human immunodeficiency virus HIV revealed that HIV-positive individuals are significantly more frequently colonized by a single BOX PCR-type *S. pneumoniae* strain for prolonged periods of time than are non-HIV-infected subjects *(8)*. Furthermore, nonserotypable pneumococci isolated in cases of epidemic conjunctivitis are demonstrated to belong to a separate lineage on the basis of BOX PCR fingerprints *(9)*. Apparently, a single clone of *S. pneumoniae* was responsible for a nationwide outbreak of conjunctivitis in the USA. BOX PCR has shown, in longitudinal studies of pneumococcal colonization of children during the first two years of life, that different colonization events could be identified and that horizontal transfer of capsular genes takes place between strains colonizing the same individual *(10)*.

The PCR methodology described in experimental detail in this chapter can be applied in routine microbiology laboratories, provided that some basic molecular biology equipment and a PCR machine are available. No special precautions or isolation procedures are required and the experimental data can be recorded readily as pictures in a straightforward manner.

2. Materials

2.1. Bacterial Strains and Cultivation

1. Todd Hewitt broth supplemented with 0.5% yeast extract (store at 4°C).
2. 1 *M* NaCl, 15% glycerol.
3. Blood agar plates.
4. Optochin susceptibility disks.
5. Sodium deoxycholate.

2.2. DNA Isolation Protocols

1. 10X TE buffer: 0.1 *M* Tris-HCl, pH 8.0, 10 m*M* EDTA.
2. Lysozyme, 10 mg/mL (store at –20°C).
3. 10% sodium dodecyl sulphate (SDS).
4. Proteinase K, 10 mg/mL in TE (Merck, Darmstadt, Germany; store at –20°C).
5. N-cetyl-N,N,N-trimethyl ammonium bromide (CTAB).
6. Chloroform isoamylalcohol (24:1).
7. Isopropanol.
8. 70% ethanol.

2.3. BOX PCR

1. 10X PCR buffer: 100 m*M* Tris-HCl, pH 9.0, 500 m*M* KCl, 25 m*M* $MgCl_2$, 0.1% gelatin, 1% Triton X-100.

2. 1 m*M* deoxyribonucleotide triphosphate mixture (0.2 m*M* final concentration) (store at –20°C).
3. *Taq* DNA polymerase at 1 U/µL (Supertaq, Sphaero Q, Leiden, The Netherlands; store at –20°C).
4. PCR machine (e.g., Biomed model 60, Theres, Germany).

2.4. Electrophoretic Analysis

1. Agarose.
2. Tris-acetate-EDTA buffer ***(11)***.
3. Molecular size markers (100 bp; Gibco-BRL LifeSciences, Breda, The Netherlands).
4. Ethidium bromide (toxic, carcinogenic; handle with care).
5. Loading buffer: 50% glycerol in water containing 1 mg/mL bromophenol blue.

2.5. Data Processing

1. Charge coupled device camera, Fujinon zoom lens (Correct, Rotterdam, The Netherlands).
2. Visionary Photo Analyst system (Progress Control, Waalwijk, The Netherlands).
3. GelCompar 3.0 (Applied Maths, Kortrijk, Belgium).

3. Methods

3.1. Bacterial Cultivation

1. Bacterial strains in a collection are stored at –80°C in solutions consisting of 1 *M* NaCl, 15% glycerol. Scrapes of these stocks are plated onto blood agar plates to check for purity and in order to obtain single colonies.
2. Pneumococci are identified by their colonial morphology on blood agar plates, gram staining, and optochin susceptibility (*see* **Notes 1** and **2**).
3. For DNA preparation, a single colony of the blood agar plate is transferred into 25 mL of fresh Todd Hewitt broth supplemented with 0.5% yeast extract. Tubes are incubated overnight in a rotary shaker at 37°C.

3.2. DNA Isolation

Chromosomal DNA is isolated using the technique described by Van Soolingen et al. ***(12)*** (*see* **Note 3**).

1. Ten mL of an overnight culture of *S. pneumoniae* is centrifuged at 2000*g* for 10 min.
2. Suspend the pellet in 500 µL TE buffer and heat for 20 min at 80°C in order to kill the cells.
3. Centrifuge the mixture again and resuspend the pellet in 500 mL fresh TE buffer.
4. Add lysozyme to a final concentration of 1 mg/mL and incubate the tube for 1 h at 37°C.
5. After incubation, add 70 µL of 10% SDS and 6 µL of proteinase K (10 mg/mL) and incubate the mixture for a further 10 min at 65°C.
6. Subsequently, add 80 µL of N-cetyl-N,N,N,-trimethyl ammonium bromide (CTAB).
7. After brief vortexing, incubate the mixture for 10 min at 65°C and add an equal vol of chloroform-isoamylalcohol.
8. After 10 s of vortexing the mixture, centrifuge for 5 min and collect the supernatant.

9. In order to precipitate the DNA, add 0.6 vol of isopropanol to the supernatant and place the tube at –20°C for 30 min.
10. After centrifugation at full speed in a microcentrifuge for 15 min, wash the pellet with 500 mL of 70% ethanol.
11. Dry the pellet in air and redissolve in 0.1X TE buffer.
12. Assess the concentration of the DNA solution by spectroscopy at 260 nm and dilute to a working stock of 100 ng/µL.

3.3. BOX PCR

1. Dispense aliquots of 50 ng of the pneumococcal DNA into microcentrifuge tubes.
2. Prepare a mastermix of the PCR reaction ingredients sufficient for the number of samples to be amplified. The final concentrations are 1X PCR buffer, 0.2 m*M* of the respective desoxynucleotide triphosphates and 0.15 U *Taq* polymerase (*see* **Note 4**) with a final volume of 50 µL (*see* **Note 5**).
3. Place the tubes in a PCR machine using the following thermocycling program: 4 min predenaturation at 94°C, 40 times (1 min 94°C + 2 min 50 or 60°C + 2 min 74°C) and a final extension step of 5 min 74°C (*see* **Note 6**).
4. Store the samples after PCR for the remainder of the overnight period at 15°C.

3.4. Electrophoretic Analysis

1. Prepare a 20 × 20 cm 1.5% agarose gel buffered in 0.5X TBE.
2. Mix approx 10 microliter of a PCR amplimer with 2 microliters of the electrophoresis sample buffer containing bromophenol blue.
3. Electrophorese the products for approx 3 h at a constant current of 100 mA.
4. Stain the gels in 0.5X TBE containing 0.5 µg ethidium bromide per liter.
5. Photograph the gels using UV transillumination.

3.5. Data Processing

The photographic image must be stored and transferred to an analytical program. This can be achieved by retaining copies of photographic images or *in silico* as a series of TIFF files. The latter files can be downloaded immediately into the analytic program GelCompar 3.0, pictures can be transferred in similar files again by scanning procedures (Hewlett Packard ScanJet, HP, Amsterdam, The Netherlands). Using GelCompar 3.0, genetic trees can be constructed after the gel pictures are normalized on the basis of the presence of the molecular size markers and visual inspection. In detail comparison of the different gel lanes is usually performed by the unweighted pair group method with arithmetic averages (UPGMA) clustering method, with the Jaccard coefficient being applied to peaks. A band tolerance setting of 1.2% is generally allowed when comparing band positions (*see* **Note 7**).

4. Notes

1. Other culture media have been described including Luria Bertani (LB) broth ***(5)*** and tryptic soy agar (TSA) medium with 5% sheep blood ***(8,9)***.

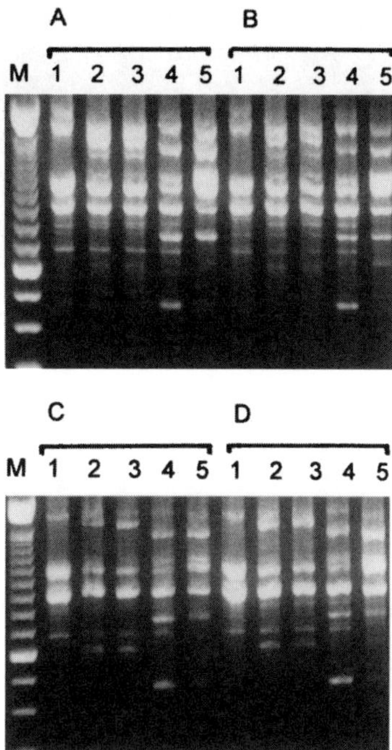

Fig. 2. BOX PCR fingerprinting using different brands of *Taq* polymerase and thermocyclers. The upper panel displays results obtained with a BioMed waterbath-based PCR machine, the lower panel displays the results obtained for the same samples in a Techne PCR machine containing a Peltier element. Each panel displays the results obtained for two times a set of five strains. Fingerprints collected under A and C are generated using Sphaero Q Tth Supertaq, those displayed under B and D are the result of amplification with Eurogentec Goldstar *Taq* polymerase. Note the increased detail in the upper panel, which also indicates that when the Biomed machine is used, yields of amplicons improve.

2. In case of discrepant results bile solubility (sodium deoxycholate testing) and, ultimately, identification of ribosomal DNA sequences on the basis of GenProbe hybridization assays can be performed.
3. Alternative DNA isolation procedures have been used *(5)*. Of importance is the fact that introduction of whole cells in the PCR mixture is a feasible option. When cells are washed in 1 *M* NaCl and suspended in distilled water at a density of 10^7–10^8, 2 µL of this suspension introduced in the PCR mixture gives rise to reproducible BOX PCR fingerprints *(8,9)*.
4. When the PCR conditions are compared, several differences are apparent. The brand of polymerase use varies from Perkin Elmer's Ampli*taq* ***(5)***, Gold Star *Taq* ***(6)***, and Supertaq ***(6,10)***. **Figure 2** illustrates that variation of PCR machines or *Taq* polymerase employed may result in differences in the banding patterns generated.

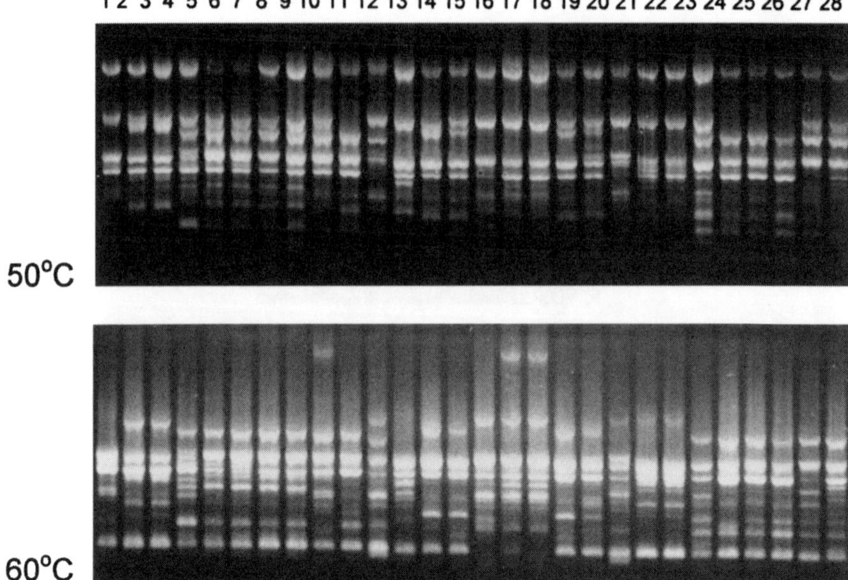

Fig. 3. Effect of the annealing temperature on pneumococcal DNA fingerprints obtained through BOX PCR. The top and bottom panels display results generated with exactly identical PCR mixtures, performed for 28 strains, but amplified using two different annealing temperatures (indicated on the left). Both pictures show the same location of the gel run after the amplification. Grossly, at higher annealing temperature the size of the PCR products decreases.

5. Sometimes 10% DMSO is added during PCR *(5,8,9)* and the dNTP concentration ranges between 0.6 to 1.5 m*M*.
6. The PCR programs share a relatively high annealing temperature (always exceeding 50°C), but differ in the number of cycles (30 in *[5]*, 40 in *[6]* for instance) and the duration of the chain extension period (8 min in *[5]*, 2 min in *[6]*). **Figure 3** demonstrates that alteration of the annealing temperature may lead to significant differences in the fingerprints produced.
7. Gel systems are quite homologous, but the software packages used for data processing may again differ widely. Available are packages from Applied Biostatistics (Simple Matching Similarity SIMQUAL, NTSYSRC 1.7 *(5)*), Applied Maths (GelCompar *(6)*) and Scanalytics (TREECON RFLP scan software package *(8)*). Inter laboratory reproducibility of PCR mediated molecular typing has not always been successful *(13,14)*. So when BOX PCR is used for multi-center application, strict adherence to a single, well-defined experimental protocol is absolutely mandatory.

References

1. Martin, B., Humbert, O., Camara, M., Guenzi, E., Walker, J., Mitchell, T., Andrew, P., Prudhomme, M., Alloing, G., Hakenbeck, R., Morrison, D. A., Boulnois, G. J., and Claverys, J. P. (1992) A highly conserved repeated DNA element located in the chromosome of *Streptococcus pneumoniae*. *Nucleic Acids Res.* **20,** 3479–3483.
2. Saluja, S. K. and Weiser, J. N. (1995) The genetic basis of colony opacity in *Streptococcus pneumoniae*: evidence for the effect of BOX elements on the frequency of phenotypic variation. *Mol. Microbiol.* **16,** 215–227.
3. Krauss, J. and Hakenbeck, R. (1997) A mutation in the D,D-carboxypeptidase penicillin-binding protein-3 of *Streptococcus pneumoniae* contributes to cefotaxime resistance of the laboratory mutant C604. *Antimicrob. Agents Chemother.* **41,** 936–942.
4. Hermans, P. W. M., Sluijter, M., Hoogenboezem, T., Heersma, H., Van Belkum, A., and De Groot, R. (1995) Comparative study of five different DNA fingerprint techniques for molecular typing of *Streptococcus pneumoniae* strains. *J. Clin. Microbiol.* **33,** 1606–1612.
5. Koeuth, T., Versalovic, J., and Lupski, J. R. (1995) Differential subsequence conservation of interspersed repetitive *Streptococcus pneumoniae* BOX elements in diverse bacteria. *PCR Meth. Appl.* **5,** 408–418.
6. Van Belkum, A., Sluijter, M., De Groot, R., Verbrugh, H., and Hermans, P. W. M. (1996) Novel BOX repeat PCR assay for high-resolution typing of *Streptococcus pneumoniae* strains. *J Clin. Microbiol.* **34,** 1176–1179.
7. Alippi, A. M. and Aguilar, O. M. (1998) Characterisation of isolates of *Paenibacillus larvae* subgr. *larvae* from diverse geographical origin by the polymerase chain reaction and BOX primers. *J. Invertebr. Pathol.* **72,** 21–27.
8. Rodrigues-Barradas, M. C., Tharapel, R. A., Groover, J. E., Giron, K. P., Lacke, C. E., Houston, E. D., Hamill, R. J., Steinhoff, M. C., and Musher, D. M. (1997) Colonisation by *Streptococcus pneumoniae* among human immuno-deficiency virus-infected adults: prevalence of antibiotic resistance, impact of immunisation, and characterisation by polymerase chain reaction with BOX primers of isolates from persistent *S. pneumoniae* carriers. *J. Infect. Dis.* **175,** 590–597.
9. Ertugrul, N., Rodrigues-Barradas, M. C., Musher, D. M., Ryan, M. A. K., Agin, C. S., Murphy, S. J., Shayegani, M., and Watson, D. D. (1997) BOX-polymerase chain reaction-based DNA analysis of non-serotypable *Streptococcus pneumoniae* implicated in outbreaks of conjunctivitis. *J. Infect. Dis.* **176,** 1401–1405.
10. Sluijter, M., Faden, H., De Groot, R., Lemmens, N., Goessens, W. H. F., Van Belkum, A., Hermans, P. W. M. (1998) Molecular characterisation of pneumococcal nasopharynx isolates collected from children during their first two years of life. *J. Clin. Microbiol.* **36,** 2248–2253.
11. Maniatis, T., Fritsch, E. F., and Sambrook, J. (1982) Molecular cloning: a laboratory manual. Cold Spring Harbor Laboratory, Cold Spring Harbor, NY.
12. Van Soolingen, D., Hermans, P. W. M., De Haas, P. E. W., Soll, D. R., and Van Embden, J. D. A. (1991) Occurrence and stability of insertion sequences in *Myco-*

bacterium tuberculosis complex strains: evaluation of an insertion sequence dependent DNA polymorphism as a tool in the epidemiology of tuberculosis. *J. Clin. Microbiol.* **29,** 2578–2586.

13. Van Belkum, A., Kluytmans, J., Van Leeuwen, W., Bax, R., Quint, W., Peters, E., Fluit, A., Vandenbroucke-Grauls, C., Van den Brule, A., Koeleman, H., Melchers, W., Meis, J., Elaichouni, A., Vaneechoutte, M., Moonens, F., Maes, N., Struelens, M., Tenover, F., and Verbrugh, H. A. (1995) Multicenter evaluation of arbitrarily primed PCR for typing of *Staphylococcus aureus* strains. *J. Clin. Microbiol.* **33,** 1537–1547.
14. Grundman, H. J., Towner, K. J., Dijkshoorn, L., Gerner-Smidt, P., Maher, M., Seifert, H and Vaneechoutte, M. (1997) Multicenter study using standardized protocols and reagents for evaluation of reproducibility of PCR-based fingerprinting of *Acinetobacter* spp. *J. Clin. Microbiol.* **35,** 3071–3077.

17

Restriction Fragment End Labeling Analysis: High-Resolution Genomic Typing of *Streptococcus pneumoniae* Isolates

Peter W. M. Hermans, Marcel Sluijter, and Alex van Belkum

1. Introduction

Streptococcus pneumoniae (pneumococcus) is one of the leading bacterial pathogens causing illness and death among young children, the elderly, and persons with certain underlying medical conditions *(1)*. Pneumococci are often part of the normal nasopharyngeal flora, especially in young children. Pneumococcal colonization is an important risk factor: children colonized with *S. pneumoniae* more often develop acute otitis media than children who are not colonized *(2–5)*.

The prevalence of penicillin resistance among pneumococci is increasing worldwide *(6–13)*. International spread of a restricted number of multiresistant pneumococcal clones has significantly contributed to this increase. Soares and coworkers have documented the spread of a multiresistant clone of serotype 6B from Spain to Iceland in the late 1980s *(14)*. This has resulted in an epidemic of this clone, which was isolated with a frequency up to 12% in 1992 *(8)*. In 1991, Muñoz and colleagues have also reported evidence for the intercontinental spread of a multiresistant clone of *S. pneumoniae* serotype 23F from Spain to the United States *(15)*. This clone has subsequently disseminated through the United States *(16)*. Gasc and colleagues have reported in 1995 the spread of a multiresistant pneumococcal clone of serotype 9V from Spain to France *(17)*. The international clones 23F and 9V have been identified in many countries all over the world *(18,19)*. Besides the international spread of the clones 6B, 23F, and 9V, novel penicillin-resistant and sometimes even multiresistant clones have been reported in former Czechoslovakia, Spain, Japan,

From: *Methods in Molecular Medicine, vol. 48: Antibiotic Resistance Methods and Protocols*
Edited by: S. H. Gillespie © Humana Press Inc., Totowa, NJ

and South Africa. These clones tend to spread easily within these countries ***(18,20–22)***.

The high incidence of pneumococcal infections and the increasing emergence of drug-resistant isolates are the major drive for epidemiological surveillance. Phenotypical and genotypical methods have been developed to assist in epidemiological investigations. These methods include serotyping ***(23–26)***, multilocus enzyme electrophoresis ***(27)***, penicillin binding protein typing ***(14–16,27)*** and pneumococcal surface protein A (pspA) typing ***(27)***, and various DNA fingerprint methods such as ribotyping ***(16,28,29)***, DNA fingerprinting of the PBP genes ***(15,28,30,31)***, and pulsed-field gel electrophoresis ***(14,32)***. Detection and reduction of transmission of drug-resistant pneumococci that are currently spreading all over the world is an important goal in the battle against pneumococcal disease. Obviously, restricted use of antibiotics remains the major defense against the epidemic dissemination of such strains. In addition, the emergence of multidrug resistant pneumococci emphasizes the need for conjugate vaccine design to efficiently protect patients at risk for pneumococcal disease such as the elderly and young children. Detailed studies on the epidemiology and epidemic behavior of resistant pneumococci will assist to identify emerging clones. To this end, close collaboration between the laboratories sharing interests in pneumococcal molecular epidemiology is of utmost importance. Extensive collaboration can be facilitated by the establishment of a freely accessible electronic network. Such a network can be used to exchange information on technical aspects of DNA fingerprinting, aiming to standardize the methodological procedures. In addition, the network can be used to construct and distribute an international data library containing DNA fingerprints of (multi)resistant pneumococcal strains. Such an approach will facilitate adequate worldwide monitoring of the epidemiology of emerging (multi)resistant pneumococcal strains.

In order to provide meaningful epidemiological information, DNA fingerprints must be different for epidemiologically unrelated strains. However, an identical pattern should be obtained for strains from a common source. For epidemiological investigations, DNA markers are needed that reflect an adequate rate of genetic rearrangements over time. Only those markers that are appropriate for answering a given epidemiological question should be used. In 1995, we have investigated the usefulness of various DNA fingerprint methods to study the molecular epidemiology of infections by *S. pneumoniae* ***(33)***. Invasive clinical isolates of *S. pneumoniae* were analyzed by:

1. Ribotyping;
2. BOX fingerprinting using the BOX repetitive DNA element ***(34)*** as a DNA probe;
3. Polymerase chain reaction (PCR) fingerprinting using a primers homologous to the enterobacterial repetitive intergenic consensus (ERIC) sequence ***(35)*** or the

pneumococcal BOX repetitive DNA element *(36)* (*see* **Chapter 16**);
4. Pulsed-field gel electrophoresis of large-size DNA restriction fragments (*see* **Chapter 18**; and
5. Restriction fragment end labeling (RFEL) analysis, which detects restriction fragment length polymorphism (RFLP) of small-size DNA fragments *(37)*.

Genetic clustering among the pneumococcal strains was independent of the DNA fingerprint technique used. However, the discriminatory power and the similarity values differed significantly between the individual techniques. BOX (PCR) fingerprinting, pulsed-field gel electrophoresis, and RFEL analysis provided the highest degree of discriminatory power. Furthermore, the ease to perform computerized fingerprint comparison also differed significantly. Ribotyping, BOX fingerprinting and restriction fragment end labeling were very suitable techniques for accurate computerized data analysis. Due to the high discriminatory potentials, and the ease of accurate analysis, we have concluded that BOX fingerprinting and restriction fragment end labeling are the most suitable techniques to type pneumococcal strains *(33,36)*.

This chapter aims to discuss the methodological details of RFEL analysis for genomic typing of *S. pneumoniae* isolates.

2. Materials

Bacterial cultivation is performed using sterile materials. DNA processing (isolation, restriction, labeling) requires DNase-free materials and conditions (for details, *see* **ref. *38***). Buffers, solutions and reagents are kept at room temperature unless otherwise stated.

2.1. Cultivation of S. pneumoniae Isolates

1. Columbia agar plates supplemented with 5% sheep blood; stored at 4°C.
2. Todd Hewitt broth supplemented with 0.5% yeast extract; THY broth can be stored for 1 month at 4°C.

2.2. Bacterial DNA Isolation

1. 1.5 mL safe-lock microcentrifuge tubes.
2. Phosphate-buffered saline (PBS).
3. 1X TE buffer: 0.01 *M* Tris-HCl, 1 m*M* EDTA (Merck), pH 8.0.
4. 10% sodium dodecyl sulphate (SDS).
5. 10 mg/mL proteinase K (Merck); store at –20°C.
6. 5 *M* NaCl (Merck).
7. 0.7 *M* NaCl containing 10% N-cetyl-N,N,N-trimethyl ammonium bromide (CTAB).
8. Chloroform/isoamylalcohol (24:1; chloroform: isoamylalcohol: Merck).
9. Isopropanol, store at –20°C.
10. 70% ethanol store at –20°C.

11. 10 mg/mL RNase A store at –20°C.
12. UV-spectrophotometer (e.g., Ultrospec III; Pharmacia, Roosendaal, The Netherlands).

2.3. DNA Restriction and Labeling

1. 1.5 mL safe-lock microcentrifuge tubes.
2. *Eco*R1 (Life technologies, Breda, The Netherlands); store at –20°C.
3. 10X buffer H (Life Technologies).
4. *Taq* DNA polymerase (Goldstar; Eurogentec, Seraing, Belgium); store at –20°C.
5. [α-^{32}P]-dATP (Amersham, Roosendaal, The Netherlands); store at –20°C.
6. 5.5 *M* ammonium acetate, pH 7.0.
7. 20 mg/mL glycogen, store at –20°C.
8. 100% ethanol, store at –20°C.
9. 70% ethanol, store at –20°C.
10. Stop solution: 98% deionized formamide in 10 m*M* EDTA containing 0.025% bromophenol blue and 0.025% xylene cyanol FF, store at –20 °C.
11. Geiger counter.

2.4. DNA Electrophoresis

1. 1X TBE buffer: 0.09 *M* Tris -borate, 1 m*M* EDTA.
2. 40% acrylamide/*bis*-acrylamide (19:1) store at 4°C.
3. 10% ammonium persulphate (APS), prepared fresh.
4. N,N,N,N-tetramethyl-ethylene diamine (TEMED).
5. Polyacrylamide gel electrophoresis equipment (Biorad, Veenendaal, The Netherlands).
6. Whatman No. 3 filter paper.
7. Vacuum dryer (e.g., HBI, Saddlebrook, NJ).
8. ECL Hyperfilm (Amersham, Roosendaal, The Netherlands).
9. Saran wrap.

2.5. Computerized Analysis of the RFEL Fingerprints

1. Imagemaster desktop scanner (Pharmacia).
2. Gelcompar 4.0 software (Applied Maths, Kortrijk, Belgium).

3. Methods

3.1. Cultivation of S. pneumoniae Isolates

1. Grow bacteria from a –80°C stock on Columbia agar plates supplemented with 5% sheep blood (overnight; 37°C; 5–10% CO_2) (*see* **Note 1**).
2. Transfer a single colony from the overnight culture to a fresh Columbia agar plate supplemented with 5% sheep blood and regrow (overnight; 37°C; 5–10% CO_2).
3. Inoculate 3-4 mL of THY broth with bacteria (a “loop-full”) from the second blood agar plate. Incubate the culture without shaking until OD_{560} = 0.3 (about 5–6 h at 37°C).

3.2. Bacterial DNA Isolation

1. Centrifuge the bacterial culture for 10 min at 3000*g*.
2. Resuspend the bacterial pellet in 1 mL of PBS and transfer to a safe-lock microcentrifuge tube. Centrifuge the bacterial suspension for 3 min at 17,000*g*.
3. Resuspend the bacterial pellet in 400 µL of 1X TE buffer, and 70 µL of 10% SDS and add 5 µL of 10 mg/mL proteinase K. Gently mix the suspension and incubate for 10 min at 65°C.
4. Add 100 µL of 5 *M* NaCl and 100 µL of 0.7 *M* NaCl containing 10% CTAB (preheated at 65°C) separately to the suspension. Mix the suspension vigorously until it turns white, and incubate for 10 min at 65°C.
5. Extract chromosomal DNA using 500 µL of chloroform/isoamyl alcohol (24:1). Mix the suspension vigorously for 10 s and centrifuge for 5 min at 17,000*g*.
6. Transfer the aqueous supernatant containing the DNA to a fresh tube, and add 400 µL of isopropanol (–20°C). Mix the solution well and precipitate the DNA for 30 min at –20°C.
7. Recover the DNA precipitate by centrifugation for 10 min at 17,000*g*, and wash the DNA pellet gently with 500 µL 70% ethanol (–20°C). Recentrifuge the pellet for 5 min at 17,000*g*). Remove the supernatant completely (pipeting, spinning, pipeting). Keep the tube open for 10 min at room temperature to permit the pellet to dry.
8. Dissolve the DNA pellet in 50 µL of 1X TE buffer containing 200 µg/mL RNase A. Subsequently, incubate the tube for 30 min at 37°C in order to facilitate dissolving of the bacterial DNA and degrading of the RNA.
9. Measure the concentration of the chromosomal DNA using a UV-spectrophotometer.

3.3. DNA Restriction and Labeling

1. Digest 1 mg of DNA in a final volume of 20 µL 1X buffer H containing 5 units of restriction enzyme *Eco*R1 incubating the solution for 2 h at 37°C (*see* **Note 2**).
2. Add 10 µL of 1X buffer H containing 0.5 units of *Taq* DNA polymerase and 1 µCi of [α-^{32}P]-dATP to the 20 µL of digested DNA, and incubate the solution for 15 min at 72°C (*see* **Notes 3** and **4**).
3. Add 100 µL of 5.5 *M* ammonium acetate; pH 7.0, 2 µL of 20 mg/mL glycogen and 400 µL of 100% ethanol (–20°C) to the solution. Mix the solution well and precipitate DNA for 30 min at –20°C.
4. Recover the DNA precipitate by centrifugation for 10 min at 17,000*g*), and wash the DNA pellet gently with 500 µmL 70% ethanol (–20°C). Recentrifuge the pellet for 5 min at 17,000*g*. Remove the supernatant completely (pipeting, spinning, pipeting). Keep the tube open for 10 min at room temperature to permit the pellet to dry.
5. Dissolve the pellet containing the radiolabeled DNA fragments in 2.5 µL H_2O supplemented with 2.5 µL of stop solution. Incubate the tube for 15 min at 60°C in order to facilitate dissolving.
6. Measure the amount of radiolabel incorporation by holding the tube close to the Geiger counter.
7. Dilute the sample with H_2O/stop solution (1:1) until an activity of 200 CPS/µL is achieved.

3.4. DNA Electrophoresis

1. Prepare a 1X TBE buffer containing 6% acrylamide/*bis*-acrylamide solution and 8 *M* urea (gel solution).
2. Add 80 µL of TEMED and 400 µL of 10% APS to 100 mL of gel solution. Subsequently, pour the gel (thickness 0.4 mm) and insert a 60-well comb. Allow the gel to polymerize for at least one hour.
3. In order to preheat the gel till 45–50°C, apply a constant power of 100 W for one hour before electrophoresis.
4. Denature the DNA samples for 5 min at 95°C and keep on ice until loading.
5. Before loading of the DNA samples, rinse the wells of the gel with 1X TBE buffer using a syringe.
6. Apply 2 µL of each radiolabeled DNA sample to the gel and run for about 4 h at 100 W until the xylene cyanol FF band has reached the bottom of the gel.
7. Transfer the gel to Whatman No 3 filter paper, cover with saran wrap and vacuum-dry for 45 min at 80°C.
8. The fragments are visualized by exposing the dried gel to an ECL Hyperfilm (overnight; room temperature; **Fig. 1A**).

3.5. Computerized Analysis of the RFEL Fingerprints

1. Scan the film at a pixel size of 190 × 190 using a desktop scanner and store the image as a TIFF file.
2. Import the TIFF file into the Gelcompar program. The DNA fragments of molecular sizes ranging from 160 bp to 400 bp are used to perform computerized comparison of the RFEL fingerprints.
3. Normalization of each lane is done by using six pneumococcal specific bands that are present in each sample (*see* arrows in **Fig. 1**).
4. Compare the patterns performed using the unweighted pair group method with arithmetic averages (UPGMA) cluster analysis and the Jaccard coefficient applied to peaks. A band tolerance setting of 1.2% is used (**Fig. 1B**).

Fig. 1. *(opposite page)* RFEL analysis of 10 clinical isolates of *S. pneumoniae*. **(A)** RFEL fingerprints visualized by X-ray. **(B)** Computerized image of the RFEL fingerprints and calculated genetic relatedness of the strains (dendrograph). The 6 arrows indicate species-specific bands that are used for computerized normalization. For methodological details, see text. Although in theory, all DNA restriction fragments are supposed to be equally labeled by this technique, in practice, additional weak bands often occur (e.g., the band marked by a closed triangle in the RFEL banding pattern of strain 1). During computerized analysis, all visible bands (strong and weak) are considered. Due to impurities in the DNA sample, dark smears may cover the RFEL fingerprints (*see* RFEL fingerprint of strain 2). Repeating the DNA isolation procedure often solves this problem.

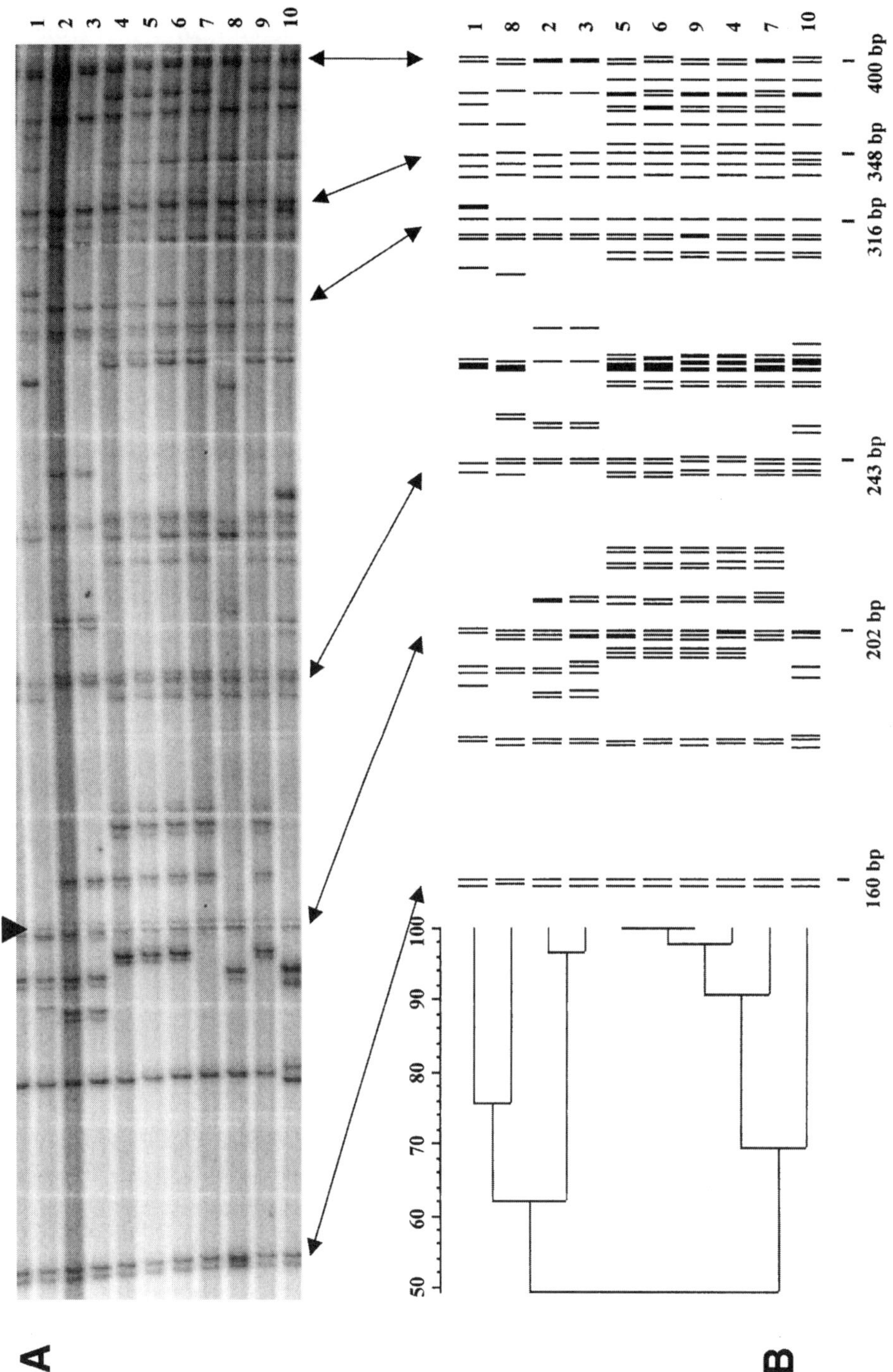
A
B
1 2 3 4 5 6 7 8 9 10
1 8 2 3 5 6 9 4 7 10
400 bp
348 bp
316 bp
243 bp
202 bp
160 bp
50 60 70 80 90 100

4. Notes

1. Small-size DNA restriction fragments representing "random" sites of the bacterial chromosome are used by RFEL analysis. Since this DNA fingerprint technique does not require detailed knowledge on the bacterial genome (e.g., gene sequence information), RFEL fingerprinting can be generally applied to various bacterial species. So far, this technique has been successfully used to identify genetic diversity in *S. pneumoniae* ***(33)***, *Escherichia coli* ***(37)***, *Actinobacillus actinomycetemcomitans* ***(37)*** and *Helicobacter pylori* ***(39,40)***.
2. The mutations detected by RFEL analysis are supposed to be primarily the result of random and "slow" evolutionary events. These cause loss or gain of restriction sites, which can result in the disappearance or appearance of small-size DNA fragments, respectively. This makes the detection of genetic diversity in highly clonal species (e.g., *Mycobacterium tuberculosis*) difficult by this technique ***(41)***. The discriminatory power of RFEL analysis can be increased by using more frequently cutting restriction enzymes (resulting in an elevated number of small-size DNA restriction fragments), or by increasing the electrophoresis time (also resulting in the appearance of more restriction fragments, albeit fragments of higher molecular size).
3. It should be noted that only restriction enzymes that create DNA fragments with 5'-protruding ends can be labeled by the methodological procedures described above. Obviously, the choice of dNTP radiolabel depends upon the base composition of the 5'-protruding ends of the restriction fragments.
4. Although we do not have experimental data available, it should also be feasible to directly label the 5' ends by using T4 polynucleotide kinase and [γ-^{32}P]-ATP irrespective of the restriction enzyme of choice.

References

1. Centers for Diseases Control (1997) Prevention of pneumococcal disease—recommendation of the Advisory Committee on Immunization Practices (ACIP). *MMWR* **46,** 1–24.
2. Zenni, M. K., Cheatham, S. H., Thompson, J. M., Reed, G. W., Batson, A. B., Palmer, P. S., Holland, K. L., and Edwards, K. M. (1995) *Streptococcus pneumoniae* colonization in the young child: association with otitis media and resistance to penicillin. *J. Pediatr.* **127,** 533–537.
3. Homoe, P., Prag, J., Farholt, S., Henrichsen, J., Hornsleth, A., Kilian, M., and Jensen, J. S. (1996) High rate of nasopharyngeal carriage of potential pathogens among children in Greenland: results of a clinical survey of middle-ear disease. *Clin. Infect. Dis.* **23,** 1081–1090.
4. Faden, H., Duffy, L., Wasielewski, R., Wolf, J., Krystofik, D., and Tung, Y. (1997) Relationship between nasopharyngeal colonization and the development of otitis media in children. *J. Infect. Dis.* **175,** 1440–1445.
5. Sluijter, M., Faden, H., de Groot, R., Lemmens, N., Goessens, W. H. F., van Belkum, A., and Hermans, P. W. M. (1998) Molecular characterization of pneu-

mococcal nasopharynx isolates in children during the first two years of life. *J. Clin. Microbiol.* **36,** 2248–2253.

6. Geslin, P., Buu-Hoi, A., Fremaux, A., and Acar, J. F. (1992) Antimicrobial resistance in *Streptococcus pneumoniae*: an epidemiology survey in France, 1970–1990. *Clin. Infect. Dis.* **15,** 95–98.
7. Koornof, H. J., Wasas, A., and Klugman, K. P. (1992) Antimicrobial resistance in *Streptococcus pneumoniae*: a South African perspective. *Clin. Infect. Dis.* **15,** 84–97.
8. Kristinsson, K. G., Hjalmardottir, M. A., and Steingrimsson, O. S. (1992) Increasing penicillin resistance in pneumococci in Iceland. *Lancet* **339,** 1606–1607.
9. Linares, J., Alonso, T., Perez, J. L., Ayats, J., Dominguez, M. A., Pallares, R., and Martin, R. (1992) Trends in antimicrobial resistance of clinical isolates of *Streptococcus pneumoniae* in Bellvitge Hospital, Barcelona, Spain (1979–1990). *Clin. Infect. Dis.* **15,** 99–105.
10. Marton, A. (1992) Pneumococcal antimicrobial resistance: the problem in Hungary. *Clin. Infect. Dis.,* **15,** 106–111.
11. Centers for Diseases Control (1995) Emergence of penicillin-resistant *Streptococcus pneumoniae*-Southern Ontario, Canada. *MMWR* **44,** 207–209.
12. Yoshida, R., Kaku, M., Kohno, S., Ishida, K., Mizukane, R., Takemura, H., Tanaka, H., Usui, T., Tomono, K., Koga, H., et al. (1995) Trends in antimicrobial resistance on *Streptococcus pneumoniae* in Japan. *Antimicrob. Agents Chemother.* **39,** 1196–1198.
13. Dagan, R., Melamed, R., Muallem, M., Piglansky, L., and Yagupsky, P. (1996) Nasopharyngeal colonization in Southern Israel with antibiotic-resistant pneumococci during the first 2 years of life: relation to serotypes likely to be included in pneumococcal conjugate vaccines. *J. Infect. Dis.* **174,** 1352–1355.
14. Soares, S., Kristinsson, K. G., Musser, J. M., and Tomasz, A. (1993) Evidence for the introduction of a multiresistant clone of serotype 6B *Streptococcus pneumoniae* from Spain to Iceland in the late 1980s. *J. Infect. Dis.* **168,** 158–163.
15. Muñoz, R., Coffey, T. J., Daniels, M., Dowson, C. G., Laible, G., Casal, J., Hakenbeck, R., Jacobs, M., Musser, J. M., Spratt, B. G., and Tomasz, A. (1991) Intercontinental spread of a multiresistant clone of serotype 23F *Streptococcus pneumoniae*. *J. Infect. Dis.* **164,** 302–306.
16. McDougal, L. K., Facklam, R. R., Reeves, M., Hunter, S., Swenson, J. M., Hill, B. C., and Tenover, F. C. (1992) Analysis of multiply antimicrobial-resistant isolates of *Streptococcus pneumoniae* from the United States. *Antimicrob. Agents Chemother.* **36,** 2176–2184.
17. Gasc, A. M., Geslin, P., and Sicard, A. M. (1995) Relatedness of penicillin-resistant *Streptococcus pneumoniae* serogroup 9 strains from France and Spain. *Microbiology* **141,** 623–627.
18. Reichmann, P., Varon, E., Günther, E., Reinert, R. R., Lüttiken, R., Marton, A., Geslin, P., Wagner, J., and Hakenbeck, R. (1995) Penicillin-resistant *Streptococcus pneumoniae* in Germany: genetic relationship to clones from other European countries. *J. Med. Microbiol.* **43,** 377–385.

19. Hermans, P. W. M., Sluijter, M., Dejsirilert, S., Lemmens, N., Elzenaar, K., van Veen, A., Goessens, W. H. F., and de Groot, R. (1997) Molecular epidemiology of drug-resistant pneumococci: toward an international approach. *Microb. Drug Resist.* **3,** 243–251.
20. Coffey, T. J., Berron, S., Daniels, M., Garcia-Leoni, E., Cercenado, E., Bouza, E., Fenoll, A., and Spratt, B. G. (1996) Multiply antibiotic-resistant *Streptococcus pneumoniae* recovered from Spanish hospitals (1988–1994): Novel major clones of serotypes 1**4,** 19F and 15F. *Microbiology* **142,** 2747–2757.
21. Smith, A. M. and Klugman, K. P. (1997) Three predominant clones identified within penicillin-resistant South-African isolates of *Streptococcus pneumoniae. Microb. Drug Resist.* **3,** 385–389.
22. Yoshida, R., Hirakata, Y., Kaku, M., Takemura, H., Tanaka, H., Tomono, K., Koga, H., Kohno, S., and Kamahira, S. (1997) Genetic relationship of penicillin resistant *Streptococcus pneumoniae* serotype19B strains in Japan. *Epidemiol. Infect.* **118,** 105–110.
23. Lund, E. and Henrichsen, J. (1978) Laboratory diagnosis, serology and epidemiology of *Streptococcus pneumoniae*, in *Methods in Microbiology*, vol. 12 (Bergan, T. and Norris, J. R., eds.), Academic Press, New York, pp. 241–262.
24. Nielsen, S. V. and Henrichsen, J. (1993) Capsular types and susceptibility to penicillin of pneumococci isolated from cerebrospinal fluid or blood in Denmark, 1983–1988. *Scand J. Infect. Dis.* **25,** 165–170.
25. Sessegolo, J. F., Levin, A. S. S., Levy, C. E., Asensi, M., Facklam, R. R., and Teixeira, L. M. (1994) Distribution of serotypes and antimicrobial resistance of *Streptococcus pneumonia* strains isolated in Brazil from 1988 to 1992. *J. Clin. Microbiol.* **32,** 906–911.
26. Shapiro, E. D. and Austrian, R. (1994) Serotypes responsible for invasive *Streptococcus pneumoniae* infections among children in Connecticut. *J. Infect. Dis.* **169,** 212–214.
27. Munoz, R., Musser, J. M., Crain, M., Briles, D. E., Marton, A., Parkinson, A. J., Sorensen, U., and Tomasz, A. (1992) Geographic distribution of penicillin-resistant clones of *Streptococcus pneumoniae*: characterization by penicillin-binding protein profile, surface protein A typing, and multilocus enzyme analysis. *Clin. Infect. Dis.* **15,** 112–118.
28. Kell, C. M., Jordens, J. Z., Daniels, M., Coffey, T. J., Bates, J., Paul, J., Gilks, C., and Spratt, B. G. (1993) Molecular epidemiology of penicillin-resistant pneumococci isolated in Nairobi, Kenya. *Infect. Immun.* **61,** 4382–4391.
29. Cherian, T., Steinhoff, M. C., Harrison, L. H., Rohn, D., McDougal, L. K., and Dick, J. (1994) A cluster of invasive pneumococcal disease in young children in child care. *JAMA* **271,** 695–697.
30. Munoz, R., Dowson, C. G., Daniels, M., Coffey, T. J., Martin, C., Hakenbeck, R., and Spratt, B. G. (1992) Genetics of resistance to third-generation cephalosporins in clinical isolates of *Streptococcus pneumoniae. Mol. Microbiol.* **6,** 2461–2465.
31. Smith, A. M., Klugman, K. P., Coffey, T. J., and Spratt, B. G. (1993) Genetic diversity of penicillin-binding protein 2B and 2X genes from *Streptococcus pneumoniae* in South Africa. *Antimicrob. Agents Chemother.* **37,** 1938–1944.

32. Lefevre, J. C., Faucon, G., Sicard, A. M., and Gasc, A. M. (1993) DNA fingerprinting of *Streptococcus pneumoniae* strains by pulsed-field gel electrophoresis. *J. Clin. Microbiol.* **31,** 2724–2728.
33. Hermans, P. W. M., Sluijter, M., Hoogenboezem, T., Heersma, H., van Belkum, A., and de Groot, R. (1995) Comparative study of five different DNA fingerprint techniques for molecular typing of *Streptococcus pneumoniae* strains. *J. Clin. Microbiol.* **33,** 1606–1612.
34. Martin, B., Humbert, O., Camara, M., Guenzi, E., Walker, J., Mitchell, T., Andrew, P., Prudhomme, M., Alloing, G., Hakenbeck, R., Morrison, D. A., Boulnois, G. J., and Claverys, J.-P. (1992) A highly conserved repeated DNA element located in the chromosome of *Streptococcus pneumoniae. Nucleic Acids Res.* **20,** 3479–3483.
35. Versalovic, J., Koeuth, T., and Lupski, J. R. (1991) Distribution of repetitive DNA sequences in eubacteria and application to fingerprinting bacterial genomes. *Nucleic Acids Res.* **19,** 6823–6831.
36. Van Belkum, A., Sluijter, M., de Groot, R., Verbrugh, H. A., and Hermans, P. W. M. (1996) A novel BOX-repeat PCR assay for high resolution typing of *Streptococcus pneumoniae* strains. *J. Clin. Microbiol.* **34,** 1176–1179.
37. Van Steenbergen, T. J. M., Colloms, S. D., Hermans, P. W. M., de Graaff, J., and Plasterk, R. H. A. (1995) Genomic DNA fingerprinting by restriction fragment end labeling. *Proc. Natl. Acad. Sci.* USA **92,** 5572–5576.
38. Sambrook, J., Fritsch, E. F., and Maniatis, T. (1989) Molecular cloning, a laboratory manual. Cold Spring Harbor Laboratory, Cold Spring Harbor, NY.
39. Debets-Ossenkopp, Y. J., Sparrius, M., Kusters, J. G., Kolkman, J. J., and Vandenbroucke-Grauls, C. M. (1996) Mechanism of clarithromycin resistance in clinical isolates of *Helicobacter pylori. FEMS Microbiol. Lett.* **142,** 37–42.
40. Van Doorn, N. E., Namavar, F., Kusters, J. G., van Rees, E. P., Kuipers, E. J., and de Graaff, J. (1998) Genomic DNA fingerprinting of clinical isolates of *Helicobacter pylori* by REP-PCR and restriction fragment end-labelling. *FEMS Microbiol. Lett.* **160,** 145–150.
41. Kremer, K., van Soolingen, D., Frothingham, R., Haas, W. H., Hermans, P. W. M., Martin, C., Palittapongarnpim, P., Plikaytis, B. B., Riley, L. W., Yakrus, M. A., Musser, J. M., and van Embden, J. D. A. (1999) Comparison of molecular epidemiologic markers for *Mycobacterium tuberculosis* complex: an interlaboratory study on differentiation and reproducibility. *J Clin Microbiol.* (In Press).

18

Pulse-field Gel Electrophoresis for Epidemiological Studies of *Streptococcus pneumoniae*

Anne-Marie Gasc

1. Introduction

Electrophoresis techniques have allowed for very effective separation of nucleic acids on the basis of molecular weight. Conventional DNA electrophoresis can only separate DNA fragments smaller than 50 kb. Above this size, DNA fragments are larger than the pore size of the matrix. They can travel through a gel matrix by deforming their shape, parallel to the field in order to pass through the pores. This mode of migration is called "reptation" and all large molecules migrate at the same rate. Shwartz et al. *(1)* were the first to introduce the concept that molecules larger than 50 kb can be separated by using two alternating electric fields, one homogeneous and the other nonhomogeneous. In pulsed field gel electrophoresis (PFGE) the electrical field is applied alternately in two directions. The orientation of DNA molecules is perturbed and they have to reorient to move efficiently in response to the new field. The time required for this reorientation has been found to be proportional to the molecular weight. Larger DNA molecules take more time to realign after the fields are switched than do smaller ones. Thus, the reorientation introduces a size dependence that is absent during simple "reptation." The timing of the electrical field in each direction is called the pulse time: too fast or too slow and no separation occurs. However molecules of DNA, whose reorientation times are less than the period of the electric pulse, will be fractionated according to size. The resolution expected from these techniques is also dependent on other parameters *(2,3)*. These include degree of uniformity of the two electric fields, the lengths of the electric pulses, the angle of the two electric fields to

From: *Methods in Molecular Medicine, vol. 48: Antibiotic Resistance Methods and Protocols*
Edited by: S. H. Gillespie © Humana Press Inc., Totowa, NJ

the gel, the relative strengths of the two electric field, but the most important parameter is the length of the molecule.

The original PFGE *(4)* method was followed by another that used two nonhomogenous electric fields and this was described by Carle et Olson *(5–6)*. These apparatuses use alternatively pulsed perpendicularly oriented electric fields and linear electrodes. The DNA skews toward the edge, with a consequent loss of resolution. To ameliorate these problems, alternative electrode configurations have been developed. Periodic inversion gel electrophoreses, or field inversion gel electrophoresis (FIGE), in which the field is periodically inverted 180°C, can also be used to separate large molecules *(7)*. In this case the field is uniform in the both directions, and the migration of DNA is in a straight tract. However, experiments revealed that the DNA molecules do not migrate as a direct function of the size for a given switch time and in certain cases, two molecules of different sizes can migrate in the same position. This problem can be minimized by progressively changing the switching interval during the run. To achieve net forward migration, FIGE employs a difference in the duration of the forward and reverse field, allowing the resolution of fragments in a certain range of sizes. The ratio between forward and reverse pulses are maintained. This technique is called switch time ramping and is commonly used. Depending of the pulse time, FIGE yields very good resolution for molecules smaller than 750 kb, and can resolve up to 2000 kb. This technology makes it possible to map the chromosomes of bacteria *(8,9)*. As the size of the *Streptococcus pneumoniae* chromosome is about 2000 kb this FIGE technique proved very convenient for mapping this organism *(10–12)*.

Another apparatus for electrophoresis, contour-clamped homogeneous field electrophoresis (CHEF) has been developed *(13–14)*. In this method the electric field is generated from multiple electrodes that are organized in a square or hexagonal contour around the horizontal gel, and are clamped to predetermined electric potentials. A square contour generates fields at 90° and a hexagonal generates fields at >120° or 60°C, depending on the placement of the gel and the polarity of the electrodes. The DNA molecules migrate in straight lanes. The range of resolution depends on switching intervals and fragments up to 5 Mb can be separated. A number of manufacturers produce apparatus based on these principles. The programs specify the range of resolution that each is able to provide and experimenters should follow the instructions provided by the manufacturer. Introducing new programs is possible, but it is difficult to improve the resolution. These techniques have provided the technology to map and to analyze several bacterial chromosomes, notably the *S. pneumoniae* R6 chromosome *(10)*. *S. pneumoniae* is a common microorganism found in the normal human respiratory flora and a major cause of morbidity worldwide. Moreover, the emergence of strains resistant to penicillin and other antibiotics, and their dissemination world wide have become a major concern. Effective means to follow the transmission to allow epidemiological surveillance are increasingly required. In comparison to other techniques: serotyping, penicillin-binding protein patterns, multilocus enzyme electrophoresis, and ribotyping, pulsed field gel electrophoresis using low-frequency cutting restriction endonucleases, provides the most efficient method to discriminate *S. pneumoniae* strains ***(11)***. The DNA of *S. pneumoniae* has an A+T content of about 61%, so the restriction enzyme with recognition sites consisting of G and C produces a reasonable number of fragments. For example, in **Fig 1A** or **B**, first lanes show Lambda ladder, second lanes, show *Sma*1 digestion of R6 chromosome. Part A and part B used different pulse time. A determination of the genetic relationships of clinical isolates from various places in the world should facilitate our understanding about the spread of pneumococcal strains, and these techniques are very useful to suggest or to infer a clonal origin for different clinical strains (for examples of this approach *see* **refs. *12,15,16***). For a good resolution, after the choice of the apparatus and pulse time, the DNA preparation is very important.

2. Materials

1. Sterile plastic culture flasks.
2. Sterile Petri dishes.
3. Sterile test tubes.
4. Autoclaved micro-centrifuge tubes (1.5 mL).
5. 200 µL and 1000 µL automatic pipet tips.
6. Plexiglass molds (50 to 100 µL).
7. Growth medium: Brain Heart Infusion.
8. NaCl, Tris HCl, EDTA.
9. Deoxycholic acid, sodium salt (DOC).
10. Sarkosyl (N-Laurylsarcosine, sodium salt).
11. Polyoxyethylene 23 Lauryl ether (Brij 35).
12. Phenylmethylsulfonyl Fluoride (PMSF).
13. Restriction enzymes were obtained from (New England Biolabs, Beverly, MA).
14. DNA size markers, e.g., Lambda DNA ladder.
15. Low-melting point agarose.
16. Normal agarose.
17. Buffer 1: 1 *M* NaCl, 10 m*M* Tris-HCl, pH 8.
18. Lysis Buffer 2: 1 *M* NaCl, 0.1 EDTA, 10 m*M* Tris-HCl, 0.5% Brij, 0.2%, DOC, 0.5% sarcosyl, pH 8.
19. Buffer 3: 0.25 *M* EDTA pH 7.8, 1% sarcosyl, 100 µg/mL proteinase K.
20. Buffer 4: 10 m*M* Tris-HCl pH 7.6, 1 m*M* EDTA, 1 m*M* PMSF (*see* **Note 1**).
21. Buffer 5 TE Buffer: 10 m*M* Tris-HCl pH 7.8, 1 m*M* EDTA.
22. Buffer 6: 100 m*M* EDTA, 10 m*M* Tris-HCl, pH 7.8.

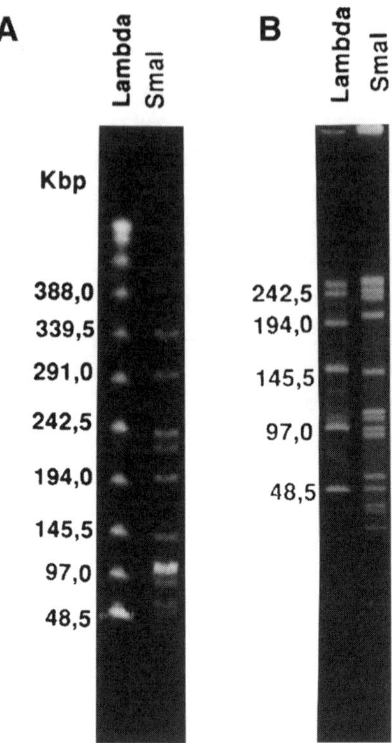

Fig. 1. FIGE profiles; First lane, Part A or B: Lambda ladder. Second lane Part A or B: SmaI restriction fragments of S. pneumoniae R6 strain. FIGE was performed in 1% (w/v) agarose for 20 h at 8°C at 5 V cm-1 in TBE buffer. Field inversion was supplied by a ramp (programmable power inverter; model PPI 200, MJ Research) that controls the time for the forward and reverse cycles. Program A was used for 0.15–12.03 s in the forward and 0.05–4.01 in the reverse direction. Program B was used for 0.3–30 s in the forward and 0.1–10 in the reverse direction.

23. TBE Buffer: Stock solution 0.45 *M* Tris-borate, 20 m*M* EDTA pH 8.0 working solution is diluted 1/10.
24. Ethidium bromide solutions:1 0 mg/mL in water, stored at 4°C in bottle wrapped in aluminium foil.

3. Methods

3.1. Growing the Cells

Inoculate 20–50 mL of Brain Heart Infusion broth and incubate until the culture reaches and O.D. of >0.3 <0.5.

3.2. Washing

1. Harvest cells by centrifugation at 5000*g* for 10 min at 4°C.
2. Resuspend the pelleted cells in 20 mL buffer 1.
3. Centrifuge again in same conditions and wash again with 10 mL buffer 1.
4. Resuspend the cells in the same buffer, and concentrate to an OD of 6.0. (Example 20 ml OD = 0.3, the final vol should be 1 mL.)

3.3. Preparation of DNA

1. Prepare low melting temperature agarose 1% in buffer 1 and cool to 42–45°C.
2. Warm the cell suspension to the same temperature.
3. Mix an equal volume of low-melting agarose and cell suspension.
4. Pipet the mix with 200 μL pipet tip and pour into the plexiglass molds.
5. Allow the mixture to set at 4°C.
6. Collect the blocks from the molds into lysis buffer 2 (5 blocks into 2 mL of buffer) (*see* **Note 2**).
7. Incubate the blocks for 2 h at 37°C (*see* **Note 3**).
8. Transfer the blocks to an equal vol of buffer 3 (proteinase K) (*see* **Note 4**).
9. Incubate the blocks 16–20 h at 50°C.
10. Transfer the blocks into 2 mL of buffer 4 (PMSF) and incubate at room temperature for 1 or 2 h with gently shaking.
11. Discard PMSF (*see* **Note 5**).
12. Wash the blocks three times in buffer 5 (TE buffer) by gentle agitation for 20 min.

3.4. Conservation of the Blocks

Blocks can be stored for a few days in buffer 5 at 4°C. If longer storage is required the blocks should be stored in buffer 6 at 4°C for up to three months.

3.5. Restriction Enzyme Digestion of DNA in Blocks

1. Blocks stored in buffer 5 can be used directly. If blocks are stored in buffer 6, remove then, add buffer 5, remove the buffer 5, add new buffer 5, and gently shake 20 min (twice).
2. Transfer the blocks into micro-centrifuge tubes.
3. Add 1X restriction buffer appropriate to the enzyme used (0.5 mL for 1 or 2 blocks.)
4. Gently shake 10 min at room temperature.
5. Remove the buffer, and perform **steps 2** and **3** again.
6. Remove the buffer carefully, add 100 μL of 1X restriction buffer and 25 units of the restriction enzyme and incubate 2 h at the optimal temperature for the enzyme.
7. Remove the buffer, add 500 μL of buffer 6 and put on ice 15 min.
8. Carefully remove buffer just before loading.

3.6. Electrophoresis

1. Prepare a 0.8–1% agarose gel in TBE buffer and cool to 15–20°C.

2. Push the block directly into the well of the gel. Alternatively, melt the blocks at 62–65°C 10 min, then add 2 mL 0.25% bromophenol blue, and immediately pipet, using cut 200 µL tips (*see* **Note 6**), 20 or 30 µL into the well.
3. Close the lid of the gel and apply the field, usually 16 to 20 h.
4. Turn off the electric current and remove the lid from the gel box.
5. Stain the gel by soaking it for 30 min in a 1 mg/mL solution of Ethidium bromide in TBE buffer (*see* **Note 7**).
6. Destain for 10 min in TBE buffer.
7. Photograph the gel with ultraviolet illumination.

4. Notes

1. PMSF, 100 m*M* stock solution in ethanol is stored at – 20°C. PMSF is extremely destructive to the mucous membrane of the respiratory tract, eyes, and skin. In case of contact immediately flush eyes or skin with copious amounts of water.
2. It is easier to collect the blocks by using a piece of silicone as large as the block to push it into a tube.
3. In some instances clinical isolates can be difficult lyse. Blocks are "white" before lysis and become " transparent " after. Sometimes lysis incubation periods need to be extended for 4–5 h. After lysis, transfer the blocks into buffer 3 as soon as possible. If you use as control strain R6, 30 min in this medium is sufficient.
4. Use a piece of sterile gauze or net above a small beaker and pour buffer, sometimes several blocks will fall down in the same time, but you can recover blocks carefully with a spatula.
5. PMSF is inactivated in aqueous solutions. The rate of inactivation increases with pH and is faster at 25°C than at 4°C. The half-life of a 20 µ*M* aqueous solution of PMSF is about 35 min at pH 8.0 *(3–17)*. Aqueous solution of PMSF can be safety discarded after they have been rendered alkaline pH 7.8, and stored several hours at room temperature.
6. To avoid DNA damage, cut yellow tip 5 to 7 mm above the extremity, and then pipet 10 to 30 µL of the melted agarose to obtain a good resolution of bands.
7. Ethidium bromide is a powerful mutagen and is moderately toxic. Gloves should be worn when using it. After this solutions should be decomtamined by usual method.

Acknowledgments

I would like to thank A. Carpousis for his kind help in preparing the manuscript.

References

1. Schwartz, D. C., Saffran, W., Welsh, J., Haas, R., Goldenberg, M., and Cantor, C. R. (1982) New techniques for purifying large DNA and studying their properties and packaging. *Cold Spring Harbor Symp. Quant. Biol.* **47,** 189–195.
2. Lai, E., Birren, B. W., Clark, S. M., Simon, M. I., and Hood, L. (1989) Pulsed field gel electrophoresis. *Biotechniques* **7,** 34–42.

3. Sambrook, J., Fritsch, E. F., and Maniatis, T. (1989) *Molecular Cloning*, 2nd ed., Cold Spring Harbor Laboratory, Cold Spring Harbor, NY, pp. 16–17, 49–62.
4. Schwartz, D. C. and Cantor, C. R. (1984) Separation of yeast chromosome-sized DNAs by pulsed field gradient gel electrophoresis. *Cell* **37,** 67–75.
5. Carle, G. F. and Olson, M. V. (1984) Separation of chromosomal DNA molecules from yeast by orthogonal-field-alternation gel electrophoresis. *Nucleic Acids Res.* **12,** 5647–5664.
6. Carle, G. F. and Olson, M. V. (1984) An electrophoretic karyotype for yeast. *Proc. Natl. Acad. Sci. USA* **82,** 3756–3760.
7. Carle, G. F., Frank, M., and Olson, M. V. (1986) Electrophoretic separation of large DNA molecules by periodic inversion of the electric field. *Science* **232,** 65–68.
8. Kauc, L. and Goodgal S., H. (1989) The size and physical map of the chromosome of *Haemophilus parainfluenzae*. *Gene* **83,** 377–380.
9. Kauc, L., Mitchell, M., and Goodgal S., H. (1989). Size and physical map of the chromosome of *Haemophilus influenzae*. *J. Bacterol.* **171,** 2474–2479.
10. Gasc, A. M., Kauc, L., Barraillé, P., Sicard, M., and Goodgal, S. (1991) Gene localization, size, and physical map of the chromosome of *Streptococcus pneumoniae*. *J. Bacteriol.* **173,** 7361–7367.
11. Lefèvre, J., Faucon, G., Sicard, A. M., and Gasc, A. M. (1993) DNA fingerprinting of *Streptococcus pneumoniae* strains by pulsed-field gel electrophoresis. *J. Clin. Microbiol.* **31,** 2724–2728.
12. Gasc, A. M., Geslin, P., and Sicard, A. M. (1995) Relatedness of penicillin-resistant *Streptococcus pneumoniae* serogroup 9 strains from France and Spain. *Microbiology* **141,** 623–627.
13. Chu, G., Vollrath, D., and Davis, R. W. (1986) Separation of large DNA molecules by contour-clamped homogeneous electric field. *Science* **234,** 1582–1585.
14. Vollrath, D. and Davis, R. W. (1987) Resolution of DNA molecules greater than 5 megabases by contour-clamped homogeneous electric fields. *Nucleic Acids Res.* **15,** 7865–7876.
15. Soares, S., Kristinsson, K. G., Musser, J. M., and Tomasz, A. (1993) Evidence for the introduction of a multiresistant clone of serotype 6B *Streptococcus pneumoniae* from Spain to Iceland in the late 1980s. *J. Infect. Dis.* **168,** 158–163.
16. Rudolph, K. M., Parkinson, A. J., Roberts, M. C. (1998) Molecular analysis by pulsed-field gel electrophoresis and antibiogram of *Streptococcus pneumoniae* serotype 6B isolates from selected areas within the United States. *J. Clin. Microbiol.* **36,** 2703–2707.
17. James, G. T. (1978) Inactivation of the protease inhibitor phenylmethylsulfonyl fluoride in buffers. *Anal. Biochem.* **86,** 574–579.

19

Outer Membrane Profiles of Clonally Related *Klebsiella pneumoniae*

Vicente J. Benedí and Luis Martínez-Martínez

1. Introduction

Antimicrobial treatment of *Klebsiella pneumoniae* infections can be complicated by the existence of multiply-antibiotic resistant (multiresistant) strains carrying plasmids coding for extended-spectrum β-lactamases (ESBLs), AmpC-type β-lactamases (ACTBLs), or aminoglycoside-modifying enzymes. This situation has become an increasingly serious problem worldwide with incidences ranging from 5% in the United States *(1)* to 16% in Europe *(2)*, and higher incidences have been reported for particular hospitals or areas due to nosocomial outbreaks *(3)*. Additionally, it should be noted that a large proportion of ESBL-producing strains are also resistant to fluoroquinolones, probably because of mutations in the genes coding for the A subunits of topoisomerases II (DNA-gyrase) and IV. When ESBLs or ACTBLs expression is accompanied by a decreased permeability of the bacterial outer membrane (OM), a major increase in the MICs of β-lactams (including carbapenems in strains expressing ACTBLs) has been observed *(4,5)*. Similarly, a reduction in permeability also causes moderate increases in the MICs of fluoroquinolones *(3,5,6)*. This decreased permeability is caused by the loss or reduced expression of porins, the nonspecific pore outer membrane proteins (OMPs), with the subsequent reductions of antibiotic influx and of access to the antibiotic target. Reduction of porin expression during antimicrobial treatment are caused by different mutations in the porin genes, including point mutations, small and large deletions, and interruption of porin genes by insertion sequences *(7)*.

The above data indicate the importance of the characterization of OMPs, particularly porins, when studying multiresistant clinical isolates. For this purpose, the OM of Gram negative lysed cells can be isolated following two groups

From: *Methods in Molecular Medicine, vol. 48: Antibiotic Resistance Methods and Protocols*
Edited by: S. H. Gillespie © Humana Press Inc., Totowa, NJ

of methods. First, since the OM is constituted by phospholipids, lipopolysaccharide (LPS) and OMPs, it can be separated in an ultracentrifuge gradient from the inner (cytoplasmic) membrane lacking LPS. Alternatively, due to their different composition, both membranes can be differentially solubilized depending on the detergent and conditions used. Interested readers are referred to the original references ***(8,9)*** and the derived protocols ***(10)***. On the other hand, porins can be isolated by methods based on their strong but noncovalent interaction with the petidoglycan and their increased, compared to other OMPs, resistance to proteases. The OMPs and porins of *K. pneumoniae* can be isolated following the above methods. For OMPs, differential solubilization in sarcosinate has been routinely used (*see* for example ***[11,12]***), since this method is faster and simpler. The porins of *K. pneumoniae* have also been isolated by a combination of differential solubilization in sodium dodecyl sulphate (SDS) and protease treatment ***(13,14)***. Three porins have been described in this species: porins OmpK37, OmpK36, and OmpK35, and they represent the homologues of *Escherichia coli* porins OmpN, OmpC, and OmpF, respectively. The role of these porins in antimicrobial resistance has also been described ***(3,5,15)***.

In this chapter we describe the methods for the isolation and analysis by electrophoresis on polyacrylamide gels containing SDS (SDS-PAGE) of *K. pneumoniae* OMPs and porins. Due to their very close molecular masses, optimal resolution of porins in this species was achieved by slight but important modifications of the usual SDS-PAGE methods. Finally, it has to be pointed out that even if an OMP is isolated following a porin isolation method and that by SDS-PAGE shows an apparent molecular mass compatible with those of the previously described porins (in the range of 35 to 40 kDa), direct proof of the porin nature of an OMP requires further experiments. When studying clonally related multiresistant isolates, clones with increased resistance can be found. Usually, the initial strain expresses only one porin, which can be isolated as described here, whereas the variant with increased resistance is deficient in the porin ***(16)***. That the lost OMP is indeed a porin can be deduced by restoring porin expression, by cloning its corresponding gene, with the subsequent decrease in MICs ***(3,5)***

2. Materials

2.1. Outer Membrane Protein isolation

1. Tris-Mg buffer: 10 m*M* Tris-HCl, 5 m*M* $MgCl_2$, pH 7.3. Store at 4°C.
2. 2% (w/v) sodium lauryl sarkosynate (SLS).

2.2. Porin Isolation

1. Tris buffer 1: 50 m*M* Tris-HCl pH 7.7.
2. Tris buffer 2: 10 m*M* Tris-HCl pH 8.0.
3. Solubilization buffer: Tris buffer 1 containing 4% SDS.

2.3. SDS-PAGE Analysis of OMPs and Porins

1. Acrylamide stock: 30% acrylamide. Filter through 0.45 µm pore filter and keep at 4°C in a dark bottle.
2. *Bis*-acrylamide stock: 1.5% *bis*-acrylamide. Filter through 0.45 µm pore filter and keep at 4°C in a dark bottle.
3. Resolving gel buffer: 1.5 *M* Tris-HCl, pH 8.8. Store at 4°C.
4. Stacking gel buffer: 0.5 *M* Tris-HCl, pH 6.8. Store at 4°C.
5. SDS stock 10% (w/v).
6. N,N,N',N'-tetramethylenediamine (TEMED). Store at 4°C.
7. 10% (w/v) ammonium persulphate (APS). Aliquot and store at –20°C. Ammonium persulphate powder is very hygroscopic: keep it in a desiccator.
8. Resolving gel overlay: Shake well a 1:1 mixture of butanol and stacking gel buffer. Let the two phases separate and use the upper phase.
9. Tank buffer: 0.025 *M* Tris-HCl, pH 8.3, 0.192 *M* glycine, 0.1% SDS.
10. Sample buffer (2X): 0.125 *M* Tris-HCl pH 6.8, 4% SDS, 20% glycerol, 10% β-mercaptoethanol, 0.004% bromophenol blue. Store aliquoted at -20°C.
11. Staining solution: 0.125% Coomassie Brilliant Blue R250 in 45% methanol-10% acetic acid.
12. Destaining solution: 45% methanol-10% acetic acid.

3. Methods

3.1. OMPs Isolation

1. Grow strains in 20 mL of Nutrient Broth overnight at 37°C in a shaker (200 rpm) (*see* **Note 1**).
2. Centrifuge at 10,000*g* for 20 min. Discard supernatant fluids.
3. Resuspend cell pellets in 20 mL of cold Tris-Mg buffer, and centrifuge as in **step 2**. Repeat resuspension and centrifugation, and finally resuspend cells in 20 mL of chilled Tris-Mg buffer.
4. Break cells using a French press. Alternatively, sonicate cell suspension, keeping samples at 4°C (*see* **Note 2**).
5. Centrifuge sonicates at 3000*g* for 10 min to eliminate unbroken cells.
6. Carefully transfer supernatant fluids (representing cytoplasmic contents and cell envelopes) to a clean centrifuge tube. Ultracentrifuge at 100,000*g* for 1 h at 4°C to pellet the cell envelopes. Discard supernatant fluids.
7. Resuspend pellets in 10 mL of 2% sodium lauryl sarcosinate in Tris-Mg buffer, and incubate for 20–30 min at room temperature.
8. Pellet outer membranes for 1 h at 70,000*g*. Eliminate supernatant fluids (cytoplasmic membranes). Repeat **steps 7** and **8**.
9. Remove completely the supernatant fluids and resuspend pellets in (depending on the pellet size) 0.1–0.2 mL of H_2O.

3.2. Porin Isolation

1. Recover cells from cultures as in **Subheading 3.1.**, **steps 1** and **2**, but start from 1 L cultures.

Table 1
Stock Solutions Needed (mL) for Resolving Gels of 11% Acryalmide and different *bis*-Acrylamide Concentrations

	mL of stock solution added for gels with *bis*-acrylamide%		
Stock solution	0.21	0.35	0.55
Acrylamide	7.3	7.3	7.3
bis-acrylamide	2.6	4.6‘	6.6
SDS	0.4	0.4	0.4
H_2O	4.6	2.6	0.6
TEMED[a]	0.04	0.04	0.04
APS[a]	0.05	0.05	0.05

[a]Mix and degas in a vacuum flask before adding TEMED and APS

2. Suspend cells in 500 mL of Tris buffer 1. Repeat **step 2**.
3. Suspend cells in 20 mL of cold Tris buffer 1 and lyse cells as in **Subheading 3.1., step 4** (*see* **Note 2**).
4. Eliminate unbroken cells as in **Subheading 3.1., step 5** and pellet cell envelopes as in **Subheading 3.1., step 6**.
5. Suspend pellets in 10 mL of Tris buffer 2. Add 0.1 mg trypsin per mg of protein and sodium azide at 0.002% final concentration to prevent bacterial growth. Incubate overnight at 37°C.
6. Add 10 mL of solubilization buffer. Incubate at 32°C for 1 h.
7. Centrifuge at 100,000*g* for 30 min.
8. Resuspend pellet in 10 mL of solubilization buffer 1:1 diluted with water. Repeat **steps 6** and **7**, and resuspend pellet in 1 mL of distilled water.
9. Porin(s) can be analyzed at this step by SDS-PAGE. They still contain tightly bound LPS, and for certain purposes, such as immunization or crystallization, one may be interested in separating LPS from porin (*see* **Note 3**).

3.3. SDS-PAGE Analysis of OMPs and Porins

1. Prepare 0.75 mm thick polyacrylamide running (resolving) gels as in **Table 1** and following the recommendations of **Note 4**. Cover gel with resolving gel overlay stock and allow gel to polymerize for 1 h.
2. Discard resolving gel overlay, rinse top of gel with water and add stacking gel. For the stacking gel mix the following mL of stock solutions: 1.34 of acrylamide, 0.66 of *bis*-acrylamide, 0.1 of SDS, 2.5 of stacking gel buffer, 5.34 of H_2O, 0.01 of TEMED, and 0.05 of APS. Remember to degas the mixture before adding APS and TEMED. Let the gel polymerize for at least 1 h (*see* **Note 5**).

3. Mix equal volumes of sample buffer (2X) and samples from **Subheading 3.1., step 9** (OMPs) or **step 8** (porins). Boil for 5 min (*see* **Note 6**).
4. Fill upper and lower reservoirs of electrophoresis apparatus with tank buffer. Load samples and run gels at 20 mA (for 8 cm long gels, such as Hoefer SE250) until the blue dye reaches the end of the gel.
5. Disassemble gels and transfer to an appropriate container. Stain for 30 min and destain until the desired background is obtained by discarding and adding destaining solution (*see* **Notes 7** and **8**).

4. Notes

1. A low osmolarity medium, such as Nutrient broth (Merck, Cat. No. 5443, 50 mosmol/kg), is used to enhance expression of porin OmpK35 (the *K. pneumoniae* homologue of *E. coli* OmpF porin). In high osmolarity media, like Luria-Bertani ***(18)***, porin OmpK36 (the homologue of *E. coli* porin OmpC) overexpresses and porin OmpK35 may not be seen in some strains due to its reduced expression.
2. Pressure lysis is more efficient than sonication. However, not all the laboratories have a French press. We routinely use these conditions for sonication: 15 cycles of 30 s each. Each cycle consists of 6 × 5 s sonication (amplitude 18–20 microns) separated by 1 s of no sonication. After completion of each cycle, leave 30 s without sonication.
3. Solubilize pellet from **Subheading 3.1., step 8** in 50 m*M* Tris (pH 7.7) containing 1% SDS, 0.4 *M* NaCl, 5 m*M* EDTA, and 0.05% β-mercaptoethanol, and load a Sephacryl-S200 column (100 cm × 2.5 cm) previously washed with the same buffer. Recover fractions of 2 mL, and determine absorbance at 280 nm. Run SDS-PAGE with protein-containing fractions and stain gels for proteins (Coomassie Blue staining) and for LPS (19). Pool LPS-free porin-containing fractions and dialyze against 3 m*M* sodium azide, first for 24 h at room temperature (SDS would crystallize in the cold) and then for 7 d at 4°C. Aliquot porins and store at –20°C.
4. Optimal resolution (separation) of porins OmpK36 and OmpK35 can be obtained, depending on the strain, on resolving gels containing 11% acrylamide and either 0.21, 0.35, or 0.55% *bis*-acrylamide ***(16)***. As a rule, we start with 0.21% gels, but if only one porin is seen, running the samples in the other two gel concentrations is advised before concluding that the studied strain expresses only one porin.
5. Gels can be polymerized overnight if covered with aluminum foil to prevent evaporation. Polymerized gels wrapped in a paper towel wetted in tank buffer can be stored for 2–3 d in a closed plastic box at 4°C.
6. Porins are trimeric proteins highly stable to detergents and salts due to their high content in β-sheet structure. This can be exploited in SDS-PAGE analysis in a phenomenon called "heat modifiability": a porin will run as a monomer if boiled for 5 min in the conditions indicated in the protocol but if it is not boiled (but solubilized in sample buffer for 1 h at 37°C) it will run as a the native trimer with its corresponding higher molecular mass compared to the monomer. An OMP, presumably a porin, can be isolated following a porin isolation method and analyzed boiled and unboiled. If in the unboiled state it runs with an apparent

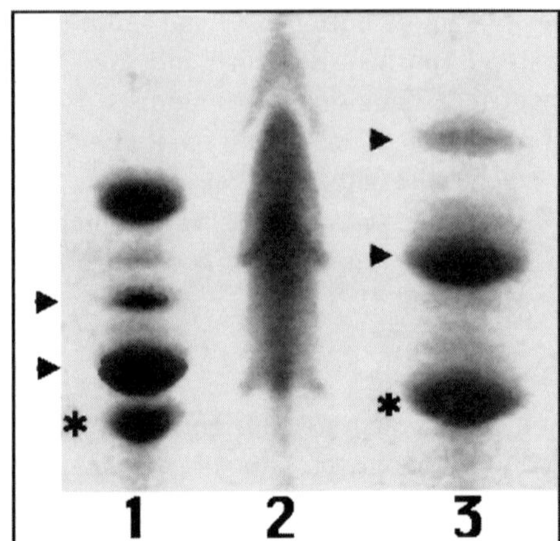

Fig. 1. SDS-PAGE analysis of OMPs from *E. coli* (lane 1) and *K. pneumoniae* (lanes 2 and 3) grown in low osmolarity medium. OMPs in lane 3 correspond to the same preparation of lane 2 but treated with phenol to remove exopolysaccharides. OmpA is labeled with an asterisk, and arrowheads indicate porins.

molecular mass of about three times that of the monomer (boiled) sample, then the isolated OMP is probably a porin.

7. Most *K. pneumoniae* clinical isolates express OmpK36 and OmpK35 ***(16)***, the two major porins of this species and the respective homologues of *E. coli* porins OmpC and OmpF. However, clinical isolates expressing ESBLs and thus with increased resistance to many β-lactams, express only porin OmpK36. OmpK35 is either very low or not expressed ***(16)***. Due to their close molecular masses, kDa for OmpK36 and 37.2 kDa for OmpK35, as deduced from their corresponding gene sequences (GenBank/EMBL accession numbers AJ011501 and Z33506), optimal resolution of the two porins required a careful investigation of the electrophoretic conditions. As shown in **Fig. 1**, when *K. pneumoniae* OMPs were analyzed in urea-containing gels ***(17)*** that resolve well *E. coli* porins produced unresolved bands. This fact may be due to a side effect of the exopolysaccharides content in OMPs preparations of *K. pneumoniae* clinical isolates, since phenol treatment of the OMPs preparation prior to electrophoresis seemed to ameliorate their resolution.
8. Another problem found with this type of analysis when applied to OMPs of *K. pneumoniae* is that isolates often differ in the electrophoretic patterns of their porin (**Fig. 2**). Independently of the expression of two or one porin, it has been observed that porins from different clinical isolates may run in the gels with different molecular masses, and for some isolates resolution of the two porins requires changing the *bis*-acrylamide content of the resolving gel. Clearly, as shown in **Fig. 2**, the same OMPs preparation analyzed in 0.21% *bis*-acrylamide gels (lane 4) shows only one porin, whereas when analyzed in 0.55% *bis*-

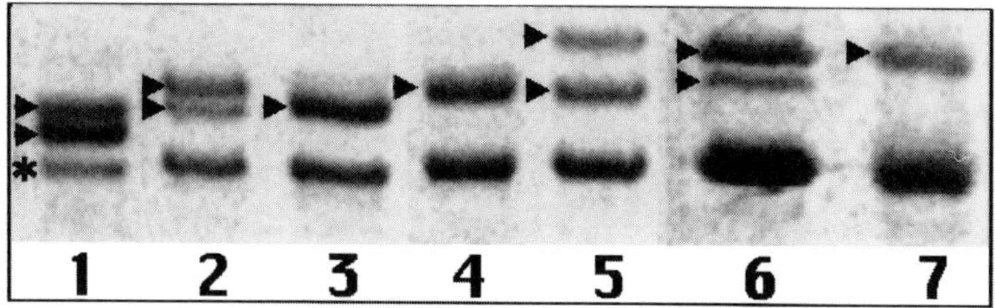

Fig. 2. SDS-PAGE analysis of OMPs preparations from clinical isolates of *K. pneumoniae* grown in low osmolarity medium. Preparations were analyzed in 11% acrylamide-0.21% *bis*-acrylamide gels as described in the protocol. The same preparation of lane 4 was also analyzed in a 11% acrylamide-0.55% *bis*-acrylamide gel (lane 5). On lanes 6 and 7, OMPs were extracted from the same isolate grown in low (lane 6) and high (lane 7) osmolarity culture media, respectively Nutrient Broth and Luria-Bertani. Porins and OmpA are labeled with arrowheads and asterisks, respectively.

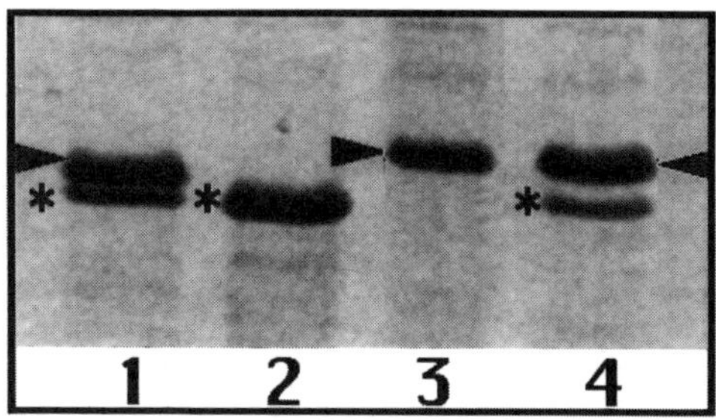

Fig. 3. SDS-PAGE analysis of two clonally related *K. pneumoniae* isolates expressing ESBLs. OMPs is lane 1 correspond to the more sensitive clone1 and lane 2 to the clone with increased resistance (clone 2). Lane 3 shows the OMP isolated from clone 1 by a porin isolation method. In lane 4, porin expression was restored in clone 2 by transformation with a plasmid containing the cloned OmpK36 porin. Porins are indicated by arrowheads, and OmpA by an asterisk.

acrylamide gels (lane 5), the two porins are resolved well. Identification of OmpK36 and OmpK35 in isolates producing both porins can be facilitated by analyzing OMPs isolated from cells grown in low and high osmolarity culture media. As shown in **Fig. 2**, the same isolate expresses both porins in low osmolarity media (lane 6), whereas in high osmolarity media OmpK35 expression is down-regulated at the expenses of porin OmpK36, the osmoporin of *K. pneumoniae* ***(14)***. As said before, when analyzing isolates expressing ESBLs, the situation is simpler because most of them express only one porin. This situation has been described before for clonally related isolates from outbreaks *(3,5)* and can also be seen in **Fig. 3**. In this type of isolates, when the initial more sensitive strain (lane 1) and the derived clone with increased resistance (lane 2) are available for analysis, comparison of their OMPs shows that an OMP, presumably a porin, is lost in the resistant clone. The porin nature of the missed OMP can be deduced from the facts that it can be isolated by a porin isolation method (lane 3) and because the resistant clone reverts its MICs for antibiotics not degraded by the ESBLs present in the isolate to the sensitive levels after porin expression from the cloned gene (lane 4).

References

1. Jacoby, G. A. (1996) Antimicrobial-resistant pathogens in the 1990s. *Annu. Rev. Med.* **47,** 169–179.
2. Sirot, D. (1995) Extended-spectrum plasmid-mediated beta-lactamases. *J. Antimicrob. Chemother.* **36,** 19–34.
3. Ardanuy, C., Liñares, J., Domínguez, M. A., Hernández-Allés, S., Benedí, V. J., and Martínez-Martínez, L. (1998) Outer membrane profiles of clonally related *Klebsiella pneumoniae* isolated from clinical samples and activity of cephalosporins and carbapenems. *Antimicrob. Agents Chemother.* **42,** 1636–1640.
4. Martínez-Martínez, L., Pascual, A., Hernández-Allés, S., Álvarez-Díaz, D., Suárez, A. I., Tran, J., Benedí, V. J., and Jacoby, G. A. (1999) Role of β-lactamases and porins in the activity of carbapenems and cephalosporins against *Klebsiella pneumoniae*. *Antimicrob. Agents Chemother.*, **43,** 1669–1673.
5. Martínez-Martínez, L., Hernández-Allés, S., Albertí, S., Tomás, J. M., Benedí, V. J., and Jacoby, G. A. (1996) In vivo selection of porin deficient mutants of *Klebsiella pneumoniae* with increased resistance to cefoxitin and third generation cephalosporins. *Antimicrob. Agents Chemother.* **40,** 342–348.
6. Martínez-Martínez, L., García, I., Ballesta, S., Benedí, V. J., Hernández-Allés, S., and Pascual, A. (1998) Energy-dependent accumulation of fluoroquinoles in quinolone-resistant *Klebsiella pneumoniae* strains. *Antimicrob. Agents Chemother.* **42,** 1850–1852.
7. Hernández-Allés, S., Benedí, V. J., Martínez-Martínez, L., Pascual, A., Aguilar, A., Tomás, J. M., and Albertí, S. (1999) Development of resistance during antimicrobial therapy caused by insertion sequence interruption of porin genes. *Antimicrob. Agents Chemother.* **43,** 937–939.
8. Osborn, M. J. and Munson, R. (1974) Separaton of the inner (cytoplasmic) and outer membranes of Gram-negative bacteria. *Methods Enzymol* **31,**642–667.
9. Filip, C., Fletcher, G., Wulf, J. L., and Earhart, C. F. (1973) Solubilization of the cytoplasmic membrane of *Escherichia coli* by the ionic detergent sodium-lauryl sarcosinate. *J. Bacteriol.* **115,** 717–722.
10. Sarvas, M. (1985) Membrane fractionation methods, in *Enterobacterial Surface Antigens. Methods for Molecular Characterisation* (Korhonen, T. K., Dawes, E. A., and Mäkelä, P. H., eds.), Elsevier, Amsterdam, pp. 111–122.
11. Tomás, J. M., Benedí, V. J., Ciurana, B., and Jofre, J. (1986) Role of capsule and O antigen in resistance of *Klebsiella pneumoniae* to serum bactericidal activity. *Infect. Immun.* **54,** 85–89.

12. Albertí, S., Marqués, G., Camprubí, S., Merino, S., Tomás, J. M., Vivanco, F., and Benedí, V. J. (1993) C1q binding and activation of the complement classical pathway by *Klebsiella pneumoniae* outer membrane proteins. *Infect. Immun.* **61,** 852–860.
13. Albertí, S., Rodríguez-Quiñones, F., Schirmer, T., Rummel, G., Tomás, J. M., Rosenbusch, J. P., and Benedí, V. J. (1995) A porin from *Klebsiella pneumoniae*: Sequence homology, three-dimensional structure, and complement binding. *Infect. Immun.* **63,** 903–910.
14. Dutzler, R., Rummel, G., Albertí, S., Hernández-Allés, S., Phale, P. S., Rosenbusch, J. P., Benedí, V. J., and Schirmer, T. (1999) Crystal structure and functional characterization of OmpK36, the osmoporin from *Klebsiella pneumoniae. Structure* **7,** 425–434.
15. Doménech-Sánchez, A., Hernández-Allés, S., Martínez-Martínez, L., Benedí, V. J., and Albertí, S. (1999) Identification and characterization of a new porin gene of *Klebsiella pneumoniae*: its role in β-lactam antibiotics resistance. *J. Bacteriol.* **181,** 2726–2732.
16. Hernández-Allés, S., Albertí, S., Álvarez, D., Doménech-Sánchez, A., Martínez-Martínez, L., Gil, J., Tomás, J. M., and Benedí, V. J. (1999) Porin expression in clinical isolates of *Klebsiella pneumoniae. Microbiology* **145,** 673–679.
17. Mizuno, T. and Kageyama, M. (1978) Separation and characterization of the outer membrane of *Pseudomonas aeruginosa. J. Biochem.* **84,** 179–191.
18. Sambrook, J., Fritsch, E. F., and Maniatis, T. (1989) Molecular cloning, Cold Spring Harbor Laboratory, Cold Spring Harbor, New York.
19. Tsai, C.-M. and Frasch, C. E. (1982) A sensitive silver stain for detecting lipopolysaccharides in polyacrylamide gels. *Anal. Biochem.* **119,** 115–119.

20

Atomic Force Microscopy

Theory and Practice in Bacteria Morphostructural Analysis

Pier Carlo Braga and Davide Ricci

1. Introduction

The production of the first "microscope" between the end of the sixteenth and the beginning of the seventeenth century was a true breakthrough in the advance of civilization *(1)*. Without the microscope, the natural, biological, medical, and other sciences would not be what they are today. After the optical microscope, a second breakthrough in the analysis of surface morphology occurred in the 1940s with the development of the scanning electron microscope (SEM). Instead of light (photons) and glass lenses, electrons and electromagnetic lenses (magnetic coils) are used to explore the sample. Optical and scanning (or transmission) electron microscopes are classified as "far field microscopes" because the distance between the sample and the point at which the image is obtained is long in comparison with the wavelengths of the photons or electrons involved. In this case, the image is a diffraction pattern and its resolution is wavelength limited *(2,3)*: in optical microscopy, resolution is determined by the Nyquist relation to the wavelength of the light used (typically about 1 μm); in a general purpose SEM, it is limited by the properties of the electromagnetic lenses (typically about 50Å) *(4)*.

In 1986, a completely new type of microscopy was proposed: without lenses, photons or electrons, it involves the mechanical scanning of samples *(5)* and opened up unexpected possibilities for the surface analysis of biological specimens. Initially called the "scanning force microscope" (SFM), it was a development of the previous "scanning tunnelling microscope" (STM) *(6)* which provided information at atomic resolution of specimens that are electrically conducing. Because SFMs involve interactions between atomic forces (about

From: *Methods in Molecular Medicine, vol. 48: Antibiotic Resistance Methods and Protocols*
Edited by: S. H. Gillespie © Humana Press Inc., Totowa, NJ

10^{-9} Newton), they are also and more frequently called "atomic force microscope" (AFMs) ***(4)***. These new types of "scanning probe microscopes" (SPMs) are based on the concept of "near field microscopy," which overcomes the problem of the limited diffraction-related resolution inherent in conventional microscopes. Located in the immediate vicinity of the sample itself (usually within a few nanometers), the probe records the "intensity" and not the "interference signal," and this greatly improves resolution ***(2)***. As shown in **Fig. 1**, AFM explores the surface of a sample not by means of a system of lenses that form an image using the diffraction patterns of rays of different wavelengths, but by means of a very small sharp-tipped probe located at the free end of a cantilever driven by the interatomic repulsive or attractive forces (van der Waals forces) between the molecules at the probe tip and those on the surface of the specimen. This can be done by scanning the sample laterally (x-y) whereas a closed loop control system keeps the tip in proximity to the surface by adjusting the z position of the sample. In most AFMs, tip movements are monitored by reflecting a laser beam from the back of the cantilever on to a position sensitive photodiode ***(7)***.

AFM is extremely useful for analyzing the tridimensional structure of the surface of biological specimens ***(8)***, particularly bacteria. Although SEM is still frequently used, the introduction of the AFM technique offers substantial benefits: real quantitative data acquisition in three dimensions, minimal sample preparation times; flexibility in ambient operating conditions (i.e., no vacuum is necessary), and effective magnifications at submicron level ***(9)***.

There are numerous definitions of bacterial resistance to antibiotics depending upon not necessarily overlapping criteria: genetic (versus the parent), biochemical (mechanism of action), microbiological (minimum inhibitory concentrations), any clinical (therapeutical effects). Investigating the surface of bacteria also offers the possibility of investigating the efficacy (mechanism of action) of antibiotics that disrupt their structure as an epiphenomenon of internal biochemical action (i.e., β-lactams) ***(10–12)***, and at the same time the possibility of investigating their lack of activity, as in the case of resistance.

2. Materials

1. Test organisms. Both Gram-positive and Gram-negative bacteria are suitable for AFM.
2. Triptic soy broth (Sigma, Milano, Italy).
3. Phosphate buffer saline (PBS) (0.02 *M* phosphate and 0.15 *M* NaCl, pH 7.3).

Fig. 1. *(opposite page)* Comparative schematic view of the elements characterizing light microscopy (LM), scanning electron microscopy (SEM) and atomic force microscopy (AFM), together with their specific technical parameters.

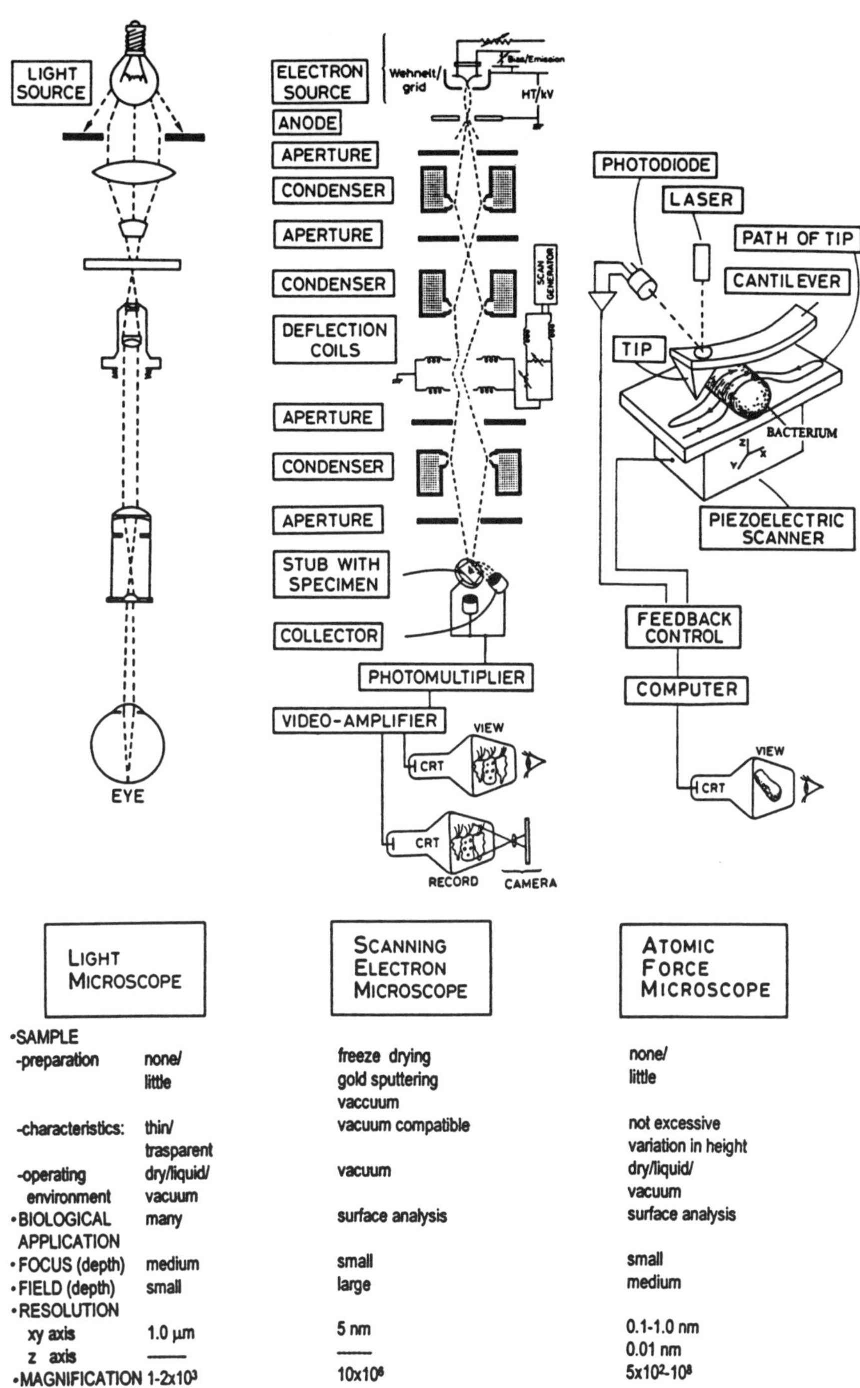

	LIGHT MICROSCOPE	SCANNING ELECTRON MICROSCOPE	ATOMIC FORCE MICROSCOPE
•SAMPLE			
-preparation	none/ little	freeze drying gold sputtering vaccuum	none/ little
-characteristics:	thin/ trasparent	vacuum compatible	not excessive variation in height
-operating environment	dry/liquid/ vacuum	vacuum	dry/liquid/ vacuum
•BIOLOGICAL APPLICATION	many	surface analysis	surface analysis
•FOCUS (depth)	medium	small	small
•FIELD (depth)	small	large	medium
•RESOLUTION			
xy axis	1.0 μm	5 nm	0.1-1.0 nm
z axis	——	——	0.01 nm
•MAGNIFICATION	$1\text{-}2 \times 10^3$	10×10^6	$5 \times 10^2\text{-}10^8$

4. Glutaraldehyde (2.5% in 0.1 *M* cacodylate buffer, pH 7.1).
5. Graded alcohols (60%, 70%, 80%, 90%, 100%).
6. Incubator.
7. Centrifuge.
8. Micropipet.
9. Round glass cover slides 6–7 mm (or mica).
10. Atomic Force Microscope included probe-tips, software for processing signals and three-dimension rendering, computer (Park Scientific Instruments, Sunnyvale, CA).

3. Methods

1. The culture of chosen microorganism is prepared according to common standard procedures.
2. Wash the test microorganism from the suspension in broth (i.e., 10^6 cells/mL) three times with PBS.
3. Resuspend the final pellet in 1–2 mL of PBS.
4. Collect 0.1 mL (or less) of this suspended bacteria using a micropipet and place it on a round glass cover slide (*see* **Note 1**).
5. Dry the cover slip in air.
6. Fix with 2.5% glutaraldehyde in 0.1 *M* cacodylate buffer (pH = 7.1).
7. Dehydrate in graded alcohols.
8. Dry the coverslip in air (*see* **Note 2**).
9. AFM observation (*see* **Notes 3** and **4**). A typical AFM imaging session begins by firmly fixing the sample cover slide to the microscope holder in order to avoid even the slightest movement (*see* **Note 5**), and then positioning it under the probe tip and locating the area of interest by moving the x-y table.
10. A good quality on-axis optical microscope is essential in order to be able to position the probe tip in the proximity of a bacterium to be imaged by AFM. As bacteria are about 1 μm in size, it is necessary to have appropriate lighting conditions to distinguish them from any debris on the slide surface. In the experiments described here a reflection optical microscope equipped with long range objectives was used. Although the cantilever bearing the probe partially obstructs the optical view of the underlying bacteria, it does allow the probe to be positioned sufficiently accurately in the area of interest (*see* **Notes 6** and **7**). Commercial AFM instrumentation coupled to a transmitted light optical microscope offers a higher degree of precision in the first approach of the probe to the sample (*see* **Note 8**).
11. Once an area has been located after the tip-to-sample approach, a first large scan (i.e., 30 by 30 μm) using a high scan speed and small number of pixels per line can be made in order to assess its exact position within the scanner coordinate system, identify the nature of the bacteria and select an interesting one. Further smaller scans may be necessary in order to position the bacterium exactly at the center of the scanning area.
12. Record high resolution images (*see* **Note 6**) using appropriate instrument settings depending on the imaging mode selected (contact, intermittent contact,

noncontact) (*see* **Note 7**). In general, accurate feedback setting is necessary in order to obtain the maximum possible gain for the resolution of bacterial surface structures although avoiding oscillation when scanning along the cell sidewalls.

13. Acquire image (typically acquired at 512 × 512 pixels) and process by means of plane fitting, high frequency filtering and three-dimensional shaded rendering (**Fig. 2**).
14. Postprocessing analysis and the spatial representation of AFM-generated data is essential in order to extract all of the available information from the image dataset. As the recorded data is an intrinsically three-dimensional digital matrix (the height of the sample recorded at each x,y coordinate), the software makes it easy to obtain numerical data of cross-sections of interesting features expressed with subnanometer accuracy (*see* **Note 8**). The same software allows three-dimensional rendering of the surface and rotation in space so that only one acquisition is needed to be able to observe the same object from many different points of view (*see* **Notes 9–11**).

4. Notes.

1. It is better to use low concentrations of bacteria because they tend to concentrate in small areas during the air drying phase, whereas a single bacterium provides a clearer image. Be sure to mark the location of your specimen on the upper surface of your round glass cover slide in order to avoid wasting time investigating the wrong side.
2. If the sample is kept dry, repeated sessions can generally be performed without any loss of resolution.
3. Bacterial sample preparation for AFM is very simple and rapid. There is no need for critical point drying, which also avoids shrinkage effects; there is no need for gold sputtering, a procedure that covers and smooths fine surface details. There is no need for vacuum conditions as with SEM.
4. A recent technical evolution has also opened up the possibility of using AFM on wet samples i.e., living cells immersed in biological fluids in culture chambers (*13,14*).
5. Care must be taken when choosing the adhesive used for fixing the glass slide to the sample holder. Avoid using thick double-sided adhesive tape, as this can expand for a long time after pressure and thus cause instability in the vertical position of the tip. The specially produced sticky tabs made by different manufacturers are fine as are thin double-sided tape obtained from the stationery store.
6. To obtain the best results, it is necessary to be thoroughly familiar with the characteristics of different cantilevers and tips, how these can be used and how they suit to the different kinds of samples investigated. For high resolution work, tip sharpness is essential: tip properties can vary significantly within the same batch of cantilevers. Fine tuning of the feedback loop and set point, together with the chosen scan speed, is critical for good surface tracking.
7. As mentioned above, AFM offers different imaging modes for investigating the sample. There is the "contact mode" in which the tip of the probe makes soft

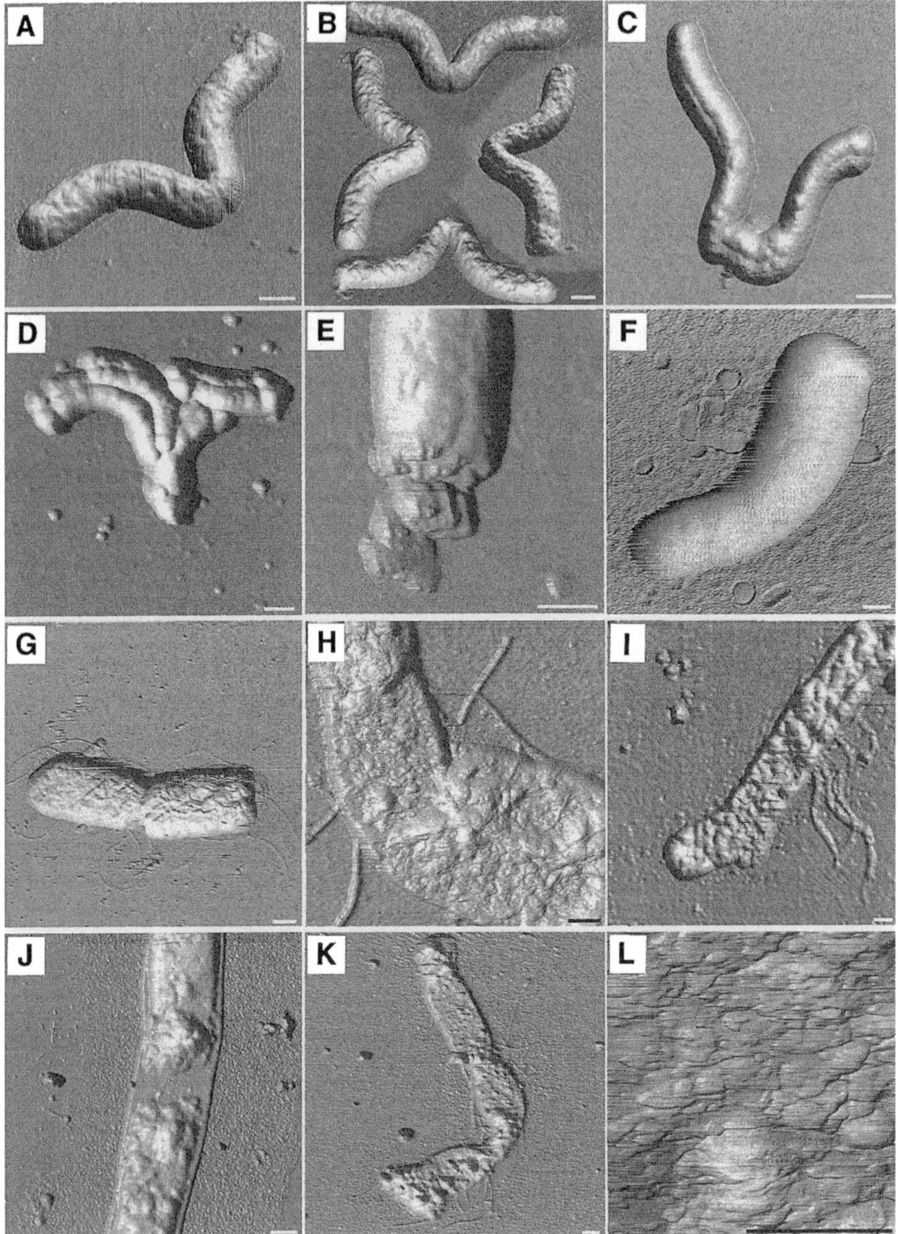

Fig. 2. Atomic force pictures of *H. pylori* and *E. coli*. The bar at the bottom right of each picture corresponds to 500 nanometers. **(A)** Common morphology of *H. pylori* without exposure to antibiotic. **(B)** Example of the different perspectives obtained by means of computer processing. **(C–E)** Different alterations induced in *H. pylori* by

"physical contact" with the sample, which should be used with harder and stiffer materials than biological samples as it can easily give rise to undesirable effects due to tip-to-sample interactions (**Fig. 2L**). Tip pressure can indent and deform the sample surface, and lateral forces can stretch the sample, drag away loosely bound fragments or even detach the whole bacterium from the substrate *(4)*. These drawbacks of the contact AFM mode are overcome by using the "intermittent-contact mode," also called "tapping mode." In this case, the AFM feedback loop constantly dampens the high frequency oscillations of the vibrating cantilever due to the tip coming into contact with the surface for a very short time *(15)*. For this reason, indentation effects are less invasive, lateral forces are greatly reduced, and a high lateral resolution can be maintained. In the third "noncontact mode," small amplitude and high frequency oscillations induced on the cantilever allow the feedback control loop to maintain the tip-to-sample distance within the range of attractive Van der Waals forces. Tip-to-sample interactions are greatly reduced, at the expense of lateral resolution and the scanning speed *(3)*. For biological specimens the noncontact and intermittent-contact are the most suitable, although the contact mode may be used for high resolution work on very small areas.

8. In order to make accurate dimensional measurements, the calibration of the AFM's piezoelectric scanner has to be periodically checked. The procedures are usually described in the instrument manual. Lateral dimension calibration is relatively straightforward, but special care must be taken when calibrating height. We used a very large scale integration (VLSI) standard calibration grid (NIST traceable) with a 100 nanometer nominal step height and an in-house developed statistical analysis procedure for calibration.
9. The images may sometimes be blurred as a result of poor washing procedures, an electrostatic charge on the specimen, improper feedback parameter settings, debris on the tip, or an eroded tip (**Fig. 2F**).
10. The images of spherical bacteria such as *S. aureus* will suffer from little lateral resolution along the perimeter, owing to the perpendicular direction of analysis. In general the shape of the tip and its lateral walls will limit the detection of steep elevated features (**Fig. 3**).
11. After image acquisition, the built-in software allows the rendering of the picture to be greatly improved by means of shadowing, rotation, different illumination, and different points of view (**Fig. 2B**).

---

exposure to sub-MICs and supra-MICs of rokitamycin. **(F)** Example of artifacts. High frequency oscillations and lack of bacterium surface detail can be due to feedback instabilities induced by an electrostatically charged sample. **(G)** Common morphology of *E. coli* without exposure to antibiotic. **(H–K)** Different alterations induced in *E. coli* by exposure to sub-MICs and supra-MICs of cefodizime. **(L)** Example of artifact produced by excessive tip-to-sample interactions in contact mode.

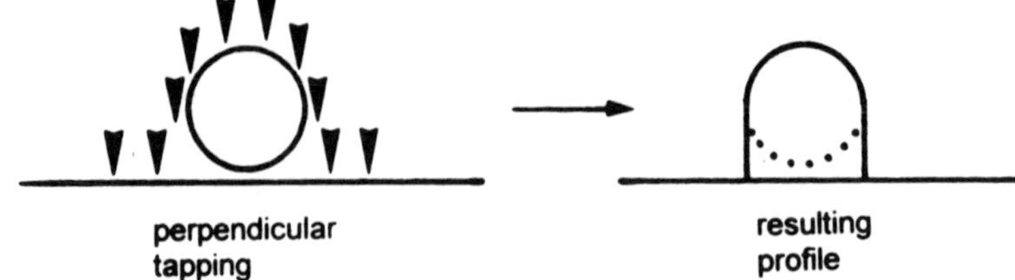

Fig. 3. Example of the AFM rendering of a spherical bacterium.

Acknowledgments

We would like to thank M. Dal Sasso and T. Zuccotti for preparing the bacterial samples. This study was partially supported by a grant from MURST (60%).

References

1. Breadbury, S. (1968) *The microscope, past and present*. Pergamon Press, Oxford.
2. Heckl, W. M. (1995) Scanning the thread of life, in *The Human Genome* (Fisher, E. P. and Klose, S., eds.), R. Piper GmbH & Co. KG, München, pp. 99–146.
3. Braga, P. C. and Ricci, D. (1998) Atomic force microscopy: Application to investigation of *Escherichia coli* morphology before and after exposure to cefodizime. *Antimicrob. Agents Chemother.* **42**, 18–22.
4. Strausser, Y. E. and Heaton, M. G. (1994) Scanning probe microscopy technology and recent innovations. *American Laboratory*, May 1–7.
5. Binning, G., Quate, C. F., and Gerber, C. (1986) Atomic force microscope. *Phys. Rev. Lett.* **12**, 930–933.
6. Binnig, G. and Rohrer, H. (1982) Scanning tunnelling microscopy. *Helv. Phys. Acta* **55,** 726–735.
7. Mc Donnel, L. and Phelan, M. (1998) The scanned cantilever AFM: a versatile tool for industrial application. *Microscopy and Analysis (European ed.)* **52**, 25–27.
8. Ratneshwar, L. and Scott, A. J. (1994) Biological applications of atomic force microscopy. *Am. J. Physiol.* **266**, C1-C21.
9. Campbell, P. A., Gordon, R., and Walmsley, D. G. (1998) Active surface modification by scanning tunnelling microscopy. *Microscopy and Analysis (European ed.)* **56**, 25–27.
10. Lorian, V. (1986) Effect of low antibiotic concentrations on bacteria: effects on ultrastructure, their virulence and susceptibility to immunodefenses, in *Antibiotics in Laboratory Medicine* (Lorian, V., ed.), Williams & Wilkins, Baltimore, pp. 596–668.
11. Lorian, V., Atkinson, B., Walushacka, A., and Kim, Y. (1982) Ultrastructure, in vitro and in vivo, of staphylococci exposed to antibiotics. *Curr. Microbiol.* **7**, 301–304.

12. Braga, P. C. and Ricci, D. (2000) Detection of rokitamycin-induced morphological alterations in *Helicobacter pylori*. *Chemotherapy* **46:** 15–22.
13. Nagao, E. and Dvorak, J. A., (1999) Developing atomic force microscope for studies of living cells. *Intern Lab.* 21–23.
14. Schaus, S. S. and Henderson, E. R., (1997) Cell viability and probe cell membrane interactions of XR1 glial cells imaged by atomic force microscopy. *Biophpys J* **73**: 1205–1214.
15. Howland, R. and Benatar, L. (1997) *A practical guide to scanning probe microscopy*. Park Scientific Instrument Ed., pp. 1–73.

IV

Biology of Resistance

21

Assessing the Activity of Bacterial Multidrug Efflux Pumps

Keith Poole and Ramakrishnan Srikumar

1. Introduction

Resistance to antibiotics in target bacterial populations has long complicated antibacterial chemotherapy. First described in the early 1980s *(1,2)*, efflux mechanism of resistance, whereby the antibiotic is actively (i.e., in an energy-dependent fashion) pumped from the bacterial cell, are being described with increasing frequency in recent years. Initial examples of bacterial antibiotic efflux systems were agent-specific, providing for export of and resistance to single agents (e.g., tetracyclines, chloramphenicol, macrolides) *(3)*. More recently, bacterial drug efflux systems of broad substrate specificity have been described *(4,5)*. These systems are able to accommodate a wide variety of structurally unrelated antibiotics, contributing to intrinsic and acquired multiple antibiotic (multidrug) resistance.

Assessment of drug efflux has traditionally relied on measurement of radiolabeled antibiotic accumulation inside the bacterial cell *(6,7)*. Alternatively, for a select few antibiotics exhibiting intrinsic fluorescence (e.g., tetracyclines and the fluoroquinolones), uptake into cells can be assessed using spectrofluorimetry *(2,8)*. In both instances, efflux activity correlates with reduced net accumulation of drug within the cell, and this low level accumulation is compromised (i.e., increased drug accumulation is observed) upon addition of an energy inhibitor. This energy-dependent "drug exclusion" is, in fact, a hallmark of drug efflux. Direct measurement of drug efflux is also possible using radiolabeled antibiotics (or fluorometry as above) *(2)*. In this instance, cells are "loaded" with the antibiotic under conditions where efflux activity is inhibited (absence of an energy source and presence of an energy inhibitor). Upon removal of the inhibitor and addition of an energy source, drug loss from the

From: *Methods in Molecular Medicine, vol. 48: Antibiotic Resistance Methods and Protocols*
Edited by: S. H. Gillespie © Humana Press Inc., Totowa, NJ

cells is measured directly, providing evidence for the presence of a drug efflux mechanism. For some efflux systems, efflux activity can also be measured in everted membrane vesicles, in which case the drug is accumulated inside the vesicles in an energy-dependent fashion ***(1)***.

The broad substrate specificity of the multidrug resistance (MDR) efflux systems, which also accommodate a range of dyes, detergents, and organic solvents ***(9,10)***, in addition to antibiotics, means that it is also possible to measure the efflux activity of such systems directly using fluorescent "dyes" as indicator substrates. Coupled with a fluorescence spectrophotometer, this permits the continuous monitoring of "drug" efflux, and doesn't require the sampling of cells at different time points to assess "drug" retention/expulsion over time, the latter being necessary when using radiolabeled antibiotics. The use of dyes to asses efflux is, obviously, limited to MDR systems which accommodate them, and cannot be used to monitor export by agent-specific efflux systems. Still, the ease of the assay, which avoids the need to separate cells from the radiolabeled drug in the growth medium (by filtration or centrifugation through silicone oil) and the attendant problems of background and low cell-associated counts, makes it an obvious choice where feasible. Acriflavine is a fluorescent molecule that is exported by a number of MDR efflux systems ***(9)***. The intrinsic fluorescence of acriflavine is significantly quenched inside cells, so that its export, via the efflux mechanism, results in an increase in fluorescence that can be measured by a fluorescence spectrophotometer. Typically, late log phase cells are used and acriflavine loading is accomplished by incubating the cells in the presence of the dye and an energy inhibitor (e.g., carbonyl cyanide *m*-chlorophenylhydrazone [CCCP]) for approx 60 min. The energy inhibitor prevents dye efflux during loading. After washing of the cells and adding an energy source (e.g., sodium formate or glucose) the release of acriflavine is assessed for 5–10 min. The protocol described here (adapted from ***[11]***) applies to *E. coli* cells and has been used in the author's laboratory to study efflux mediated by *P. aeruginosa* efflux systems cloned into *E. coli*.

2. Materials

1. For cultivation of bacteria, use a rich medium such as Luria-Bertani (LB) broth.
2. Sodium N-2-hydroxy-ethyl piperazine-N'-2-ethanesulfonate (HEPES): 20 m*M*, pH 7.0. Store at room temperature.
3. Acriflavine-HCl: 2 m*M* in 20 m*M* HEPES, pH 7.0. Store at room temperature in the dark.
4. Carbonyl cyanide *m*-chlorophenylhydrazone (CCCP): 10 m*M* in 50 % (v/v) ethanol. Make fresh and keep on ice. Can be stored overnight at –20°C.
5. Sodium formate: 1 *M*. Store at room temperature.
6. Fluorescence spectrophotometer.

3. Methods

1. Culture bacteria overnight in liquid culture (5 mL) with aeration. Dilute the overnight culture 1/100 into fresh medium (100 mL) and grow to an absorbance at 600 nm (A_{600}) of 1.0.
2. Harvest cells by centrifugation (6000*g* for 10 min at 4°C), wash twice with 50 mL of HEPES and resuspend the final cell pellet in 10 mL HEPES (*see* **Note 1**).
3. Add 100 µL acriflavine (20 µ*M* final concentration) and 20 µL CCCP (20 µ*M* final concentration), mix and incubate for 1 h at 37°C (*see* **Note 2**).
4. Harvest cells by centrifugation as above and resuspend in HEPES to an A_{600} of 10.
5. Add 1.86 mL HEPES to 40 µL of cells in a fluorescence spectrophotometer cuvet (1 cm path length) to promote mixing, and place cuvet into a fluorescence spectrophotometer hooked up to a chart recorder or other recording device. Using an excitation wavelength of 447 nm and an emission wavelength of 502, monitor fluorescence for 1–5 min to ensure that it is stable over time.
6. Initiate efflux by the addition of 100 µL sodium formate (*see* **Note 3**). Mix by pipeting up and down, and monitor the increase in fluorescence for 5–10 min. Typically, if efflux is observed (increase in acriflavine fluorescence with time the experiment is repeated and an energy inhibitor (e.g., CCCP at 20 µ*M* final concentration) is added at **step 5**, prior to the addition of the formate. This should inhibit efflux, thereby providing evidence that the efflux previously observed was, as expected, energy-dependent (*see* **Note 4**).

4. Notes

1. Bacterial cells used for the efflux assay can be prepared ahead of time. After completion of **steps 2** or **4**, cells can be stored on ice for up to 12–16 h before being used in the assay.
2. The assay can also be carried out using ethidium bromide in place of acriflavine, in which case ethidium bromide and CCCP are added to the cells at a final concentration of 10 and 20 µ*M*, respectively (**step 3**). 1.7 mL HEPES is ultimately added to 200 µL of cells (**step 5**) and the excitation and emission wavelengths are set at 467 nm and 580 nm, respectively. Because ethidium fluorescence is maximal inside cells, fluorescence is initially high and efflux is seen as a decrease in fluorescence over time. CCCP included prior to the addition of formate at the start of the efflux assay (for the purpose of assessing the energy-dependence of any efflux seen) is at a final concentration of 100 µ*M*. Additional fluorescent substrates have also been used to monitor the efflux activity of MDR efflux systems, including proflavin ***(11)*** and 1-(4-trimethylammoniumphenyl)-6-phenyl-1,3,5-hexatriene-*p*-toluenesulfonate (TMA-DPH) ***(12)***. Proflavine has enhanced intrinsic fluorescence over acriflavine, making the assay much more sensitive.
3. Other energy sources can be used in place of sodium formate, including glucose (at a final concentration of 50 m*M*).
4. The assay described was originally developed for use in *E. coli* but we have adapted it to assess the efflux activity of MDR efflux systems of *P. aeruginosa* by cloning the *P. aeruginosa* efflux genes into *E. coli* ***(13)***. In this instance the

use of an *E. coli* strain lacking its endogenous MDR efflux system acrAB, (e.g., KZM120) ***(14)*** is required, and the antibiotic appropriate for maintaining the efflux gene-containing plasmid must be included in the growth medium. Direct measurement of efflux activity of MDR efflux systems can also be made directly in the host from which the systems originates and, indeed, efflux assays have been described for organisms other than *E. coli*, including *P. aeruginosa* ***(12)***.

References

1. McMurry, L., Petrucci, R. E., and Levy, S. B. (1980) Active efflux of tetracycline encoded by four genetically different tetracycline resistance determinants in *Escherichia coli. Proc. Natl. Acad. Sci. USA* **77**, 3974–3977.
2. Ball, P. R., Shales, S. W., and Chopra, I. (1980) Plasmid-mediated tetracycline resistance in *Escherichia coli* involves increased efflux of the antibiotic. *Biochem. Biophys. Res. Commun.* **93**, 74–81.
3. Levy, S. B. (1992) Active efflux mechanisms for antimicrobial resistance. *Antimicrob. Agents Chemother.* **36**, 695–703.
4. Paulsen, I. T., Brown, M. H., and Skurray, R. A. (1996) Proton-dependent multidrug efflux systems. *Microbiol. Rev.* **60**, 575–608.
5. Bolhuis, H., van Ven, H. W., Poolman, B., Driessen, A. J. M., and Konings, W. N. (1997) Mechanisms of multidrug transporters. *FEMS Microbiol. Lett.* **21**, 55–84.
6. McMurry, L. M., George, A. M., and Levy, S. B. (1994) Active efflux of chloramphenicol in susceptible *Escherichia coli* strains and in multiple-antibiotic-resistant (Mar) mutants. *Antimicrob. Agents Chemother.* **38**, 542–546.
7. Li, X.-Z., Nikaido, H., and Poole, K. (1995) Role of MexA-MexB-OprM in antibiotic efflux in *Pseudomonas aeruginosa. Antimicrob. Agents Chemother.* **39**, 1948–1953.
8. Chapman, J. S. and Georgopapadakou, N. H. (1988) Fluorometric assay for fleroxacin uptake by bacterial cells. *Antimicrob. Agents Chemother.* **33**, 27–29.
9. Nikaido, H. (1996) Multidrug efflux pumps of Gram-negative bacteria. *J. Bacteriol.* **178**, 5853–5859.
10. Li, X.-Z., Zhang, L., and Poole, K. (1998) Role of the multidrug efflux systems of *Pseudomonas aeruginosa* in organic solvent tolerance. *J. Bacteriol.* **180**, 2987–2991.
11. Turner, R. J., Taylor, D. E., and Weiner, J. L. (1997) Expression of *Escherichia coli* TehA gives resistance to antiseptics and disinfectants similar to that conferred by multidrug resistance efflux pumps. *Antimicrob. Agents Chemother.* **41**, 440–444.
12. Ocaktan, A, Yoneyama, H, and Nakae, T. (1997) Use of fluorescence probes to monitor function of the subunit proteins of the MexA-MexB-OprM drug extrusion machinery in *Pseudomonas aeruginosa. J. Biol. Chem.* **272**, 21,964–21,969.
13. Srikumar, R., Kon, T., Gotoh, N., and Poole, K. (1998) Expression of *Pseudomonas aeruginosa* multidrug efflux pumps MexA-MexB-OprM and MexC-MexD-OprJ in a multidrug-sensitive *Escherichia coli* strain. *Antimicrob. Agents Chemother.* **42**, 65–71.
14. Ma, D., Cook, D. N., Alberti, M., Pon, N. G., Nikaido, H., and Hearst, J. E. (1995) Genes *acrA* and *acrB* encode a stress-induced system of *Escherichia coli. Mol. Microbiol.* **16**, 45–55.

22

The Use of a Continuous Culture System to Study the Antimicrobial Susceptibility of Bacteria in Biofilm

J. Keith Struthers

1. Introduction

The classical method for determining the minimum inhibitory concentration (MIC) and minimum bactericidal concentration (MBC) of an antibiotic is the tube test. Details of this test are well known and recognized methods are published *(1)*. The recent development of the E-test (AB Biotest, Solna, Sweden), has been a significant development in the determination of MIC. This system is straightforward to perform and is suitable for larger scale work.

1.1. The Characteristics of Biofilm Growth

The question arises as to whether the MIC and MBC values determined by current methods are relevant to interpreting the action of an antibiotic in an in vivo system. Determination of the MIC is performed in nutritionally rich media and the bacteria will undergo a single growth cycle in the tube multiplying logarithmically. In contrast, biofilms are considered to be a dynamic system of adherent and planktonic bacteria interacting within a continuous culture system. The growth conditions, rate of growth and availability of nutrients are likely to be very different from those found in broth culture in nutrient rich laboratory medium *(2)*. It is known that bacteria growing in a biofilm are less susceptible to antimicrobial agents than planktonic cells grown in broth culture and a number of workers have investigated this phenomenon *(3–6)*. This apparent resistance has been attributed to factors such as extracellular matrix production, simple physical barriers due to the biofilm itself and the accumulation of antibiotic inactivating enzymes such as β-lactamase *(7)*. Other factors may also influence the activity of antibiotics: phenotypic variation occurring

From: *Methods in Molecular Medicine, vol. 48: Antibiotic Resistance Methods and Protocols*
Edited by: S. H. Gillespie © Humana Press Inc., Totowa, NJ

through the depth of a biofilm may lead to the dominance of relatively sessile cells (organisms that are sedentary, attached either to a solid surface, or other organisms within the biofilm) at the base of the biofilm *(2)*. It is recognized that nutrient limitation affects both the growth rate and physiology of such cells *(8)*. A useful model for this is presented by Anwar et al. *(9)*, who detail the range of bacteria that may be found in a biofilm. Those on the surface of the biofilm will have properties, including antibiotic susceptibility, similar to planktonic bacteria. The accumulation of antibiotic inactivating enzymes within the biofilm matrix may protect physiologically susceptible bacteria. The nutritional deficiency of bacteria attached to a surface at the base of the biofilm may make these cells physiologically resistant to antibiotics.

1.2. The Biofilm Eradicating Concentration (BEC)

With the Sorbarod filter system described here, an established biofilm can be exposed to a single antibiotic concentration for a given period of time. After this, effluent containing planktonic bacteria can be collected, and the biofilm filter subsequently disintegrated by vortex mixing. The suspension of bacteria from both the biofilm and effluent can then be quantified *(10)*. The effluent MBC can be determined, as well as the biofilm eradicating concentration (BEC). The BEC is defined as the lowest concentration of an antibiotic that eliminates bacterial growth from a biofilm *(11)*.

1.3. Biofilm Models

A number of biofilm systems have been developed for laboratory use; these include the constant thickness biofilm fermenter *(12)* and the perfused biofilm fermenter *(13)*, both examples of continuous growth models. Details of various biofilm models have been reviewed previously *(14)*.

1.4. The Requirements of a Biofilm System for Antimicrobial Susceptibility Testing

In order for a biofilm system to have a use in routine antimicrobial susceptibility testing, it must be able to fulfill a number of criteria. These are:

1. The system must be reproducible.
2. There must be sufficient individual biofilms available in one experiment to cover a meaningful range of antibiotic concentrations.
3. There must be a simple system for delivery of media to, and collection of effluent from all of the biofilms.
4. The number of connections that are involved in the system must be minimal, so as to minimize the possibility of contamination during assembly of the system.

5. Inoculation of the system must be designed to minimize the chance of contamination.
6. Retrograde bacterial growth from the biofilm along the broth feed tubes to the stock feed bottles must be prevented by a simple mechanism.
7. It should be possible to collect effluent fluid containing planktonic bacteria at any time before the biofilm is sacrificed and titrated.

1.5. The Sorbarod Filter System

As a system, the Sorbarod filter model is able to satisfy these criteria and its use is described here. The initial work defining the Sorbarod biofilm system showed that the system maintained both *Staphylococcus aureus* and *Pseudomonas aeruginosa* at concentrations of 10^8–10^9 cfu/mL for up to 100 h ***(15)***. The system has been used for the growth of other bacteria. Budhani and Struthers ***(16)*** showed that the Sorbarod system maintained *Streptococcus pneumoniae* for at least 96 h, where the number of recoverable cfu/filter was in excess of 10^{12} from 24 h after inoculation of the filters. The titer of the planktonic bacteria in effluent was in the order of 10^8 cfu/mL. Muli and Struthers ***(17,18)*** achieved similar titers in their studies of the growth of *Gardnerella vaginalis* and *Lactobacillus acidophilus*. Similar titers were obtained with *Enterococcus faecalis*, whereas *Candida albicans* achieved biofilm concentrations of 10^9 cfu/filter ***(19)***.

1.6. The Use of the Sorbarod Biofilm System in Antimicrobial Susceptibility Testing

As the Sorbarod biofilm system satisfies the criteria for a useful system set out above, it has been adapted to investigate the antimicrobial susceptibilities of several organisms ***(16,18,20)***. The system employs a 12 channel peristaltic pump, enabling 12 Sorbarod filters to be run in one experiment. This allows for 1 or 2 control biofilms to be run in conjunction with 10 or 11 test biofilms, each exposed to a different concentration of an antibiotic. The Sorbarod system has been used to investigate the susceptibility of *S. pneumoniae* to the β-lactam antibiotics benzyl penicillin, amoxycillin, co-amoxiclav, and cefuroxime; with this organism it was shown that this biofilm mode of growth did not reduce its susceptibility ***(16)***. The system was also used to examine the protective effect of β-lactamase producing *Moraxella catarrhalis* in being able to "rescue" penicillin sensitive pneumococcus from the effects of benzyl penicillin and amoxycillin ***(20)***. The antibiotic susceptibility of *G. vaginalis* and *L. acidophilus* with the Sorbarod system has also been investigated ***(18)***. These workers were also able to assess the spatial arrangement of organisms within the filter, as the filters were processed by being embedded in wax, sectioned, and gram stained.

2. Materials

2.1. General Requirements

In order to run an experiment with the Sorbarod system, sufficient materials must be prepared for 12 filters, and the following items are needed.

1. Sorbarod cellulose filters 20-mm length × 10-mm diameter (Ilacon, Tonbridge UK).
2. Autoclavable silicone tubing cut into twelve 10-cm lengths. The internal diameter of this housing tubing must be 10 mm.
3. A12 channel peristaltic pump with drive unit #205U or 205S (Watson-Marlow, Falmouth, UK).
4. Silicon manifold tubing (#982.0063.000 Watson-Marlow).
5. Straight polypropylene connectors for tubing with an internal diameter of 0.5 to 0.8-mm (#999.2008.000 Watson Marlow).
6. T polypropylene connectors for tubing with an internal diameter of 0.5 to 0.8-mm (#999.3008.000 Watson Marlow).
7. Silicon connecting tubing internal diameter 0.8-mm (#910.0008.016 Watson-Marlow).
8. Automatic pipet.
9. Disposable pipet tips: 200 μL.
10. Disposable tips (polypropylene clear) volume range 2–10 mL.
11. 12-mm aluminum test tube caps (Oxoid).
12. Sterile 150 mL medical white flint glass bottles, with white plastic tops ("medical flats").
13. Two 2 L Duran media bottles with plastic tops.
14. Twelve 250 mL Duran media bottles without tops.
15. Aluminum foil.
16. Autoclave tape.
17. Brain heart Infusion broth (BHI) or other broth suitable for susceptibility testing.
18. 37°C incubator of sufficient size to take all the assembled apparatus (*see* **Note 1**)

2.2. Items Needed to Assemble One Sorbarod Filter System with Delivery Tubing and Effluent Collection

In order to prepare one complete filter system the following is needed:

1. Three lengths of silicone connecting tubing; A: 45-cm, B:25-cm, C: 30-cm (*see* **Fig. 1**).
2. One T connector.
3. One manifold tubing.
4. One straight connector.
5. One metal cap.
6. One yellow tip. Cut off and discard the 10-mm tip section.
7. 10-cm length silicone housing tubing with internal diameter of 10 mm.
8. One 2–10 mL volume tip. Cut off and discard top and bottom 30 mm. Central section is retained.

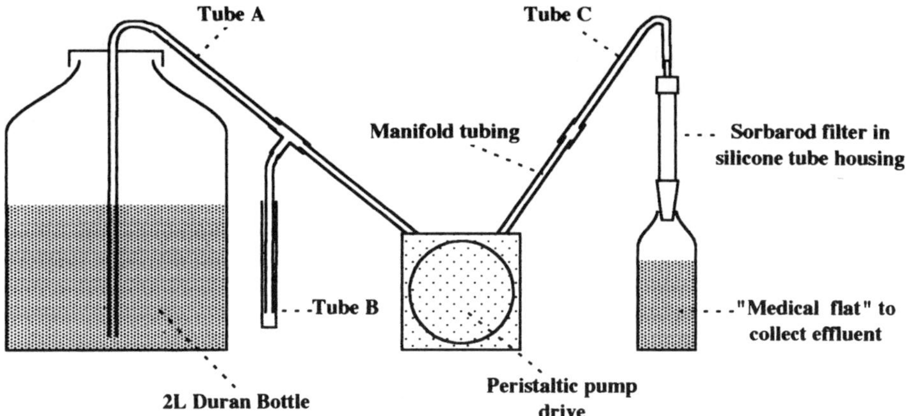

Fig. 1. Diagrammatic representation of a complete filter unit. "Feed" broth from the 2 L Duran bottle is delivered to the filter system by tube A, the pump manifold tube and tube C. Once a biofilm is established, the aluminum foil sleeve on tube B is removed and the end of this tube placed in a 250 mL Duran bottle with antibiotic containing broth. A clamp on tube B is moved to clamp off tube A.

9. One white plastic cap of "medical flat" bottle. A central hole with a diameter of 10-mm must be cut.
10. Removable tube clamps (e.g., Bibby clamp).
11. One Sorbarod filter.

3. Methods

3.1. General Preparation

1. Using suitable workshop equipment, make holes in the tops of the plastic and metal caps. For each plastic Duran cap, two holes that can take three silicone connecting tubes (A), should be made. Holes with a diameter of about 8 mm are sufficient.
2. Make a hole with a diameter of 4 mm in the center of the Oxoid metal cap. The hole should be punched from the inside out.
3. Make a 10-mm hole in the plastic tops that fit the 150 mL "medical flat" bottles.

3.2. Assembly of One Complete Sorbarod Filter System

There is a separate assemble for each Sorbarod filter (*see* **Fig. 1**).

1. Insert one end of tube A into the hole made for three tubes in the top of the Duran bottle. This tube is fed into the cap to a length of about 25 cm.
2. Insert the next two tube As in the same way.
3. Seal the three tubes placed through one hole of this cap with autoclave tape to ensure that there are no routes for external contamination of the system after autoclaving.

4. Repeat this process for the second set of three tubes and the second Duran bottle.
5. Connect each Tube A to the manifold tubing by the T connector.
6. Attach each Tube B to the side arm of the T connector.
7. Wrap the far end of this tube in a sleeve of aluminum foil with a length of 20 cm. This aluminum sleeve is tethered to the tubing by a piece of autoclave tape.
8. Clamp this tube adjacent to the T connector.
9. Attach Tube C to the other end of the manifold tube by the straight connector.
10. Insert the free end of this tube into the upper end of the cut yellow plastic tip (*see* **Notes 2** and **3**).
11. Place the tip into the hole made in the Oxoid metal cap.
12. Seal the two resulting joints with autoclave tape.
13. Insert a Sorbarod filter is inserted into one end (lower) of the 10-cm length silicone housing tube so that the lower end of the filter is 2 cm from the end of this tube.
14. Insert the cut 2–10 mL volume tip over the lower end of the silicone tube, and insert the free end of this tip into the hole in the white plastic "medical flat" bottle.
15. Seal the two joints with autoclave tape.
16. Attach a "medical flat" into position.

The separate parts for the assembly of the Sorbarod filter in the silicone tubing housing are shown in **Fig. 2**.

3.3. Assembly of the Complete System for Autoclaving

Flow rates of 6 mL/hour/filter have been used for experiments with a number of bacteria in the Sorbarod system ***(16–18,20)***. Each filter will thus require about 150 mL broth over 24 h, therefore each 2 L Duran bottle should have at least 1 L of medium to "feed" 6 filters for a 24 h period.

1. Place the prepared media in the Duran bottles with the free ends of the six "A" tubes free at the bottom of the bottle.
2. Adjust the length through the autoclave tape seal to rectify any positioning problems.
3. Tighten the cap of the bottle.
4. Place the metal capped end of tube C over the top of the 10-cm silicon tube housing the Sorbarod filter and fix by a short piece of autoclave tape.
5. Once all 12 filter systems have been assembled autoclave the entire apparatus consisting of 2 × 2 L Duran bottles and 12 complete filter systems.

3.4. Final assembly and Inoculation of the Filters

3.4.1. Attaching the Peristaltic Pump

1. Following removal of the apparatus from the autoclave and subsequent cooling, insert the 12 manifold tubes into the cassettes of the peristaltic pump.
2. Clamp the tubes onto the drive shaft and pump the media through the tubing until it is seen running through tube C. This step is essential to ensure that all the

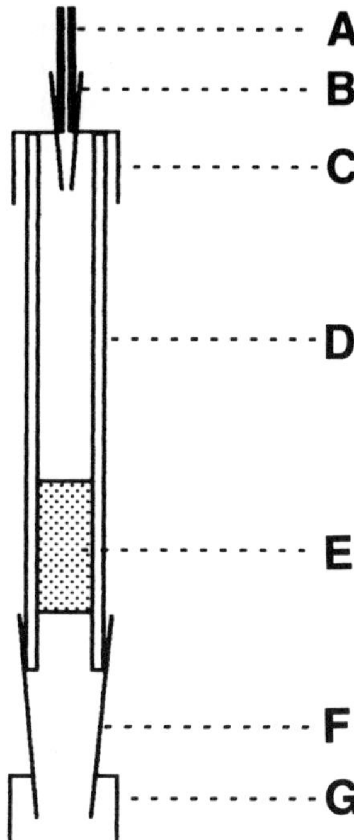

Fig. 2. Diagrammatic representation of the Sorbarod filter assembly. **(A)** silicone connecting tube delivering broth; **(B)** cut yellow tip; **(C)** metal cap; **(D)** silicone housing tubing; **(E)** Sorbarod filter; **(F)** cut 2–10 mL tip; **(G)** plastic cap of "medical flat" bottle.

delivery systems are functioning and that any blocked systems are identified prior to inoculation. An outline of the completely assembled system is shown in **Fig. 1**.

3.4.2. Preparation of the Inoculum

Prepare an exponential phase broth culture. For bacteria such as *P. aeruginosa*, *E. faecalis, M. catarrhalis, G. vaginalis*, and *L. acidophilus* broth cultures incubated overnight at 37°C are suitable ***(17–20)***. For *S. pneumoniae* broth cultures were incubated for 4–6 h before inoculation of the filters ***(16)*** (*see* **Note 4**).

3.4.3. Inoculation of the Filters

1. Remove the autoclave tape joined between the metal cap and silicone tube housing and soak each filter with 3–5 mL of the "feed" broth prior to inoculation of each biofilter film.
2. Dispense 3 mL of the exponential phase broth culture of the test organism onto each filter (*see* **Note 5**).

3. Seal the metal cap and silicone tubing housing with parafilm.
4. Loosen the cap on each 150 mL "medical flat" one half turn.
5. Deliver "feed" broth at the required rate to each filter.
6. Place the entire apparatus on a trolley in a 37°C "walk in" incubator (*see* **Notes 6–8**).

3.5. Determination of the Biofilm Eradicating Concentration

3.5.1. General

Determination of the BEC by the Sorbarod filter system is by the method reported previously ***(16,18,20)***.

1. Twenty four hours after inoculation, when steady-state growth is established, collect the effluent in the 150 mL "medical flat" and check for growth; no turbidity indicates that a biofilm has not been established on the filter (*see* **Note 9**).
2. If growth is evident, replace the bottles with empty sterile bottles.
3. In order to expose each established biofilm to a particular antibiotic concentration, carefully remove the aluminum foil sleeve from tube B, and place the end of this tube in a 250 mL Duran bottle containing one antibiotic concentration made up in 150 mL of the appropriate broth. The required number of these bottles are prepared prior to the experiment.
4. Replace the plastic cap with an aluminum foil cover that allows easy insertion of the side arm tubing B, thus maintaining the sterile environment. The aluminum foil top is carefully crimped over the tubing and sealed down with autoclave tape.
5. Shut off the broth "feed" from the 2 L Duran bottle and feed the antibiotic containing broth at the same flow rate onto each biofilm for 18 h.

3.5.2. Collection of Effluent and Harvesting the Biofilm

1. In order to obtain an effluent MBC at the end of the 18 h exposure period, place a new collection bottle and collect effluent for a fixed period such as 10 or 15 min.
2. Remove each filter unit by pulling out the end of tube C fitting into the yellow tip. Seal the exposed end of the yellow tip by crimping the autoclave tape at this site.
3. After the autoclave tape is removed from the base of the silicone tube housing, disconnect the tube and remove the filter with sterile tweezers.
4. Tear the paper sleeve and place each filter in 5 mL BHI in a sterile 30 mL standard container.
5. Mix by vortexing for 2 min to disintegrate the cellulose fibers. There is no need to separate off the fibers.

3.5.3. Titration of the Vortexed Biofilm and the Effluent

Both the effluent and biofilm vortex broths are titrated ***(10)***. The lowest concentration of the antibiotic that prevents bacterial growth in the effluent determines the effluent MBC. The concentration that sterilizes an established biofilm, determines the BEC. Titers for biofilm effluent are expressed as cfu/mL, in most cases the biofilm titer is expressed as total recoverable cfu/filter. This is obtained by multiplying the cfu/mL by a factor of 6.57. This takes into account the volume of the 20-mm length × 10-mm diameter filter plus the 5 mL of BHI added before vortex mixing.

3.6. Reuse of Equipment

Apart from the Sorbarod filters and the yellow plastic tips, the remainder of the apparatus may be recycled.

1. Place the cap, silicone tubing holder, and large tip overnight in a suitable laboratory disinfectant, then thoroughly clean and dry before reassembly (*see* **Notes 10** and **11**).
2. Remove the delivery tubing from the Duran cap and bottles, and run 10 mL of 70% ethanol, followed by 50 mL water through the tubing by means of the peristaltic pump.

4. Notes

1. A "walk in" incubator with all the equipment on a trolley is the best system.
2. The aperture at the cut end of the yellow tip must be greater than the 0.8 mm internal diameter of the silicone connecting tubing. A smaller aperture will create unnecessary resistance to flow, creating leaks.
3. Using the cut 200 µL tip to deliver "feed" broth to the filter, no back growth of a variety of organisms was observed ***(16–20)***. Other methods for the delivery of broth to the filter can also be considered ***(15)***.
4. It is clearly important to determine the growth characteristics of an organism on this filter system prior to any further experimental work with antibiotics. Previous workers ***(17)*** used the 12 filter system to examine the growth of *G. vaginalis* and *L. acidophilus* over a 96 h period. Such experiments determine the time taken for a particular organism to establish itself at a constant titer.
5. For inoculating the Sorbarod filters, it is always important to characterize the optimum growth conditions in broth culture of the organism being examined. Failure of the organism to "take" on the filter may be due to compromised viability.
6. All the equipment should be assembled and experiments performed on a trolley; incubation should preferably be done in a "walk in" incubator. Conducting experiments in a standard size incubator is at best difficult. If "feed" is delivered to the filters from a pump outside the incubator, there must be final assembly of the system inside the incubator. This leads to an increased chance of contamination.
7. After inoculation of the filters, it is worthwhile to place all the "medical flat" bottles in wire basket lined with an autoclavable plastic bag. On occasion "medical flats" or the autoclave tape seals may leak, and this procedure localizes spills and minimizes subsequent problems of decontamination.
8. Always check the system at the end of the working day to ensure that "feed" broth is being delivered to all the filters. This is done by checking the level of effluent broth accumulating in the "medical flats". This check is also important to ensure that the pump has not been turned off by mistake.

9. Recurrent problems with contamination by the coagulase negative staphylococci may occur. Scrupulous adherence to sterile technique, including stringent hand washing, usually resolves the situation. A worker soon becomes familiar with the appearance of the turbidity for a particular organism in the effluent bottles. If there is any doubt, it is always worthwhile to perform a gram stain on broth from effluent bottles before conducting a BEC experiment.
10. Always label the pot being used for decontamination of the reusable material clearly. Other laboratory staff may inadvertently discard useful materials.
11. Always identify a delivery system that is blocked. After the experiment, the entire tube and connectors should be dismantled and cleaned. Blockage is usually due to particulate matter from the feed broth blocking the upstream side of the T connector.

References

1. Holt, A. and Brown, D. (1989) Antimicrobial susceptibility testing, in *Medical Bacteriology: A Practical Approach* (Hawkey, P. M. and Lewis, D. A., eds.), IRL Press at Oxford University Press, Oxford, pp. 167–194.
2. Gander, S. (1996) Bacterial biofilms: resistance to antimicrobial agents. *J. Antimicrob. Chemother.* **37,** 1047–1050.
3. Prosser, B. L., Taylor, D., Dix, B. A., and Cleeland, R. (1987) Method of evaluating effects of antibiotics on bacterial biofilms. *Antimicrob. Agents Chemother.* **31,** 1502–1506.
4. Evans, D. J., Allison, D. G., Brown, M. R. W., and Gilbert, P. (1990) Susceptibility of bacterial biofilms to tobramycin: role of specific growth rate and phase in the division cycle. *J. Antimicrob. Chemother.* **25,** 585–591.
5. Duguid, I. G., Evans, E., Brown, M. R. W., and Gilbert, P. (1992) Effect of biofilm culture on the susceptibility of *Staphylococcus epidermidis* to tobramycin. *J. Antimicrob. Chemother.* **30,** 803–810.
6. Nichols, W. W. (1991) Biofilms, antibiotics and penetration. *Rev. Med. Microbiol.* **2,** 177–181.
7. Foley, I. and Gilbert, P. (1996) Antibiotic Resistance of Biofilms. **10,** 331–346.
8. Brown, M. R. W. and Williams, P. (1985) Influence of substrate elimination and growth phase to sensitivity to antimicrobial agents. *J. Appl. Bacteriol. Suppl.* **15A,** 7–14.
9. Anwar, H., Strap, J. L., and Costerton, J. W. (1992) Establishment of ageing biofilms: possible mechanism of bacterial resistance to antimicrobial therapy. *Antimicrob. Agents Chemother.* **36,** 1347–1351.
10. Miles, A. A., Misra, S. S., and Irwin. J. D. (1938) The estimation of the bactericidal power of blood. *J. Hyg.* **38,** 732–749.
11. Anwar, H. and Costerton, J. W. (1990) Enhanced activity of combination of tobramycin and piperacillin for eradication of sessile biofilm cells of *Pseudomonas aeruginosa. Antimicrob. Agents Chemother.* **34,** 1666–1671.
12. Wimpenny, J. W. T., Peters, A., and Scourfield, M. (1989) Modeling spatial gradients, in *Structure and Function of Biofilms* (Charackalis, W. G., and Wilderer, P. A., eds.), John Wiley, Chichester, UK, pp. 111–127.

13. Gilbert, P., Allison, D. G., Evans, D. J., Handley, P. S., and Brown, M. R. W. (1989) Growth rate control of adherent bacterial populations. *Appl. Environ. Microbiol.* **55,** 1308–1311.
14. Brown, M. R. W. and Gilbert, P. (1993) Sensitivity of biofilms to antimicrobial agents. *J. Appl. Bacteriol. Suppl.* **74,** 87S–97S.
15. Hodgson, A. E., Nelson, S. M., Brown, M. R. W., and Gilbert, P. (1995) A simple *in vitro* model for growth control of bacterial biofilms. *J . Appl. Bacteriol.* **79,** 87–93.
16. Budhani, R. K. and Struthers, J. K. (1997) The use of Sorbarod biofilms to study the antimicrobial susceptibility of a strain of *Streptococcus pneumoniae. J. Antimicrob. Chemother.* **40,** 601–602.
17. Muli, F. M. and Struthers, J. K. (1998) The growth of *Gardnerella vaginalis* and *Lactobacillus acidophilus* in Sorbarod biofilms. *J. Med. Microbiol.* **47,** 401–405.
18. Muli, F. W. and Struthers, J. K. (1998) The use of a continuous culture biofilm system to study the antimicrobial susceptibilities of *Gardnerella vaginalis* and *Lactobacillus acidophilus. Antimicrob. Agents Chemother.* **42,** 1428–1432.
19. Struthers, J. K. (personal observations).
20. Budhani, R. K., and Struthers, J. K. (1998) Interaction of *Streptococcus pneumoniae* and *Moraxella catarrhalis*: investigation of the indirect pathogen role of β-lactamase producing moraxellae by use of a continuous culture biofilm system. *Antimicrob. Agents Chemother.* **42,** 2521–2526.

23

Estimation of Mutation Rates in Antibiotic Research

Owen J. Billington and Stephen H. Gillespie

1. Introduction

Luria and Delbruck identified that the frequency of mutation was subject to considerable fluctuation. They argued that the large fluctuation in the number of organism surviving exposure to bacteriophage meant that resistance was acquired through mutation rather than a physiological adaptation to the bacteriophage. Mutations that arose early in the broth culture would give rise to a "Jackpot culture" *(1)*. Thus the size of a lineage of mutant cells depends on when the mutation occurred. It is said that the original idea came to Luria while he was observing a slot machine in Bloomington, IN *(2)*. Early mutations are rare (like jackpots with a slot machine) thus when a series of cultures are compared the numbers of mutants would have "a distribution with an abnormally high variance" *(1)*.

The failure of a series of cell survivor counts to obey a Poisson distribution indicated that there is a mutation event affecting the outcome. A result influenced by a mutation will produce a variance to mean ratio of greater than one.

The mutation rate to form a single specific base change in the *rpo*B gene in *Mycobacterium tuberculosis* occurs with a mutation rate of approx 10^{-10} per cell per division *(3)*. If this is the average rate at which all bases and the genome of *M. tuberculosis* is 4.4 Mb long *(4)* then a mutation will occur once in each 2000 divisions. A broth started from a single cell that is grown to produce 10^6 cells will contain approx 400 individual base changes.

The growth rate of mutant cells will be higher than the mutation rate. This means that the frequency of mutant cells in a broth will increase with time. Estimates of mutant frequencies (mutants per cell in culture) will be dependant on the mutation rate and the size of both (in CFU) used. C. J. Crane et al. *(5)*

From: *Methods in Molecular Medicine, vol. 48: Antibiotic Resistance Methods and Protocols*
Edited by: S. H. Gillespie © Humana Press Inc., Totowa, NJ

produced a simple formula relating both size and the number of mutants from which the mutation rate can be estimated.

Point mutation will produce one base change or step change in the original DNA sequence. The mycobacterium tuberculosis genome is 4.4 Mb long. For each base in that sequence there are three alternative bases, leading to a possible $3 \times 4.4 \times 10^6$ possible one step mutations. The number of two step mutations is this figure squared. The number of possible base changes that can happen increases logarithmically as the number of steps rises linearly. This produces a vast number of possible gene sequences. This is gene space containing all possible sequences of bases 4.4 Mb long each sequence separated from its neighbors by a single base change. It is impossible for any culture to fully explore the entirety of this gene landscape.

The quasi-species theory uses the differential growth of mutants to explain the search of gene space in an almost intelligent fashion, concentrating on those regions producing the greatest benefit. The production of a mutant in a haploid population with no gene recombination will produce a new lineage. This lineage must compete to survive with all other lineages, including its parental lineage. Those mutants able to grow will produce larger lineages, and these are then more likely to produce further mutant lineages.

A selective pressure, such as antibiotic at an inhibitory, but not lethal concentration, will enable more rapid growing, low-level resistant cells to predominate. From this low-level resistant population further mutations can develop that produce high-level resistance. This has been used to explain the development of expanded spectrum β-lactamase ***(8)***.

The evolution of antibiotic resistance is now an important subject for study. Many organisms develop resistance through point mutation notable *M. tuberculosis*, where resistance to rifampin, quinolones isoniazid, and pyrazinamide are mainly mediated through point mutations in the bacterial chromosome ***(6)***. The method described here has been developed to investigate rifampin resistance in *M. tuberculosis* but can be readily adapted for other organisms where resistance develops through point mutations in chromosomal genes, e.g., quinolone resistance.

2. Materials

1. Tween albumin broth: 0.2% bovine fatty acid free albumin, 0.01% Tween-80. Dissolve in deionized distilled water and filter sterilize.
2. Middlebrook 7H9 Broth supplemented with Albumin Dextrose Catalase (ADC) and Tween-80.
3. Middlebrook 7H10 agar to which OADC (Oleic acid ADC) supplement is added. It should be distributed in 20-mL aliquots in Petri dishes.
4. *M. tuberculosis* H37Rv ATCC 9360 (*see* **Notes 1** and **2**).
5. Automatic pipets with 100-µL tips.

6. Sterile plastic Pasteur pipets.
7. A 200-mL culture vessel.
8. Small glass containers (e.g., bijou bottles).
9. Insulin syringe (28G Monojet).
10. Antibiotic, e.g., rifampin.

3. Methods

The purpose of this experiment is to estimate the mutation rate for antibiotic resistance. To conduct this experiment it is necessary to grow a suitable large number of bacteria, so that mutation to resistance will have occurred and then to estimate the number of mutants present and the total number of cells.

3.1. Growth in the Absence of Selection Pressure

A sufficiently large number of cells must be grown to have a chance of observing a mutation event. Mutation to resistance will have occurred by chance as the cells divide. The more cell divisions the higher the probability that a resistance mutation event will occur. The size of the broth will depend on the frequency of mutation: if mutation rates are low, a large broth must be grown whereas if mutation rates are large (e.g., streptomycin) a smaller broth will be satisfactory.

1. From a Lowenstein-Jensen slope with a good healthy growth of *M. tuberculosis*, inoculate a 4-mL Middlebrook 7H9 broth (0.01% Tween-80) (*see* **Note 3**).
2. Incubate for 2–3 wk at 37°C without agitation to produce a visible growth.
3. Inoculate 100-mL Middlebrook 7H9 broth (0.01% Tween-80) with 100 mL taken from the 4 mL broth.
4. Incubate for 3–4 wk so that a large cell deposit is formed.

3.2. Concentration of Cells

The purpose of this stage is to concentrate all of the cells grown in the 100-mL broth. This volume of the original culture is known and the total number of bacterial cells is estimated by a conventional plate count.

1. Ensuring that the lid of the bottle is firmly in place, swirl the vessel to resuspend the cell deposit. Make sure that the lid does not become contaminated at any point with the broth culture.
2. Pour the broth culture into suitable large centrifuge tubes (50-mL centrifuge tubes or 20-mL universals).
3. Centrifuge for 30 min at 2000*g*.
4. Pour the supernatant into a liquid disinfectant (e.g., Hycolin).
5. Resuspend the deposit using a plastic Pasteur pipet in a small volume of fresh 7H9 Middlebrook broth.
6. Pool all of the deposit into a single container.
7. The volume of the deposit can be estimated to within 0.1 mL using a 10-mL pipet.

3.3. Plate Count

The aim of this plate count is not to screen for antibiotic resistance, but to measure the total number of cells in the cell deposit. This is achieved by preparing a series of log dilutions from 1:10 to 1:10^9 of the cell deposit. These dilutions are then inoculated as a single drop onto the surface of an agar plate. The number of colonies forming from the drop and the dilution enables a calculation of the colony forming units per milliliter (mL) of cell deposit.

M. tuberculosis tends in culture to form large clumps of cells. Ideally each colony-forming unit should be a single cell. It is necessary therefore to break down these clumps. Tween-80 can reduce the size of clumps both in culture broth and in the Tween-Albumin broth. Shearing forces can be used to further break down clumps.

1. Distribute Tween-Albumin broth in 0.9-mL vol in a series of sterile bijoux.
2. Vortex the cell concentrate to ensure an even distribution of cells. Add 0.1 mL of the cell concentrate to a bijou containing 0.9-mL Tween-Albumin broth. This is the first log dilution (dilution of cell deposit 1:10).
3. *M. tuberculosis* clumps must be broken down in this dilution. This can be achieved by passing the cell dilute ten times through a fine fixed needle insulin syringe (28G Monojet). This step is very likely to produce aerosols, and like all of the steps described here must be carried out in a biosafety exhaust protective cabinet within a biosafety three room.
4. Vortex the first log dilution of cell deposit and transfer 0.1-mL from this to a second bijoux containing 0.9-mL Tween-Albumin broth (this is the second log dilution). Continue in this way to produce nine log dilutions of the cell concentrate.
5. Place Middlebrook 7H10 agar plates into an incubator at 37°C with the agar face down and the lid removed for 15 min. This will dry the surface and ensure the drops inoculated will soak into the agar.
6. Inoculate 50 µL of the log dilutions onto the surface of the agar plates. The log dilutions you need to inoculate will depend on the amount of bacteria you have grown. There should be at least 10^6 cells so the sixth to ninth log dilution can be inoculated. These counts should be performed at least in triplicate.
7. Seal the plates and incubate at 37°C.
8. Count colonies formed at 3 and 4 wk. If over one hundred colonies are counted record the count as >100.
9. Find the dilution at which a low number of individual countable colonies are present (between 10 and 50). Calculate the average number of colonies (n) formed per 50 µL of diluted cell concentrate.
10. Calculate the concentration of bacteria cells in the cell deposit using the formula.

$$\text{CFU/mL} = \text{n} \times 20 \times \text{log dilution counted}$$

11. Calculate the total number of cells present by multiplying the CFU/mL by the volume in the deposit.

3.4. Screening for Antibiotic Resistant Cells

The aim of this procedure is to kill all sensitive cells. Leaving a few isolated resistant colonies. The resistant colonies are those which have acquired a resistance mutation. A very heavy inocula will allow sensitive cells to survive. The idea of using varying volumes of cell concentrate is to find the cell volume where all sensitive cells are killed and where resistant colonies grow as separate isolated colonies. Repetition of the experiment will produce varying numbers of these resistant colonies; as such it is advisable to use both low volumes of cell concentrate as well as high volumes to enable cultures to increase the range of mutants that can be counted.

1. Prepare a set of Middlebrook 7H10 agar plates with antibiotic present (e.g., Rifampin 5 mg/mL (*see* **Note 4**). Inoculate the plates with varying volumes of the cell concentrate.
2. Spread the cell concentrate evenly over the surface of the agar plate. A bent glass rod can be used or an inoculating loop. If a loop is used make sure that an even distribution of cells is achieved. Do not use a sterile cotton wool bud. The cotton wool will absorb an unknown amount of cells; the volume inoculated must reflect the number of cells challenged by the antibiotic.
3. Incubate at 37°C for 24 h with the agar face up to ensure none of the cell concentrate runs off the agar. After 24 h the plates may be placed in the normal fashion agar face down. Incubate the plates for 4 wk and then count the number of separate individual colonies on each plate (*see* **Notes 5** and **6**).
4. Count only those plates where single isolated colonies are seen.

3.5. Calculation of Mutation Rate.

1. The total number of mutants that are present in the broth must be calculated (M).

   M = number of mutants counted/proportion of deposit plated

   The median number of mutants found in a number of broths (Me) is used to calculate the most likely number of mutations that have occurred.
2. Number of mutation events (γ)

   $$\gamma = \text{Me- } 0.693/\text{Ln(Me)} + 0.367 \quad (1)$$

3. Mutation rate (β)

   $$\beta = \gamma/\text{Median broth size} \quad (2)$$

3.6. Example

Seven broths with a median cell count of 4×10^{10} CFU produce 72, 96, 118, 124, 219, 444, and 1220 mutants resistant to rifampin. The median number of mutants is 124 leading to an estimate of 23.7 mutation events using formula 1. The total mutation rate is 6×10^{-10} mutants per cell per division using formula 2 *(5)*.

4. Notes

1. *M. tuberculosis* is a hazard category 3 pathogen, aerosols are a particular hazard and should be avoided. Force the liquid out of the syringe slowly, make sure that the needle is beneath the surface of the broth liquid so that the broth is not striking a flat surface. Attempt not to introduce bubbles into broths, as when these burst they can produce aerosols.
2. We have successfully adapted this method for *Streptococcus pneumoniae* to investigate quinolone resistance using wild-type strains.
3. It is important that no resistant mutants are inoculated into the 100-mL broth in **step 3.1.** To check that mutants have not occurred the 4-mL broth can be screened for antibiotic resistant mutants (*see* Screening for Antibiotic Resistant Cells, **Subheading 3.4.**).
4. The amount of antibiotic is crucial. This concentration must be high enough so that all sensitive cells are killed. Any resistant mutations that lead to resistance below the antibiotic level used will be missed. A series of concentrations doubling from the minimum inhibitory concentration can be used. Alternatively use an antibiotic concentration twice the concentration used to define resistance clinically or two and four times the MIC. It may be necessary to prove mutations have occurred for example by checking that a poisson distribution is not followed in frequency of cells between tests.
5. Plates should be incubated in sealed plastic bags. This prevents any possibility of contamination of fingers with open plates. The plates should be placed into these bags while still in a biosafety cabinet.
6. The growth conditions of the inocula are critical. Culture under a selective pressure will make advantageous mutants accumulate faster and make two step mutants available. This will lower the calculated mutation rate.

References

1. Luria, S. A. and Delbrook, M. (1943) Mutations of bacteria from virus sensitivity to virus resistance. *Genetics* **28,** 491–511.
2. Foster, P. L. (1999) Sorting out mutation rates. *Proc. Natl. Acad. Sci. USA* **96,** 7617–7618.
3. Billington, O. J., McHugh, T. D., and Gillespie, S. H. (1999) Physiological cost of Rifampin resistance induced in vitro in *Mycobacterium tuberculosis. Antimicrob. Agents Chemoth.* **43,** 1866–1869.
4. Cole, S. T., Brosch, R., Parkhill, J., Garnier, T., Churcher, C., Harris, D., et al. (1998) Deciphering the biology of *Mycobacterium tuberculosis* from the complete genome sequence. *Nature* **393,** 537–544.
5. Crane, C. J., Thomas, S. M., and Jones, M. E. (1996) A modified Luria-Delbrück fluctuation assay for estimating and comparing mutation rates. *Mutat. Res.* **354,** 171–82.
6. Ramaswamy, S. and Musser, J. M. (1998) Molecular genetic basis of antimircobial resistance in *Mycobacterium tuberculosis*: 1998 update. *Tuber. Lung Dis.* **79,** 3–29.
7. Koch, A. L. (1993) Genetic response of microbes to extreme challenges. *J. Theoret. Biol.* **160,** 1–21.
8. Baquero, F. and Negri, M. C. (1997) Selective compartments for resistant microorganisms in antibiotic gradients. *BioEssays* **19,** 731–736.

24

In Vitro Assessment of the Fitness of Resistant *M. tuberculosis* Bacteria by Competition Assay

Stephen H. Gillespie

1. Introduction

Bacteria become resistant by a number of different mechanisms, and these include mutation in chromosomal genes *(1)*, acquisition of plasmids *(2)*, insertion of bacteriophage, transposon or insertion sequence DNA *(3–5)*, or gene mosaicism *(6)*. There is a dogma that bacteria that become resistant pay a significant physiological price and that if antimicrobial prescribing is controlled it will result in the eradication of resistant organisms. There are only very few studies that investigate the physiology of resistance acquisition and these do show that a physiological price is paid for this change *(7,8)*. Once an organism acquires resistance through mutation, acquisition of resistance genes via plasmids, transposons and bacteriophages the initial physiological defect is compensated by the antibiotic selective pressure, which balances the physiological deficit imposed by the resistant mutation or additional DNA *(8,9)*.

Many studies have shown that plasmids have a deleterious effect on bacterial fitness and the plasmid is soon lost if the selective pressure that retains it is removed. For example, in substrate limited chemostat cultures *E. coli,* K12 carrying the plasmid TP120, loses resistance to tetracycline, ampicillin, sulfonamide, and chloramphenicol with a resulting increase in growth rate *(7)*.

The fitness deficit imposed by resistance determinants can be overcome by bacterial adaptation in a study of plasmid borne resistance, the introduction of the plasmid pACYC 184 into *E. coli* confers resistance to tetracycline and chloramphenicol and consequently reduces bacterial fitness in comparison with the isogenic plasmid-free strain. When grown for 500 generations under chloramphenicol selective pressure, the plasmid bearing strain adapted to the

From: *Methods in Molecular Medicine, vol. 48: Antibiotic Resistance Methods and Protocols*
Edited by: S. H. Gillespie © Humana Press Inc., Totowa, NJ

experimental regimen and the presence of the plasmid increased the fitness of its host relative to that of the plasmid-freed segregant *(7)*. More recently studies of streptomycin resistant *E. coli* have indicated that after the metabolic burden imposed by streptomycin resistance, as measured by chain elongation rate, was rapidly reversed *(8)*. Similar results have been obtained in *Mycobacterium tuberculosis* resistant to rifampin *(9)*. To develop our understanding of the evolution of drug resistance simple in vitro methods to measure bacterial fitness are required to investigate the physiological cost of resistance and the mechanism whereby resistant organisms adapt. The method described here is simple to perform and can be adapted to many different species.

2. Materials

2.1. Bacteria

1. *M. tuberculosis* H57RV ATCC9360 National Collection of Type Culture, Central Public Health Laboratory, London, UK and resistant mutant strains derived from this species.
2. Lowenstein Jensen media.
3. Middlebrook 7H9 broth with added 0.1% Tween-80.
4. Automatic pipet.

2.1. Viable Count Determination

1. Plastic disposable loops.
2. 1-mL insulin syringe (28 gage).
3. Tween albumin broth: 0.2% bovine albumin, 0.01% Tween-80.
4. Middlebrook 7H10 agar containing either 5 mg rifampin or no drug (*see* **Notes 1** and **2**).

3. Methods

3.1. Preparation of Inocula

1. Using a plastic disposal loop inoculate colonies of the test or control organisms into 7H9 broth (0.1% Tween-80)
2. Incubate susceptible and resistant broth cultures for 3–4 wk.
3. Prepare a 10-fold dilution of the susceptible broth culture and a 100-fold dilution of the resistant culture using automatic pipet.
4. Mix a 550 μL sample of each of these dilutions and inoculate into 4 mL of fresh Middlebrook 7H9 broth to create a mixed culture of rifampicin susceptible and resistant cells.
5. Incubate the mixed broth cultures at 37°C for 2–3 wk.

3.2. Estimation of Viable Count

1. Take an aliquot of the culture for viable count.
2. Pass the aliquot of the broth culture 8–10 times through a 1 mL fine needle insulin syringe prior to dilution (*see* **Note 2**).

3. Serially dilute the dispersed broth culture in fresh Tween albumin broth in a dilution series 10^{-1} to 10^{-7}.
4. Mix the dilutions by vortexing briefly three times.
5. Inoculate 20 µL of each dilution in triplicate onto Middlebrook 7H10 containing either rifampicin 5 mg/L or no drug.
6. Seal the plates and incubate them at 37°C for 2–3 wk.
7. Count the number of colonies on each dilution spot on the drug free medium taking the average of the spots on which the colonies are separate and easy to count (*see* **Note 3**).
8. Calculate the number of resistant colonies and susceptible colonies taking into account the volume of the inoculum and the dilution. The number of susceptible colonies is obtained by subtracting the total count from the number of resistant colonies.

3.3. Calculation of Relative Fitness

1. Calculate the number of generations grown by the susceptible and resistant strains using the formula g = log B - log A ÷ by log 2, where g is the number of generations grown, A is the number of CFU per mL at time 0 and B is the number of CFU per mL at the end of the culture period.
2. The relative fitness of each strain pair is calculated from the ratio of the number of generations grown by the resistant strain to the rifampicin susceptible strains.

4. Notes

1. *M. tuberculosis* is a hazard group three organism (P3) and all procedures with viable organisms must be performed in a suitably equipped category 3 laboratory or equivalent.
2. The method presented here is for *Mycobacterium tuberculosis* and rifampin. It can be readily adapted by substituting different antibiotics in the Middlebrook 7H10. Also, this method can be adapted to other organisms by changing the relevant growth conditions, for example, *Streptococcus pneumoniae* can be grown using Brain Heart Infusion broth and inoculated onto solid medium such as Columbia agar with 5% lysed horse blood.
3. A characteristic of *M. tuberculosis* is that it naturally forms cords and these must be disrupted if an accurate count is to be obtained.
4. It is important to choose the correct dilution when measuring the viable count. The spots containing approximately twenty colonies are the most suitable for counting. Do not attempt to count very large numbers as this will produce an inaccurate result.

References

1. Ramaswamy, S. and Musser, J. M. (1998) Molecular genetic basis of antimicrobial resistance in *Mycobacterium tuberculosis*: 1998 update. *Tubercle. Lung Dis.* **79,** 3–29.

2. Lenski, R. E., Simpson, S. C., and Nguyen, T. T. (1994) Genetic analysis of a plasmid-encoded, host genotype-specific enhancement of bacterial fitness. *J. Bacteriol.* **176,** 3140–3147.
3. Hyder, S. L. and Steitfeld, M. M. (1978) Transfer of erythromycin resistance from clinically isolated lysogenic strains of *Streptococcus pyogenes* via their endogenous phage. *J. Infect. Dis.* **138,** 281–286.
4. Poyart, C., Pierre, C., Quesne, G., Pron, B., Berche, P., and Trien-Cust, P. (1997) Emergence of vancomycin resistance in the genus *Streptococcus*: characterization of a *vanB* transferable determinant in *Streptococcus bovis*. *Antimicrob. Agents Chemother.* **41,** 24–29.
5. Lemaitre, N., Sougakoff, W., Truffot-Pernot, C., and Jarlier, V. (1999) Characterization of new mutations in pyrazinamide-resistant strains of *Mycobacterium tuberculosis* and identification of conserved regions important for the catalytic activity of the pyrazinamidase PncA. *Antimicrob. Agents Chemother.* **43,** 1761–1763.
6. Tomasz, A. (1997) Antibiotic resistance in *Streptococcus pneumoniae*. *Clin. Infect. Dis.* **24(Suppl. 1),** 585–588.
7. Gillespie, S. H. and McHugh, T. D. (1997) The biological cost of antimicrobial resistance. *Trends Microbiol.* **5,** 337–339.
8. Schrag, S. J., Perrot, V., and Levin, B. R. (1997) Adaptation to the fitness costs of antibiotic resistance in *Escherichia coli*. *Proc. Roy. Soc. Lond. – Series B: Biol. Sci.* **264,** 1287–1291.
9. Billington, O., McHugh, T. D., and Gillespie, S. H. (1999) The physiological cost of rifampicin resistance induced *in vitro* in *Mycobacterium tuberculosis*. *Antimicrob. Agents Chemother.* **43,** 1866–1869.

25

Purification of DNA Topoisomerases and Inhibition by Fluoroquinolones

John T. George and Ian Morrissey

1. Introduction

Fluoroquinolones act by inhibiting the essential type II topoisomerases, DNA gyrase and topoisomerase IV *(1)*. DNA gyrase is a tetramer composed of 2 A subunits and 2 B-subunits encoded for by *gyrA* and *gyrB*, respectively. This enzyme is the only enzyme known that is capable of negatively supercoiling DNA *(2)*, a process essential for the bacterium to contain its DNA within the confines of the cell. Topoisomerase IV is also a tetramer composed of 2 C subunits and 2-E subunits encoded for by the *parC* and *parE* genes. This enzyme is involved in the unlinking of daughter chromosomes following replication *(3)*.

Investigations into the action of fluoroquinolones directly against topoisomerases comprises two main tasks: purification of the enzyme, and inhibition of topoisomerases by quinolones.

1.1. Purification of the Enzyme

This can be achieved by either traditional column chromatography techniques using native enzyme or by gene cloning and subsequent recombinant protein over-expression. Traditional chromatography methods can be time consuming and achieving a pure protein can be very difficult. However, once achieved the advantage is that all of the results are generated with native enzyme. Gene cloning on the other hand is relatively quick and by using the most appropriate cloning vector results in the purification of large amounts of enzyme. This method can only be used once the sequence of the genes that encode the enzyme of interest has been determined. For a large number of organisms the sequence of DNA gyrase and topoisomerase has already been

From: *Methods in Molecular Medicine, vol. 48: Antibiotic Resistance Methods and Protocols*
Edited by: S. H. Gillespie © Humana Press Inc., Totowa, NJ

determined, therefore, most researchers interested in the action of fluoroquinolones on topoisomerases should use this route to purify them.

There are a number of commercial vectors available for use in the overproduction of protein, however, this chapter focuses on the use of the pMAL-c2 cloning vector (New England Biolabs, Hertfordshire). The pMAL-c2 vector is a protein fusion vector that fuses the protein under investigation to the maltose binding protein (MBP). It allows simple protein purification via amylose affinity chromatography. Once pure protein is obtained the MBP "tag" is removed by restriction with factor Xa, and is then separated from the protein under investigation by further amylose resin chromatography.

1.2. Inhibition of Topoisomerases by Quinolones

By far the most common method of assessing the inhibition of DNA gyrase or topoisomerase IV is to measure the drug concentration at which enzyme catalysis is inhibited by 50% (IC_{50}). Here a standard amount of enzyme (usually 1 U) is exposed to various fluoroquinolone concentrations. Since both type II topoisomerases alter DNA topology, inhibition assays have been designed to exploit these functions. For topoisomerase IV kinetoplast DNA is widely used as enzyme substrate. Kinetoplast DNA, isolated from trypanosomal mitochondria, contains a number of linked circular plasmids that collectively have a very high molecular weight. Topoisomerase IV has the ability to unlink this DNA into individual plasmid monomers that have a low molecular weight and can therefore be separated from the high molecular weight DNA by agarose gel electrophoresis.

DNA gyrase has the unique ability of being able to supercoil relaxed plasmid DNA. Therefore, in order to assay for DNA gyrase activity one measures the conversion of relaxed DNA into a supercoiled form. Since supercoiled DNA migrates through agarose gels at a faster rate than the relaxed form the two topologies can be distinguished by agarose gel electrophoresis.

By exposing these topoisomerase assays to a range of fluoroquinolone concentrations it is possible to measure the percentage inhibition of the enzyme and thereby calculate the IC_{50}.

2. Materials

1. Oligonucleotide primers. Obtainable from a number of commercial sources.
2. Polymerase chair reaction (PCR) reagents: *Taq* polymerase and buffer, mixed deoxyribonucleotides (dNTPs), $MgCl_2$.
3. pMAL -c2 over-expression vector (New England Biolabs).
4. Amylose resin (New England Biolabs).
5. Maltose.
6. Competent host strain *E. coli* (e.g., DH5 α prepared using standard techniques Sambrook et al., 1989).

7. Isopropyl β-D-thiogalactoside (IPTG).
8. Ampicillin.
9. LB broth (10 g tryptone, 5 g yeast extract , 10 g NaCl per L).
10. Agarose.
11. Agarose gel running buffer (TBE): 45 m*M* Tris-borate, 1 m*M* EDTA.
12. Stop solution: 0.04% bromophenol blue, 0.04% xylene cyanol and 5% glycerol.
13. 10% SDS-PAGE gels.
14. SDS-PAGE running buffer: 25 m*M* Tris, 250 m*M* glycine pH 8.3, 0.1% SDS.
15. SDS-PAGE loading buffer: 50 m*M* Tris-HCl (pH 6.8), 100 m*M* dithiothreitol (DTT), 2% SDS, 0.1% bromophenol blue, 10% glycerol.
16. Topoisomerase inhibition assay buffer; 40 m*M* Tris-HCl\, 0.5 m*M* ATP, 5 m*M* $MgCl_2$, 20 m*M* KCl, 50 μg/mL BSA, 1 m*M* DTT, and 0.4 μg kinetoplast DNA (Topogen, O).

3. Method

3.1. Polymerase Chain Reaction

1. After isolation of DNA from the organism under study, using standard techniques *(4)* amplify the gene of interest by PCR. Since the success of PCR is dependent on the optimization of all the reagents used in this technique it is impossible to provide a recipe that will work every time. However, a convenient starting point is 2 U of *taq*, 1 μg chromosomal DNA, 1 μ*M* of each primer, 200 μ*M* dNTPs, 5 m*M* $MgCL_2$ (*see* **Note 1**). The thermal cycles of the PCR reaction are also dependent on a number of variables such as the size of the gene you are amplifying and the melting temperature of the oligonucleotides (*see* **Note 2**).
2. Following amplification of the target gene, load 10% of the PCR reaction onto a 1% agarose gel along with an appropriate molecular marker (*see* **Note 3**). Subject the gel to electrophoresis for 1 h at 100 V. Stain the gel using ethidium bromide (50 μg/mL) for 30 min and visualize by UV illumination (Ethidium bromide is a carcinogen, appropriate safety clothing should be used: UV light is also dangerous and specialist screens should be used to protect the scientist).
3. If the size of the PCR product falls within the expected size for the topoisomerase gene of interest then one can proceed to clone the gene into the pMAL -c2 vector.
4. Purify the PCR product by using Gene-Clean kit (Bio-Rad, Hertfordshire, UK) according to the manufacturer's instructions.

3.2. Cloning DNA Topoisomerase

1. Treat the purified PCR product with 1 U T4 polymerase along with each dNTP at a final concentration of 100 μ*M*.
2. Incubate at 37°C for 5 min, stop the reaction by heating to 75°C for 10 min (*see* **Note 4**).
3. Restrict 1 μg of the pMAL-c2 vector with 1 U XmnI for 1 h at 37°C. Remove the restriction enzyme by using the Gene-Clean kit (Bio-rad) (*see* **Note 5**).
4. Add the PCR product to the restricted vector and treat with 1 U of T4 DNA ligase in ligation buffer. Incubate overnight at 4°C (*see* **Note 6**).

5. Thaw a 200 µL aliquot of competent cells on ice. Add 10 ng of DNA from the ligation mixture and swirl gently to mix (do not pipet). Incubate on ice for 30 min.
6. Heat the tube at 42°C for 1 min, place on ice for 2 min to cool. Add 1.5 mL of LB broth and incubate at 37°C for 1 h.
7. Spread 100–200 µL of the transformation mixture or an appropriate dilution onto agar plates containing the appropriate antibiotic selection. In this case the plates contain 50 µg/mL of ampicillin. Incubate the plates at 37°C overnight.
8. Pick off 12 colonies using a sterile toothpick and touch a fresh agar plate, then dip the toothpick into 10 mL of LB broth containing 50 µg/mL ampicillin.
9. Incubate the plate overnight at 37°C. Incubate the broths until an absorbance of 0.2 is reached at an optical density of 600 nm (usually 3 h).
10. Add IPTG to a final concentration of 0.1 m*M*. Incubate the broths for a further 3 h.
11. Take a 1.5 mL aliquot of each tube and centrifuge. Discard the supernatant and add 20 µL of SDS loading buffer. Load the 20 µL samples onto a 10% SDS-PAGE gel along with an appropriate molecular marker. Subject the samples to electrophoresis for 1 h at 200 V.
12. Stain the SDS-PAGE gel for 30 min using coomassie blue protein stain. Destain the gel by washing the gel in 10% acetic acid, 10% methanol solution.
13. Clones which are over-expressing the topoisomerase subunit will have a strong protein band at the approximate molecular weight for that subunit (remember that the topoisomerase subunit is still fused to the maltose binding protein, so the subunit will be c. 45 kDa larger than it should be).
14. Select one clone which is over-expressing the topoisomerase subunit for large scale purification.
15. The precise method for the large scale purification is provided in the manufacturer's instructions provided with the pMAL-C2 system, therefore, it will be outlined only briefly here. The transformed *E. coli* are grown in a large volume (4 × 200 mL) of LB broth and fusion protein over-production is induced. The bacteria are washed and lysed to release cellular proteins. The fusion protein is separated from the rest of the cellular proteins by one-step affinity chromatography. The MBP is then cleaved from the topoisomerase subunit and purified by further affinity chromatography. In this manner pure protein is produced. **Figure 1** illustrates an example of the purification procedure as observed by SDS-PAGE.

3.3. Enzyme Inhibition Studies

3.3.1. Topoisomerase IV Inhibition Assays

1. Mix the test protein with the Topoisomerase assay buffer.
2. Incubate for 1 h at 37°C.
3. Stop the reaction by the addition of stop mix (5 µL).
4. Examine the sample by agarose gel electrophoresis and stain with ethidium bromide for 30 min.
5. Examine the gel under UV illumination.
6. Capture an image of the gel using a gel documentation system, e.g., Gel Doc 1000 (Bio-Rad). A typical gel image is shown in **Fig. 2**. The brighter the mono-

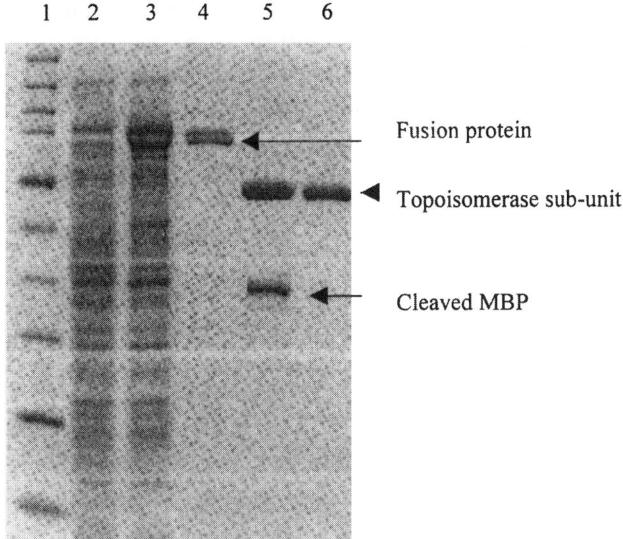

Fig. 1. SDS-PAGE of purification procedure. Lane 1, Molecular marker. Lane 2, uninduced cell extract. Lane 3, induced cell extract. Lane 4, purified fusion protein. Lane 5, cleaved fusion protein. Lane 6, pure topoisomerase subunit.

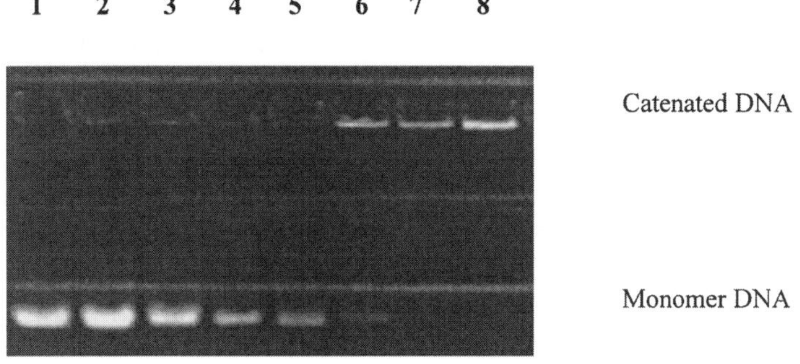

Fig. 2. Decatenation of kinetoplast DNA by topoisomerase IV.

mer DNA band the greater the decatenating activity. Lanes 2–8 show decreasing decatenating activity.

7. Make serial dilutions of one subunit in the presence of undiluted opposing subunit. The last dilution which fully decatenates 0.4 µg of DNA is taken to contain 1 U of activity. This is repeated to determine 1 U of the remaining subunit.
8. Optimize the condition of ATP, KCl, $MgCl_2$. Once optimum conditions have been reached, readjustment of the *par*C/*par*E levels required to give 1 U may be necessary.

9. Perform inhibition studies using test drug over a range of concentrations, making sure one tube is kept drug free (this will act as the control).
10. Perform electrophoresis, staining, and image capture and calculate the amount of decatenated product in each of the conditions compared to the control. The gel shown in **Fig. 2** is actually the result of an inhibition assay, lane 1 is the drug free control and lanes 2–8 contain increasing concentrations of ciprofloxacin.
11. Determine the concentration of monomer DNA using specialized gel documentation software such as multianalyst (Bio-Rad).
12. Because one of the samples (lane 1 in **Fig. 2**) contains no drug then the amount of each product (in lanes 2–8) can be compared to the amount in the drug free control and therefore, it is possible to determine the percentage inhibition of the enzyme at each of the drug concentrations.
13. The percentage inhibition against drug concentration should then be plotted (as shown in **Fig. 3**). From this plot the IC_{50} can be interpolated.
14. The activity of any number of compounds can be compared by calculating the IC_{50} in the same manner.

3.3.2. Inhibition of DNA Gyrase

DNA gyrase inhibition is measured in exactly the same fashion as for topoisomerase IV, however, the catalytic activity of DNA gyrase is to supercoil relaxed DNA. Therefore, before any assays can be performed relaxed plasmid DNA must be prepared as the assay substrate.

1. Incubate 1 µg of pBR322 with 1 U of topoisomerse I (GIBCO, UK), in the presence of 50 m*M* KCl, 50 m*M* Tris (pH 7.5), 10 m*M* $MgCl_2$, 0.1 m*M* EDTA and 30 µg/mL BSA for 1 h at 37°C (*see* **Note 7**).
2. Add an equal volume of phenol/chloroform solution and mix gently. (Phenol/chloroform is toxic so adequate safety precautions should be taken.)
3. Centrifuge at 10,000*g* for 5 min.
4. Remove the upper aqueous layer and add to an equal volume of ice-cold isopropynol. Pellet the DNA by centrifugation at 10,000*g* for 10 min.
5. Resuspend in 50 µL of sterile distilled water.
6. Assays can then be performed as shown above with topoisomerase IV except traditionally 0.2 µg of this relaxed DNA is used in the presence of Tris-HCl, KCl, $MgCl_2$, BSA, DTT, ATP, spermidine, and t-RNA.
7. The supercoiling reaction of DNA gyrase is shown in **Fig. 4**. This time inhibition is measured by the reduction in the supercoiled DNA band. The intensities of these bands are used to calculate the IC_{50}.

4. Notes

1. It is important to realize that *Taq* polymerase may incorporate errors into the PCR product. If this occurs in the early stages of PCR then a majority of the amplified gene will differ from the native gene. Any errors in the PCR product will be expressed in the protein. As the purpose of this technique is to perform

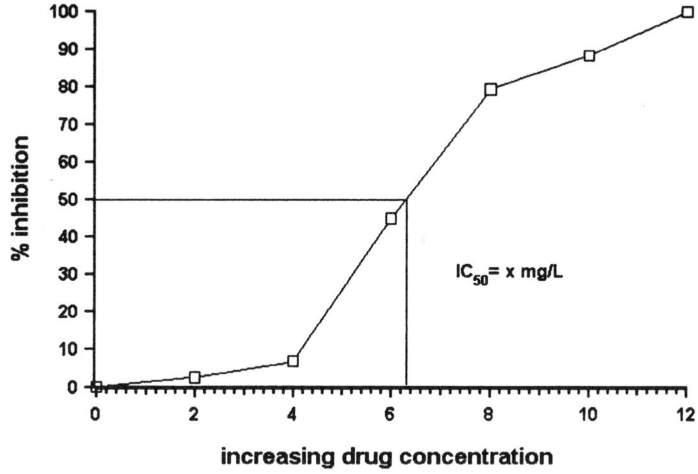

Fig. 3. Inhibition of topoisomerase IV by test compound.

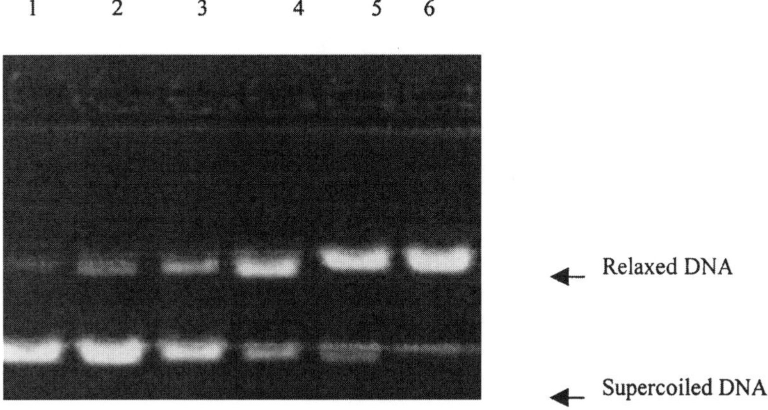

Fig. 4. Inhibition of DNA gyrase by a fluoroquinolone.

assays on the protein it is important, therefore, that the amplified gene is error free. This can be achieved by using a proofreading polymerase, a number of which are commercially available.

2. A useful way to determine the melting temperature of your oligonucleotides is to assign A and T nucletides a value of 2°C and assign G and C nucleotides a value of 4°C. The sum of these can then be used as a starting point in the annealing step of PCR. It is also worth incubating the oligonucleotides with T4 polynucleotide kinase in the presence of buffer prior to PCR. This is a necessary step if you intend to clone blunt ended PCR fragments as this method describes.

3. Topoisomerase genes are generally in the region of 1200–2000 bp, therefore, the molecular marker chosen to estimate the size of these products should have optimal separation between that range.
4. A common but rarely mentioned feature of *Taq* polymerase is that it incorporates an extra A nucleotide at the 3' end of the DNA fragment. In order to clone the PCR fragment in a blunt end fashion this "A" overhang has to be removed by T4 polymerase. Be sure to obtain the correct concentration of dNTPs in the reaction buffer, as if the supply of dNTPs is exhausted the T4 polymerase will start to degrade the double-stranded DNA as well.
5. To improve the efficiency of the blunt end ligation of the fragment into the restricted vector it helps to remove the phosphates from the vector. This can be done by the enzyme Calf Intestinal phosphatase. Once the phosphates have been removed the vector is unable to religate back together.
6. The vector insert ratio is extremely important for a successful ligation. The calculation in order to achieve this is as follows:

$$\frac{\text{ng vector} \times \text{kb size of insert}}{\text{kb size of vector}} \times \text{molar ratio (in this case 3:1)} = \text{ng insert.}$$

7. It is useful to check whether all of the supercoiled DNA has been converted into relaxed DNA, by running samples on a gel at intermittent times.

References

1. Drlica, K. and Zoah, X. (1997) DNA gyrase and topoisomerase IV, and the 4-quinolones. *Microbiol. Mol. Biol. Rev.* **61,** 377–392.
2. Gellert, M., Mizuuchi, K., O'Dea, M. H., and Nash, H. A. (1976) DNA gyrase: an enzyme that introduces superhelical turns into DNA. *Proc. Natl. Acad. Sci. USA* **73,** 3872–3876.
3. Kato, J., Nishima, Y., Imamura, R., Niki, H., Higari, S., and Suzuki, H. (1990) New topoisomerase essential for chromosome segregation in *E. coli. Cell* **63,** 393–404.
4. Sambrook, J., Fritsch, E. F., and Maniatis, T. (1989) Molecular cloning. Second edition. Cold Spring Harbor Laboratory, Cold Spring Harbor, NY.

26

Site-Directed Mutagenesis to Determine Structure Function Relationships in *Streptococcus pneumoniae* Penicillin-Binding Protein Genes

Victoria A. Barcus and Christopher G. Dowson

1. Introduction

β-lactam resistance in clinical isolates of *Streptococcus pneumoniae* arises by only one route, the reduction of the affinity of the penicillin-binding proteins (PBPs) for β-lactams. The pneumococcus possesses five high molecular weight PBPs (PBP1A, 1B, 2A, 2B, and 2X) which are involved in the final crosslinking stages of peptidoglycan synthesis in the bacterial cell wall. β-lactam antibiotics are structural analogs of the natural cell wall peptide substrates of the PBPs. The antibiotic binds to the active site within the transpeptidase domain of these PBPs, forming an acyl-enzyme complex which is far more stable than the transient enzyme-substrate complex that normally occurs. In this way, the β-lactams block the crosslinking in what is essentially an irreversible manner. The result is a cessation in cell growth and, depending on the PBP inhibited, lysis.

Low affinity PBPs in the pneumococcus have initially evolved as a result of interspecies gene transfer rather than simply by point mutation. DNA encoding PBPs from related, resistant streptococcal species may be taken up by the naturally-transformable pneumococcus and incorporated into the chromosome via homologous recombination. The resulting mosaic genes encode chimaeric PBPs with reduced affinity for β-lactam antibiotics. Such mosaic genes have been documented for the *pbp1a*, *pbp2b,* and *pbp2x* genes of resistant pneumococcal strains ***(1–4)***. However, it is also apparent that selective pressure applied by the therapeutic use of different β-lactams can result in subsequent mutation

From: *Methods in Molecular Medicine, vol. 48: Antibiotic Resistance Methods and Protocols*
Edited by: S. H. Gillespie © Humana Press Inc., Totowa, NJ

of mosaic genes conferring increased levels of resistance to penicillins or cephalosporins *(5)*.

Low, intermediate, or high level resistance to different classes of β-lactams can arise through alterations of different combinations of PBPs. Low level resistance to penicillins and isoxoylpenicillins such as oxacillin and intermediate level resistance to the third generation cephalosporins may be conferred by low affinity forms of PBP2X alone *(6,7)*. Altered PBP2X and PBP1A are necessary to confer high level resistance to the third generation cephalosporins *(5)* though this has no further effect on resistance to the other two groups of β-lactam antibiotics. A low affinity PBP2B is required, in addition to altered PBP1A and PBP2X for high level penicillin resistance, and in conjunction with a low affinity 2X for high level oxacillin resistance (6,8). An altered PBP2B alone is sufficient to confer piperacillin resistance *(9)*.

The roles of PBP2A and PBP1B in clinical resistance to β-lactams are less well known. Alterations to PBP2A have been noted in laboratory mutants *(10)*, and transformation of susceptible pneumococci in the laboratory with chromosomal DNA from very highly penicillin resistant streptococcal species has also implicated PBP1B and PBP2A in very high level resistance *(11,12)*. The sequences of *pbp2a* and *pbp1b* are now available *(12)* for further studies.

Sequence comparisons between the *pbp* genes of β-lactam susceptible and resistant isolates highlight the acquired blocks of sequence, and the amino acid differences specific to resistant PBPs. Sequence comparisons between the *pbp* genes of resistant isolates help to identify blocks from different donor species and on this basis help divide mosaic genes into different classes *(1,13)*. There is little evidence as to which of the many alterations found in mosaic *pbp* genes may be responsible for the development of resistance, though some individual substitutions in different PBPs have been shown to be important *(1,12,14)*. Structure function analyses such as those described in these papers are central to determining the importance of the individual amino acid substitutions.

Structure function analyses can be used to identify amino acids involved in catalysis and specifically those that may be substituted leading to the development of resistance. Residues involved in substrate specificity for different β-lactams may also be pinpointed, as well as those that influence levels of resistance. Mutagenesis, whether random or site-directed, is a powerful tool in the study of such structure function relationships. The next sections outline a number of methods suitable for these sort of mutagenic studies of PBPs.

1.1. Mutagenesis

1.1.1. Random Polymerase Chain Reaction (PCR) Mutagenesis

The error-prone nature of *Taq* polymerase during DNA amplification may be used to create random point mutations in a gene. Grebe and Hakenbeck *(9)* made use of this method to select for PBPs with reduced affinity for β-lactams. Following PCR amplification of *pbp2x* or *pbp2b* using normal conditions for the amplification of these genes (*see* **Subheading 3.2.**), β-lactam susceptible recipients were transformed with these products to increased levels of resistance by selection on antibiotic-containing plates. Using this method, only those mutations that do not severely affect the essential in vivo function of the enzyme will be found. Repeated rounds of PCR amplification and transformation may result in greater levels of resistance, as further mutations are introduced. Sequencing *pbp* genes from the resistant transformants will reveal the position(s) of the introduced mutation(s).

1.1.2. Random Replacement Mutagenesis

Palzkill and his colleagues ***(16–19)*** used random mutagenesis of the entire *bla* gene to determine amino acid residues critical for the structure and function of the TEM-1 β-lactamase. This was done by randomizing three contiguous codons at a time to create a random plasmid library containing all possible amino acid substitutions for that region. Functional mutants may then be selected by plating out the library. Amino acids that are not tolerant to substitution are likely to be critical for structure and function, for example by being directly involved in catalysis or making important interactions in the active site. By using antibiotic selection in the screening of the library, it is possible to identify residues involved in substrate specificity. Furthermore, it may also reveal acceptable substitutions that are not yet seen in natural isolates but which may appear under continued antibiotic selection. This could be a major factor to be considered in the development of new antibiotics that target PBPs. Optimally, such antibiotics should interact with highly constrained residues and avoid those where substitution is more readily tolerated.

1.1.3. Site Directed Mutagenesis Using "Overlap Extension"

This method of mutagenesis, first described in 1988 ***(20,21)***, enables the introduction of specified nucleotide substitutions anywhere along a DNA template, using PCR in three rounds of amplification with four primers (*see* **Fig. 1**). Two internal, mutagenic primers are designed in such a way as to be complementary and overlapping. Each mutagenic primer is used in a PCR with a flanking primer that hybridizes to one end of the target sequence. The result is two overlapping DNA fragments each carrying the desired mutation. The two fragments are mixed together, denatured, and allowed to anneal. The overlapping DNA strands can then act as primers for each other, resulting in the formation of the full-length duplex containing the desired mutations. Addition of the two flanking primers results in the amplification of the full-length product.

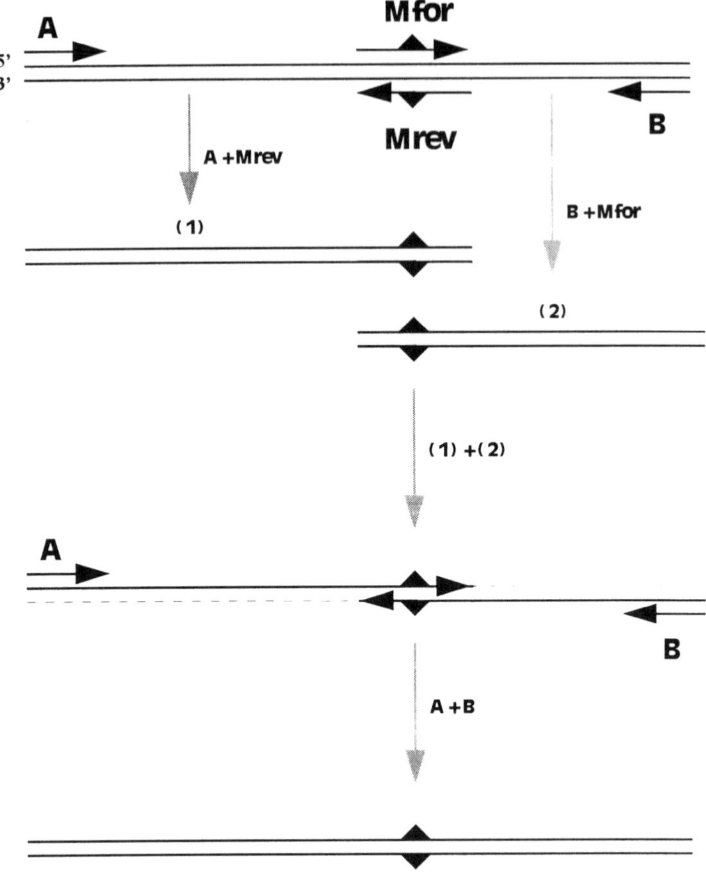

Fig. 1. Schematic diagram of PCR-mediated site-directed mutagenesis by overlap extension. The flanking primers, **A** and **B,** and the mutagenic oligos Mfor and Mrev are shown as arrows, indicating the 5' to 3' orientation. The solid triangles in the mutagenic oligos represent the site of mutagenesis. The double-stranded products resulting from the first round of amplification, (1) and (2), are melted and reannealed with results in the denatured DNA fragments annealing at the overlap. This primes DNA extension by polymerase (dotted lines). Addition of primers A and B further amplifies the mutant fusion products. Adapted from Ho et al. *(21)*.

1.1.4. "Megaprimer" PCR Mutagenesis

Another method of PCR-mediated introduction of nucleotide substitutions into a target sequence is the so-called 'megaprimer' method originally described by Landt et al. *(22)* and Sarkar and Sommer *(23)*. Like the overlap extension method, the megaprimer method does not require initial cloning of the gene in an appropriate vector, and can in fact be performed on chromosomal DNA. Because the megaprimer method utilizes three oligonucleotide primers and two rounds of amplification to create the mutation(s), it is perhaps less likely than overhang extension to introduce spurious mutations. In the megaprimer method, an internal mutagenic primer with the desired substitutions is used in conjunction with a flanking primer in a round of PCR amplification (*see* **Fig. 2**). The resulting DNA fragment is then used as a primer, or "megaprimer", in a second round of PCR, using the second flanking primer to amplify the entire target sequence with the mutations incorporated.

Prior to the secondary PCR, the megaprimer is usually purified to remove the initial oligonucleotide primers, avoiding unwanted priming by the first round primers resulting in production of wild-type sequence. Some research groups have developed methods to by-pass the purification step without excessive production of wild-type sequence, allowing the entire mutagenesis reaction to be carried out in one Eppendorf tube. These include staggered addition of the primers *(24)*, or choosing flanking primers each having a significantly different T_m, so that the second PCR may be carried out at an annealing temperature sufficiently high that the low T_m flanking primer from the first amplification does not continue priming *(25)*. A third method omitting purification requires use of different restriction enzymes to cleave the template prior to each of the PCR reactions with the result that only the full-length product possesses the desired substitutions *(26)*.

A frequently-encountered problem associated with the megaprimer method is poor yield of product after the secondary PCR. This is due to inefficient priming by the megaprimer, particularly when using long (>300bp) megaprimers. The long megaprimers may reanneal preferentially to annealing to the DNA template, or they may adopt secondary structures that interfere with the polymerization reaction. Remedies for this include increasing the template concentration to microgram rather than nanogram levels *(27)*, though this could lead to contamination of mutant product with wild-type sequence when using large templates *(28)*. Alternatively, rendering the megaprimer single-stranded prior to secondary amplification will circumvent the problem of reannealing, though this adds extra steps to the protocol (*see* **Subheading 3.3.1**). A further method, incorporating five cycles of asymmetric PCR with only the megaprimer added *(29)* is now widely used and is described below .

Smith and Klugman *(14,28)* successfully used the megaprimer method to create substitutions in the *pbp1a* gene of *S. pneumoniae* for structure function studies. Using *pbp1a*-specific flanking primers and two mutagenic primers with the whole of *pbp1a* as the template, they investigated the effects of amino acid substitutions at two sites on the level of resistance to penicillin. These poten-

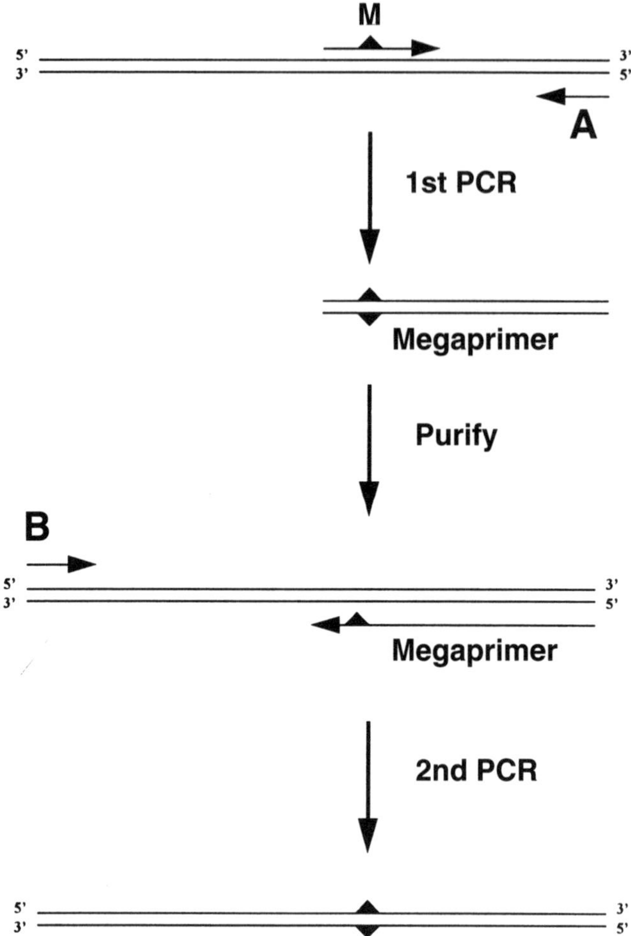

Fig. 2. Schematic outline of the "megaprimer" method of site-directed mutagenesis. **A** and **B** represent the flanking primers, whereas *M* designates the mutagenic primer. Arrows show the direction of priming, and the site of the mutation is marked with a black triangle. The template DNA is designated by double lines, with numbers designating the 5' to 3' orientation. Following the first PCR, the double-stranded megaprimer is purified. This is then used as a primer in a secondary PCR with the other flanking primer to produce the full-length mutated PCR product. Adapted from Ke and Madison *(25)*.

tially important amino acid residues had previously been identified by DNA sequence comparisons of *pbp1a* genes from susceptible and resistant isolates of *S. pneumoniae*. Using *pwo* polymerase for primer extension, and incorporating five cycles of asymmetric PCR using only the megaprimer, they were

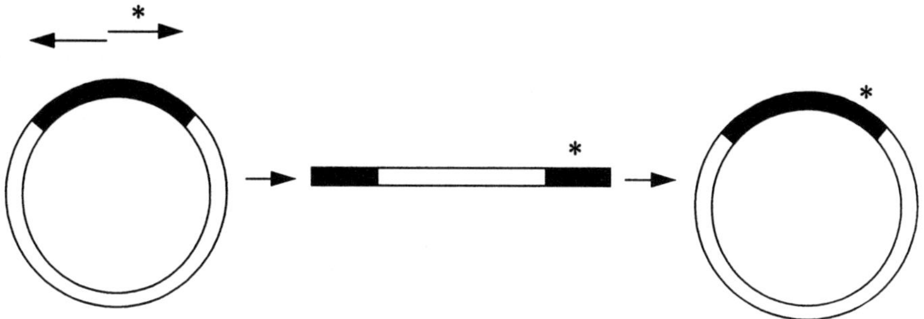

Fig. 3. Diagrammatic representation of inverse PCR-mediated site directed mutagenesis. The solid box represents cloned DNA. Arrows designate the orientation of the back-to-back primers. One of these primers includes the mutagenic site (shown as an asterisk). Inverse PCR results in amplification of a linear product. This is then religated to produce the intact plasmid with the mutation introduced. Adapted from Dorrell et al. ***(33)***.

able to create mutant *pbp1a* genes with megaprimers of 370 or 980 nucleotides in length. Therefore, the megaprimer method has been shown to be appropriate for site-directed mutagenesis of the pneumococcal *pbp* genes.

1.1.5. Primer-Directed Mutagenesis by Inverse PCR

Sequence-specific point mutations, or indeed randomized codons similar to those described in random replacement mutagenesis, may be introduced into a gene cloned in any plasmid using an adaptation of inverse PCR ***(30,31)***. Amplification is directed by two primers in a back-to-back configuration on opposing DNA strands (*see* **Fig. 3**). One primer contains one or more mismatches that will produce the desired mutation(s), whereas the other primer is complementary to the wild-type template. PCR results in the amplification of a linear molecule, and subsequent ligation produces covalently closed circular plasmid carrying the mutated gene. The concentration of template DNA required for the inverse PCR is very low (10 fmol), so that the amount of wild-type DNA after mutagenesis is expected to be negligible. This method allows introduction of mismatches anywhere along the length of a gene. One limiting factor in this method of mutagenesis is the size of the plasmid; as the plasmid increases in size, the PCR reaction conditions become more demanding.

Since the initial description of inverse PCR-directed mutagenesis, modifications have been reported to improve the method. Polymerases specific for long range PCR are now commercially available (e.g., Expand™ Long-Template PCR; Roche Diagnostics, Lewes, East Sussex, UK). These generally also have some degree of proofreading ability. Proofreading polymerases will improve the fidelity of the PCR amplification, as well as provide blunt ends for ligating *(32)*. It has also been reported that open circular (nicked) forms such as the DNA isolated by plasmid "minipreps" make better template for inverse PCR than highly pure, supercoiled plasmid *(30)*. Alternatively, the plasmid DNA may be treated to alkaline denaturation, which should result in the introduction of single-stranded nicks in the DNA *(33)*.

1.1.6. Site-Directed Mutagenesis in Plasmids Using Commercially Available Kits

If the other methods of mutagenesis are not feasible, an alternative method is site-directed mutagenesis of the gene cloned in specially-designed plasmids. A number of kits are commercially available that allow the generation of one or more point mutations in the gene of interest. Generally, these kits are fairly fail-safe, if time-consuming. In our laboratory, we have had success using the Altered Sites™ in vitro Mutagenesis System (Promega, Southampton, UK) to introduce point mutations into *pbp* genes.

In this kit, the gene of interest is introduced into the pALTER plasmid which has two antibiotic resistance markers, ampicillin and tetracycline. The ampicillin resistance gene has been inactivated, so that introduction of the gene to be mutated is selected by tetracycline resistance. A mutagenic primer, plus the ampicillin "repair oligo" are used to prime the synthesis of the mutant strand of DNA (the plasmid may be double-stranded if the strands are first separated by alkaline denaturation). Simultaneous use of the tetracycline "knockout oligo" provides a further screen, as well as selection in further rounds of mutagenesis, if desired. Following synthesis of the mutant DNA strand by T4 DNA polymerase, the mutant plasmids are recovered in ES1301 *mutS E. coli* cells to prevent repair of the mismatch. Concomitant introduction of a helper phage releases the plasmid into the surrounding medium for direct transformation of a suitable host for long-term maintenance. Purification of the plasmid from the strain allows identification of mutants by restriction or sequencing (or transformation of a suitable pneumococcal recipient to observe changes in minimum inhibotory concentration [MIC]).

The obvious advantage of using such a system is the enhanced efficiency of recovery of mutated DNA. Antibiotic selection for the mutated strand yields a high percentage of mutants, and recovery in a *mutS* strain suppresses repair of the introduced mutation to wild-type. Furthermore, in this system multiple simultaneous mutations may be introduced by annealing additional mutagenic oligonucleotide primers to the DNA insert. Subsequent mutagenesis may also be carried out, by simultaneously inactivating the alternate antibiotic resistance marker on the mutagenesis plasmid although selecting for repair of the primary antibiotic resistance. The disadvantages of the system are the number of steps involved, and, of course, the expense. However, the efficiency of recovery of mutants means that use of these kits should not necessarily be dismissed.

2. Materials

2.1. Growth and Transformation of Pneumococci, and Preparation of Chromosomal DNA

1. Brain heart infusion (BHI) broth.
2. BHI agar.
3. BHI blood agar.
4. BHI plus catalase (10 U ctalase per mL agar; *see* **Note 1**).
5. Mueller Hinton broth.
6. C+y medium. *See below.*
7. $CaCl_2$, 1% (w/v).
8. Bovine serum albumin (BSA), 10% (w/v).
9. Competence Stimulating Peptide (CSP). 10 mg/mL in sterile water.
10. Mueller Hinton agar.
11. 50 m*M* Tris-HCl, 20 m*M* EDTA, pH 7.5.
12. Sodium deoxycholate, 5% (w/v).
13. Proteinase K, 2.5 mg/mL.
14. Sodium dodecyl sulphate (SDS), 10% (w/v).
15. Phenol:chloroform:isoamyl alcohol (25:24:1).
16. 3 *M* ammonium acetate.
17. Ethanol. 100%, 70% (v/v).

3.2. Amplification of pbp Genes and Mutagenesis

1. 20 m*M* dNTPs: 20 m*M* dATP, dCTP, dGTP, dTTP in sterile water.
2. Loading buffer: 0.25% (w/v) bromophenol blue, 0.25% (w/v) xylene cyanol FF, 30% (v/v) glycerol in water. Store at 4°C.
3. Ethidium bromide, 10 mg/mL.
4. 50X TAE buffer: 242g Tris, 57.1 mL glacial acetic acid, 100 mL EDTA pH 8.0.

2.3. Phosphorylation of Primers, Digestion by λ Exonuclease, and Addition of "A" Overhangs

50 m*M* ATP.

2.4. C+y-Medium (34)

PreC (*see* below)	160 mL
Supplement	5.2 mL
Glutamine (1 mg/mL)	4 mL
Adams III	4 mL
Pyruvate	2 mL
1 *M* Phosphate buffer	6 mL
5% Yeast extract	3.6 mL

Filter sterilize and keep in a dark bottle at 4°C.

Unless otherwise stated, chemicals were supplied by Sigma (Poole, Dorset, UK).

1. PreC

Sodium Acetate (anhydrous; BDH, Merck, Lutterworth, UK)	1.23 g
Casamino acids (Difco, Detroit, MI)	5 g
L-tryptophan	5 mg
L-cysteine	50 mg

Make up to 1 L with distilled water. Titer pH to 7.4–7.6 using 10 *N* NaOH and 1 *M* NaOH. Autoclave, and store at room temperature.

2. Adams I

Biotin (2 mg/mL)	7.5 µL
Nicotinic acid	15 mg
Pyridoxine HCl	17.5 mg
Calcium pantothenate	60 mg
Thiamine HCl	16 mg
Riboflavin	7 mg

Make up to 100 mL with distilled water, filter sterilize and store in a dark bottle at 4°C.

3. Adams II

$FeSO_4{\cdot}7H_2O$	50 mg
$CuSO_4{\cdot}5H_2O$	50 mg
$ZnSO_4{\cdot}7H_2O$	50 mg
$MnCl_2{\cdot}4H_2O$	20 mg
Concentrated HCl	1 mL

Make up to 100 mL with distilled water and filter sterilize.

4. Adams III

Adams I	48 mL
Adams II	12 mL
Asparagine	600 mg
Choline chloride	60 mg
0.1 *M* $CaCl_2$ (BDH)	480 µL

Make up to 300 mL with distilled water. Filter sterilize and store in a dark bottle at 4°C.

5. Glutamine 1 mg/mL. Filter sterilize, store at 4°C.
6. 2% Pyruvate. Filter sterilize and store at 4°C.
7. 5% Yeast extract. Filter sterilize.
8. 1 *M* Phosphate buffer.
9. Supplement

"3 in 1" Salts	15 mL
20% Glucose (BDH)	30 mL
50% Sucrose (BDH)	1.5 mL
Adenosine (2 mg/mL)	15 mL
Uridine (2 mg/mL)	15 mL

Filter sterilize, store at 4°C.

10. "3 in 1" Salts

$Mg\ Cl_2{\cdot}6H_2O$	100 g

$CaCl_2 \cdot 2H_2O$ 0.66 g
0.1 *M* $MnSO_4 \cdot 4H_2O$ 0.2 mL
Make up to 1 L with water, autoclave.

3. Methods

3.1. Growth of Bacteria and Preparation of Pneumococcal DNA

1. Spread bacteria from a frozen culture on the surface of a BHI+catalase plate to obtain single colonies. Incubate overnight at 37°C in an atmosphere of 5% CO_2/95% air.
2. The following morning, pick a single colony and spread onto a fresh plate to make a "patch" approx the size of a postage stamp. Incubate again at 37°C in an atmosphere of 5% CO_2/95% air over the course of the day.
3. At the end of the day, use the growth from the patch to spread over the surface of a wet BHI+catalase agar plate. Incubate overnight at 37°C in an atmosphere of 5% CO_2/95% air.
4. Harvest the plate into 400 µL 50m*M* Tris/10 m*M* EDTA pH 8.0.
5. Add 80 µL of 5% w/v sodium deoxycholate to the resulting milky suspension and invert a few times to mix. The suspension should begin to lyse after 5–10 min at room temperature with frequent inversion.
6. Add 50 µL 10% w/v sodium dodecyl sulphate, invert to mix, and leave at room temperature for 5 min.
7. Add 100 ng proteinase K (10 µL of a 10 mg/mL solution) to finish the lysis. Incubate at 37°C for 10 min, preferably with slow mixing. At this stage, the solution should be clear. If not, add extra deoxycholate.
8. Add an equal vol (540 µL) of phenol/chloroform/isoamyl alcohol (25:24:1) and mix the phases thoroughly by inversion, until the solution appears milky. Spin at maximum speed in a microfuge for 5 min.
9. Carefully remove the aqueous (top) layer.
10. Repeat the extraction.
11. Add a one-tenth vol of 3 *M* sodium acetate (pH 5.4) to the aqueous layer, and two volumes of 100% ethanol. Mix by inversion and place at –20°C for at least two hours (or on dry ice for 30 min).
12. Spin the DNA sample at maximum speed for 30 min at room temperature. Discard the ethanol. Wash with 70% ethanol and dry the pellet in a vacuum.
13. Resuspend the DNA pellet in 50 µL sterile water. Store at –20°C.
14. Check approximate concentration of DNA by running 1 µL undiluted, and 1 µL of a 1:10 dilution on an agarose gel.

3.2. Amplification of pbp Genes

Of the five high molecular weight PBPs, three of the genes (*pbp1a, pbp2x, pbp2b*) are routinely amplified by PCR. The primers used are listed in **Table 1**. Using these primers, the 1.5 kb amplified fragment of the *pbp2b* gene includes all of the penicillin-binding transpeptidase domain. The 2 kb fragment of *pbp2x*

Table 1
Primers Used to Amplify *pbp* Genes from *Streptococcus pneumoniae*

Primer	Sequence (5'-3')[a]
pbp2b up	CTA CGG ATC CTC TAA ATG ATT CTC AGG TGG
pbp2b down	CAA TTA GCT TAG CAA TAG GTG TTG G
pbp2x up	CGT GGG ACT ATT TAT GAC CGA AAT GG
pbp2x down	AAT TCC AGC ACT GAT GGA AAT AAA CAT ATT A
pbp1a up	GGT AAA ACA TGA AYA ARC C
pbp1a down	TGG ATG ATA AAT GTT ATG GTT G

[a]IUB codes: Y = C or T; R = A or G

includes all but the first 80 bp of the coding region. The entire *pbp1a* gene is amplified as a fragment of 2.1 kb.

1. Make a 100 µL reaction mix including 10 µL of 10X buffer (supplied with polymerase enzyme), 40 µ*M* dNTPs (store frozen at –20°C as a 2 m*M* stock), 1.25 m*M* $MgCl_2$, 1 µ*M* each primer, and 1 ng template. For routine amplification of *pbp* genes, *Taq* polymerase is used. However, for mutagenesis, a proofreading enzyme is preferable (*see* **Note 2**).
2. The PCR program typically consists of an initial denaturation step at 96°C for 5 min followed by cooling (1°C/10 s) to the annealing temperature (usually 58°C for *pbp2b*; 55°C for *pbp1a* or *pbp2x*). The reaction is held at the annealing temperature for approx 2 min so that the polymerase may be added (1 U) in a "hot start." An initial extension at 72°C for 2 min is carried out prior to commencement of the cycling. Twenty-five cycles of amplification follow, consisting of denaturation at 96°C for 1 min, annealing for 2 min, and then extension (1 min/kb template) at 72°C. After the final cycle, an additional step of 72°C for 10 min allows completion of extension.
3. A 5 µL aliquot of the PCR product is loaded next to a size marker onto a 0.7% agarose gel for viewing.

3.3. Mutagenesis Methods

3.3.1. Megaprimer Mutagenesis

This method falls into several main stages. The first is a PCR that makes the megaprimer, and this is carried out under the same conditions described in "Amplification of *pbp* genes" (*see* **Note 2**) except that one of the primers will be the mutagenic primer. The choice of the other primer depends on the position of the desired substitution in the gene. Although megaprimers need only be 200–500 nt shorter than the whole gene in order to allow differentiation of the two on an agarose gel, long megaprimers tend to work less efficiently.

Thus, whether the "up" or "down" primer is used should depend on the position of the mutation (*see* **Note 3**).

Purification of the megaprimer prior to the second amplification is highly recommended. This will remove the primers from the first PCR and thus reduce the frequency with which wild-type gene is amplified. Purification may be done by gel purification, most easily using a kit such as the Qiagen Gel Extraction Kit (Crawley, West Sussex, UK) according to the manufacturer's instructions. Alternatively, if the megaprimer appears as the only band when electrophoresed through an agarose gel, cleanup may be done by filtration, for example using Centricon 100 (Amicon, Witten, Germany) or a kit such as the Qiagen PCR Cleanup Kit. Optional: Generation of single-stranded megaprimer (*see* below)

For the second PCR, initial 5 cycles of asymmetric PCR using just the megaprimer has been shown to improve the yield of the final mutated product, especially when using large megaprimers. (>300 bp ***[29]***).

1. Make a 100 µL reaction mixture containing 1X PCR buffer, 1.25 m*M* $MgCl_2$, 1 ng template, 200 µ*M* dNTPs (*see* **Note 4**), the recommended amount of polymerase (6 µL ULTma™), and all of the megaprimer produced in the first reaction (*see* **Note 5**).
2. Perform 5 cycles of asymmetric PCR (94°C 1 min, 72°C 3min). While the tube is at 72°C for the last time, add the other flanking primer at a concentration of 1 µ*M*.
3. Continue the PCR using the same program as that for the first amplification.
4. A 5 µL aliquot is electrophoresed through a 0.7% agarose gel to determine approximate concentration.

3.3.2. Optional: Generation of Single-Stranded Megaprimer

A common complaint in using the megaprimer method of PCR mutagenesis is a poor recovery of product after the secondary PCR, particularly when using large megaprimers. This may be because of inefficient priming as a result of the two strands of the megaprimer reannealing. One way of coping with this problem is to render the megaprimer single-stranded using λ exonuclease. This enzyme selectively digests from the 5' end of a phosphorylated double-stranded DNA molecule, resulting in a single-stranded megaprimer. Preparation of the phosphorylated primer is achieved using T4 polynucleotide kinase on the single-stranded primer prior to the first PCR amplification. Treatment of the PCR product with λ exonuclease gives the single-stranded megaprimer for the second amplification.

1. Add:
   a. 20 µg primer
   b. 6 µL 10X buffer (supplied with enzyme)
   c. 2 µL 50m*M* ATP

d. 2 µL T4 Polynucleotide Kinase
e. Sterile distilled water to 60mL.
2. Incubate for 1 h at 37°C.
3. Inactivate the enzyme by freezing at –20°C.
4. Perform a PCR reaction using the conditions described above.
5. Perform a suitable PCR cleanup to remove primers.
6. Keep aside 5 µL as "pre-exo" to run on gel after treatment.
7. Make volume of PCR product up to 53 µL with water.
8. Add 6 µL 10X exonuclease buffer (supplied with enzyme).
9. Add 1 µL l exonuclease.
10. Incubate at 37°C for 1 h.
11. Inactivate enzyme by heating at 75°C for 10 min.
12. View pre- and postexonuclease samples on a 0.7% agarose gel. The single-stranded DNA should migrate faster than the double-stranded form, and appear considerably fainter.

3.4. Site-Directed Mutagenesis by Overlap Extension

3.4.1. Primary PCR Amplifications

1. The overlapping mutagenic primers should be designed to have at least 12 nucleotides either side of the mutagenic region.
2. Conduct two PCR reactions, each with one mutagenic primer and the corresponding flanking primer, using the conditions described in **Subheading 3.2.** (*see* **Note 6**).

3.4.2. Gel Purification

Gel purify the resulting two PCR products to remove internal primers and the original wild type template.

3.4.3. Combinatorial PCR

1. Set up a PCR reaction containing the two PCR products, ideally in equimolar ratio totalling 200 ng of DNA, and the other components (except the polymerase) required for PCR as described in **Subheading 3.2.**
2. Heat at 96°C for 2 min to separate the DNA strands, then cool to room temperature to allow annealing.
3. Add the polymerase and heat to 72°C for 2 min for extension of the overlapping primers using the complementary "primer" strand as a template.
4. Add the two flanking primers and heat at 96°C for 1 min; continue PCR using the conditions required for amplification of *pbp* DNA using the flanking primers.
5. The amplified product may then be cloned for further analysis.

3.5. Preparation of DNA for Cloning

Unlike *Taq*, which adds an untemplated "A" to the 3' ends of the amplified DNA, most proofreading polymerases produce a PCR product that has blunt ends. For cloning purposes, it is possible to do a blunt-ended ligation to a vector that has been digested with a restriction enzyme that generates blunt ends, such as *Eco*RV. Perhaps more simply, addition of "A" overhangs allows cloning in one of the many available TA vectors, such as pCRII (Invitrogen, The Netherlands) or pGEM T (Promega, Southampton, UK).

1. To 1 μg PCR product, add 2 m*M* dATP and 1U *Taq*.
2. Incubate at 72°C for 2 h.
3. Remove *Taq*, either by phenol extraction and ethanol precipitation, or by PCR cleanup (e.g., Qiagen PCR Cleanup Kit).

3.6. Cloning and Transformation of E. coli *Cells*

Choice of the plasmid vector governs the method of cloning and *E. coli* transformation. Most commercially available cloning kits give detailed protocols for plasmid cloning and transformation of the appropriate cells (including preparation of competent cells). Otherwise, Sambrook et al. ***(35)*** provide valuable information. Purification of transformed colonies is recommended to avoid multiple copies or variants of plasmids within cells.

3.7. Transformation of Pneumococcal Cells

3.7.1. Preparation of Competent Cells

Pneumococcal cells are routinely made competent in the laboratory by growing in C+y medium at 37°C until they reach a density at which competence is induced. Unfortunately, the state of competence is only transitory. Thus, samples of the growing cells must be taken and frozen at intervals throughout exponential growth, to be checked afterward in a test transformation.

1. Resuspend overnight growth from a BHI blood plate in 5 mL C+y medium. Incubate at 37°C until turbid, approx 2–4 h. Add glycerol to 15% and freeze at –80°C in aliquots for future use as "C-adapted" cells.
2. Inoculate 5–10 mL of C+y medium with 100 μL C-adapted cells.
3. Incubate cells at 37°C. When culture begins to appear turbid, start sampling at 10 min intervals and freezing as 500 μL aliquots in 15% glycerol at –80°C. Keep aside a 20 μL aliquot from each time point to test for competence. Generally, cells will become competent some time within 2.5 h of commencing sampling.
4. To test for competence, a trial transformation must be carried out for each time point. This is most easily done using pneumococcal chromosomal DNA from a strain carrying an antibiotic resistance marker such as rifampin, spectinomycin, or even a β-lactam, and selecting for resistant transformants on antibiotic-containing BHI-blood agar.
5. To the 20 μL aliquots of cells add 380 μL C+y medium and approximately 2 μg chromosomal DNA.
6. Mix and then incubate at 30°C for 30 min.

Table 2
Amino Acid Sequences of Competence Stimulating Peptides 1 and 2 from *S. pneumoniae*

Competence Stimulating Peptide (CSP)	Amino Acid Sequence
CSP 1	E M R L S K F F R D F I L Q R K K
CSP 2	E M R I S R I I L D F L F L R K K

7. Transfer to 37°C for 150 min to allow expression of antibiotic resistance.
8. Spread aliquots of the transformation mixture onto BHI-blood plates with and without (as a viability control) selective antibiotic. Four time points can easily be tested on one agar plate if only 30 µL aliquots are plated.
9. Incubate the plates overnight at 37°C in an atmosphere of 5% CO_2/95% air.

The time points with the most colonies growing on the antibiotic-containing agar (you should expect 1000 or more for the 30 µL plated) should be used for the transformations. These competent cells will generally keep at –80°C for months.

3.7.2. Transformation

The actual volume of the transformation reaction will depend on the number of antibiotic concentrations to be tested.

1. Dilute the competent cells 1:20 in C+y medium (10^5–10^6 cells/mL).
2. Add DNA to a final concentration of 4 µg/mL for chromosomal DNA or 1 µg/mL for plasmid DNA. A "cells-only" control with no added DNA should also be prepared.
3. Incubate initially at 30°C for 30 min and then move to 37°C for 150 min.
4. Spread 100 µL vol onto BHI-blood agar plates containing the appropriate concentration of antibiotic. Be sure to spread on agar plates without antibiotic as well to test for viability.
5. Incubate for 24 h at 37°C in an atmosphere of 5% CO_2/95% air.

3.7.3. Transformation Using Competence Stimulating Peptide

In *Streptococcus pneumoniae*, competence is induced by the action of the 17-amino acid competence stimulating peptide (CSP), the product of the *comC* gene. Though a number of *comC* alleles are found amongst *S. pneumoniae* and related oral streptococci the most common are *comC1* and *comC2* ***(36,37)***. The corresponding CSP1 and CSP2 peptides, chemically synthesized from the predicted amino acid sequences (**Table 2**), are able to stimulate competence when added to growing cells ***(38)***. This provides an alternative, potentially quicker method for making cells competent for genetic transformation.

1. Streak out culture for single colonies on BHI-blood agar plates and incubate overnight at 37°C in an atmosphere of 5% CO_2/95% air. Pick a single colony and restreak it on BHI-blood agar; incubate overnight.

2. Inoculate bacteria in C+y medium to an initial optical density of OD_{600} = 0.01. Incubate at 37°C.
3. Monitor OD after approx 3 h. Cultures are expected to become responsive to CSP approx 2–3 generations before they reach stationary phase, but we take samples at intervals from when the cultures have reached an OD of 0.1 until OD of 0.5, if they reach this level.
4. For the transformation, frozen cells are diluted 1:20 in C+y medium containing 0.16% Bovine Serum Albumin (BSA), 0.01% $CaCl_2$, CSP (10–100 ng/mL) and transforming DNA (1 µg/mL for plasmids, 4 µg/mL chromosomal DNA).
5. The transformation is held at 37°C for 150 min, and then spread on antibiotic selective agar.

4. Notes

1. Filter sterilization of the catalase prior to making BHI-catalase plates is recommended. Catalase comes as a suspension and has a tendency to precipitate out of solution. This can cause problems during filtration, as the filter may become blocked and tear. Warming the catalase at 37°C encourages the precipitate to resuspend. Additionally, we add sterile water (approx 1.5 mL to 0.5 mL catalase) prior to filtration, which also improves resuspension.
2. The early reports of the use of the megaprimer method utilized *Taq* polymerase for primer extension. As a result, they suffered misincorporation of nucleotides leading to unwanted mutations. Furthermore, *Taq* displays terminal transferase activity, generally adding an extra "A" to the 3' ends of amplified double stranded DNAs. This further decreases fidelity and efficiency of the PCR. To avoid this, it is best to choose a proofreading polymerase where possible. The authors used ULTma polymerase (Perkin Elmer) and describe the protocol suitable for this enzyme, though apparently this is no longer available. Other authors have reported success with *Pwo* (Roche Diagnostics, Lewes, East Sussex, UK) and *Pfu* (Stratagene, Cambridge, UK).
3. Flanking primers may be vector sequence if the gene is cloned.
4. Most groups tend to use a high concentration of dNTPs (200 µ*M*) for the primary and secondary PCR. This could potentially cause problems in the first PCR if using *Taq* polymerase, as it encourages the addition of untemplated nucleotides to the 3' ends of the PCR product, resulting in a megaprimer with a mutation at its 5' end. For this reason, Landt and colleagues ***(22)*** recommended 50 µ*M* dNTPs for the primary PCR, and 200 µ*M* for the second. However, this should not be a problem when using proofreading polymerases.
5. Smith and Klugman ***(14)*** reported that a high ratio of megaprimer to template gave the best results when mutagenizing the *pbp1a* gene. They found that 6 µg megaprimer to 5 ng template was optimal, with no product evident when using less than 2 µg megaprimer. A number of groups have reported success using less megaprimer (e.g., 50 ng megaprimer ***[29,39]***). However, we would recommend using all of the megaprimer recovered from the initial PCR.
6. It is recommended to use a proofreading polymerase such as *Pfu* (Stratagene) to avoid introduction of errors. PCR errors may also be limited by using a large

amount of template (500 ng), allowing fewer cycles of amplification to be done (no more than 20).

References

1. Dowson, C. G., Hutchison, A., Brannigan, J. A., George, R. C., Hansman, D., Liñares, J., Tomasz, A., Maynard Smith, J., and Spratt, B. G. (1989) Horizontal transfer of penicillin-binding protein genes in penicillin-resistant clinical isolates of *Streptococcus pneumoniae. Proc. Natl. Acad. Sci. USA* **86,** 8842–8846.
2. Laible, G., Spratt, B. G., and Hakenbeck, R. (1991) Interspecies recombination events during the evolution of altered PBP2X genes in penicillin-resistant clinical isolates of *Streptococcus pneumoniae. Mol. Microbiol.* **5,** 1993–2002.
3. Martin, C., Briese, T., and Hakenbeck, R. (1992) Nucleotide sequences of genes encoding penicillin-binding proteins from *Streptococcus pneumoniae* and *Streptococcus oralis* with high homology to *Escherichia coli* penicillin-binding proteins 1A and 1B. *J. Bacteriol.* **174,** 4517–4523.
4. Sibold, C., Henrichsen, J., Koenig, A., Martin, C., Chalkley, L., and Hakenbeck, R. (1994) Mosaic *pbpX* genes of major clones of penicillin-resistant *Streptococcus pneumoniae* have evolved from *pbpX* genes of a penicillin-sensitive *Streptococcus oralis. Mol. Microbiol.* **12,** 1013–1023.
5. Coffey, T. J., Daniels, M., McDougal, K. K., Dowson, C. G., Tenover, F. C., and Spratt, B. G. (1995) Genetic analysis of clinical isolates of *Streptococcus pneumoniae* with high-level resistance to expanded-spectrum cephalosporins. *Antimicrob. Agents Chemother.* **39,** 1306–1313.
6. Dowson, C. G., Johnson, A. P., Cercenado, E., and George, R. C. (1994) Genetics of oxacillin resistance in clinical isolates of *Streptococcus pneumoniae* that are oxacillin resistant and penicillin susceptible. *Antimicrob. Agents Chemother.* **38,** 49–53.
7. Muñoz, R., Dowson, C. G., Daniels, M., Coffey, T. J., Martin, C., Hakenbeck, R., and Spratt, B. G. (1992) Genetics of resistance to third-generation cephalosporins in clinical isolates of *Streptococcus pneumoniae. Mol. Microbiol.* **6,** 2461–2465.
8. Barcus, V. A., Ghanekar, K., Yeo, M., Coffey, T. J., and Dowson, C. G. (1995) Genetics of high level penicillin resistance in clinical isolates of *Streptococcus pneumoniae. FEMS Microbial. Lett.* **126,** 299–304.
9. Grebe, T. and Hakenbeck, R. (1996) Penicillin-binding proteins 2b and 2x of *Streptococcus pneumoniae* are primary resistance determinants for different classes of β-lactam antibiotics. *Antimicrob. Agents Chemother.* **40,** 829–834.
10. Laible, G. and Hakenbeck, R. (1987) Penicillin-binding proteins in β-lactam-resistant laboratory mutants of *Streptococcus pneumoniae. Mol. Microbiol.* **1,** 355–363.
11. Reichmann, P., Koenig, A., Liñares, J., Alcaide, F., Tenover, F. C., McDougal, L., Swidinski, S., and Hakenbeck, R. (1997) A global gene pool for high-level cephalosporin resistance in commensal *Streptococcus* species and *Streptococcus pneumoniae. J. Inf. Dis.* **176,** 1001–1012.
12. Hakenbeck, R., Koenig, A., Kern, I., Van Der Linden, M., Keck, W., Billot-Klein, D., LeGrand, R., Schoot, B., and Gutmann, L. (1998) Acquisition of five high-M_r

penicillin-binding protein variants during transfer of high-level β-lactam resistance from *Streptococcus mitis* to *Streptococcus pneumoniae. J. Bacteriol.* **180,** 1831–1840.

13. Dowson, C. G., Coffey, T. J., Kell, C., and Whiley, R. A. (1993) Evolution of penicillin resistance in *Streptococcus pneumoniae*; the role of *Streptococcus mitis* in the formation of a low affinity PBP2B in *S. pneumoniae. Mol. Microbiol.* **9,** 635–643.
14. Smith, A. M. and Klugman, K. P. (1998) Alterations in PBP 1A essential for high-level penicillin resistance. *Antimicrob. Agents Chemother.* **42,** 1329–1333.
15. Asahi, Y. and Ubukata, K. (1998) Association of a Thr–371 substitution in a conserved amino acid motif of Penicillin-Binding Protein 1A with penicillin resistance of *Streptococcus pneumoniae. Antimicrob. Agents Chemother.* **42,** 2267–2273.
16. Palzkill, T. and Botstein, D. (1992a) Probing β-lactamase structure and function using random replacement mutagenesis. *Proteins: Struct., Funct., Genet.* **14,** 29–44.
17. Palzkill, T. and Botstein, D. (1992b) Identification of amino acid substitutions that alter the substrate specificity of TEM–1 β-lactamase. *J. Bacteriol.* **174,** 5237–5243.
18. Palzkill, T., Le, Q.-Q., Venkatachalam, K. V., LaRocco, M., and Ocera, H. (1994) Evolution of antibiotic resistance: several different amino acid substitutions in an active site loop alter the substrate profile of β-lactamase. *Mol. Microbiol.* **12,** 217–229.
19. Huang, W., Petrosino, J., Hirsch, M., Shenkin, P. S., and Palzkill, T. (1996) Amino acid determinants of β-lactamase structure and activity. *J. Mol. Biol.* **258,** 688–703.
20. Higuchi, R., Krummel, B., and Saiki, R. K. (1988) A general method of *in vitro* preparation and specific mutagenesis of DNA fragments: study of protein and DNA interactions. *Nucleic Acids Res.* **16,** 7351–7367.
21. Ho, S. N., Hunt, H. D., Horton, R. M., Pullen, J. K., and Pease, L. R. (1989) Site-directed mutagenesis by overlap extension using the polymerase chain reaction. *Gene* **77,** 51–59.
22. Landt, O., Grunert, H.-P., and Hahn, U. (1990) A general method for site-directed mutagenesis using the polymerase chain reaction. *Gene* **96,** 125–128.
23. Sarkar, G. and Sommer, S. S. (1990) The "megaprimer" method of site-directed mutagenesis. *BioTechniques* **8,** 404–407.
24. Picard, V., Ersdal-Badju, E., Lu, A., and Bock, S. C. (1994) A rapid and efficient one-tube PCR-based mutagenesis technique using *Pfu* DNA polymerase. *Nucleic Acids Res.* **22,** 2587–2591.
25. Ke, S. H. and Madison, E. L. (1997) Rapid and efficient site-directed mutagenesis by single-tube 'megaprimer' PCR method. *Nucleic Acids Res.* **25,** 3371–3372.
26. Seraphin, B., and Kandels-Lewis, S. (1996) An efficient PCR mutagenesis strategy without gel purification step that is amenable to purification. *Nucleic Acids Res.* **24,** 3276–3277.
27. Barik, S. and Galinski, M. S. (1991) "Megaprimer" method of PCR: increased template concentration improves yield. *BioTechniques* **10,** 489–490.

28. Smith, A. M. and Klugman, K. P. (1997) "Megaprimer" method of PCR-based mutagenesis: the concentration of megaprimer is a critical factor. *BioTechniques* **22,** 438–442.
29. Datta, A. K. (1995) Efficient amplification using 'megaprimer' by asymmetric polymerase chain reaction. *Nucleic Acids Res.* **23,** 4530–4531.
30. Hemsley, A., Arnheim, N., Toney, M. D., Cortopassi, G., and Galas, D. J. (1989) A simple method for site-directed mutagenesis using the polymerase chain reaction. *Nucleic Acids Res.* **17,** 6545–6551.
31. Eisinger, D. P. and Trumpower, B. L. (1997) Long-inverse PCR to generate regional peptide libraries by codon mutagenesis. *BioTechniques* **22,** 250–254.
32. Hidajat, R. and McNicol, P. (1997) Primer-directed mutagenesis of an intact plasmid by using *Pwo* DNA polymerase in long distance inverse PCR. *BioTechniques* **22,** 32–34.
33. Dorrell, N., Gyselman, V. G., Foynes, S., Li, S.-R., and Wren, B. W. (1996) Improved efficiency of inverse PCR mutagenesis. *BioTechniques* **21,** 604–608.
34. Tomasz, A. and Hotchkiss, R. D. (1964) Regulation of the transformability of pneumococcal cultures by macromolecular cell products. *Proc. Natl. Acad. Sci. USA* **51,** 480–487.
35. Sambrook, J., Fritsch, E. F., and Maniatis, T. (1989) *Molecular Cloning: A Laboratory Manual.* Cold Spring Harbor Laboratory, Cold Spring Harbor, NY, pp. 1.53–1.83.
36. Pozzi, G., Masala, L., Iannelli, F., Manganelli, R., Håvarstein, L. S., Piccoli, L., Simon, D., and Morrison, D. A. (1996) Competence for genetic transformation in encapsulated strains of *Streptococcus pneumoniae*: two allelic variants of the peptide pheromone. *J. Bacteriol.* **178,** 6087–6090.
37. Whatmore, A. M., Barcus, V. A., and Dowson, C. G. (1999) Genetic diversity of the streptococcal competence (*com*) gene locus. *J. Bacteriol.* **181,** 3144–3154.
38. Håvarstein, L. S., Coomaraswamy, G., and Morrison, D. A. (1995) An unmodified heptadecapeptide induces competence for genetic transformation in *Streptococcus pneumoniae. Proc. Natl. Acad. Sci. USA* **92,** 11,140–11,144.
39. Barretino, D., Feigenbutz, M., Valcarcel, R., and Stunnenberg, H. G. (1993) Improved methods for PCR-mediated site-directed mutagenesis. *Nucleic Acids Res.* **22,** 541–542.

27

Detection of Low Affinity Penicillin-Binding Protein Variants in *Streptococcus pneumoniae*

Regine Hakenbeck

1. Introduction

Penicillin-resistance in *Streptococcus pneumoniae* is mediated by altered penicillin-target enzymes, the penicillin-binding proteins or PBPs. PBPs interact with β-lactam antibiotics by forming an active penicilloyl-PBP complex via an active site serine. This complex is enzymatically inactive, and stable enough so that it can be visualized by incubating cells, cell lysates or membrane fractions with radioactive β-lactam, followed by SDS-polyacrylamide-gel electrophoresis (PAGE) and fluorography. The increasing frequency of β-lactam resistant isolates necessitates techniques for describing such strains. PBP profile analysis allows the detection of the variation in six proteins simultaneously and thus each PBP profile is basically a fingerprint of the strain, allowing to assign hundreds of isolates into distinct clonal groups ***(1,2)***.

The purpose of this Chapter is to describe conditions for the labeling procedure and for the protein separation on SDS gels to enable detection of low affinity PBPs in *S. pneumoniae.*

Streptococcus pneumoniae contains six PBPs that are grouped into class A high molecular weight (hmw) PBPs 1a, 1b, and 2a, class B hmw PBPs 2x and 2b, and the single low molecular weight (lmw) PBP 3 (for reviews, *see* **refs. *3*** and ***4***). Low affinity variants have been described for all six PBPs. PBP2x and PPB2b are primary resistance determinants, i.e., low affinity variants confer resistance in the absence of any other altered PBP (5). The other PBPs are apparently secondary targets, i.e., they function only as a resistance determinant in a strain that carries already either a low affinity PBP2x or PBP2b or both. Resistance to third generation cephalosporins is mediated by altered

From: *Methods in Molecular Medicine, vol. 48: Antibiotic Resistance Methods and Protocols*
Edited by: S. H. Gillespie © Humana Press Inc., Totowa, NJ

PBP2x and PBP1a only, since PBP2b is not a target for this class of antibiotics *(6,7)*.

In clinical isolates, PBP2x, PBP2b, and PBP1a appear to be primarily involved with PBP1a being responsible for high resistance levels. Low affinity PBP2a have been described on various occasions, but only recently it was confirmed that indeed, it can function as a resistance determinant in β-lactam resistant laboratory mutants, and by using a high level β-lactam resistant *S. mitis* strain as donor in transformation experiments with the susceptible laboratory R6 strain as recipient *(8,9)*. PBP3 was affected in one particular laboratory mutant *(10)*, and although a low affinity PBP1b has been described, experimental proof that it confers resistance still has to be obtained *(8)*. The apparent M_r of the PBPs range between approx 92 kDa to 43 kDa according to their electrophoretic mobilities, numbers that do not reflect the actual M_r as calculated from the deduced peptide sequence. The two clusters of PBP1a and PBP1b on one hand, and PBP2x, 2a, and 2b on the other hand, are often difficult to separate. In addition, PBP profiles of penicillin-resistant isolates pose the problem that especially PBP1a and PBP2x frequently have electrophoretic mobilities distinct from those of the penicillin-susceptible isolates whose PBP profile is generally fairly uniform *(1,2)*. Methods will be described here that allow identification and separation of the PBPs.

The kinetic parameters characterizing the interaction between PBPs and β-lactams are estimated on the basis of the three step model *(11)*.

$$E + I \xrightarrow{K} E \cdot I \xrightarrow{k_2} E\text{-}I^* \xrightarrow{k_3} E + P$$

where K is the dissociation constant of E • I and E-I* is the acyl-enzyme. For most studies, exact determination of these parameters is not required. However, this formula should be kept in mind in order to set up appropriate concentrations of the antibiotics to be tested.

Detailed kinetic studies on isolated, soluble PBP derivatives have not been considered here. Examples include a variety of PBPs tested with β-lactams as well as with substrate analogues *(12)*; for PBP2x and derivatives (*see* **ref.** ***13***).

2. Materials

2.1. Growth of Bacteria

1. Growth medium.
2. Nephelometer.
3. Microcentrifuge tubes.
4. Microcentrifuge.

2.2. Labeling of Penicillin-Binding Proteins

1. Sodium phosphate buffer: 20 m*M*, pH 7.2.
2. Triton X100: 0.4% (w/v).
3. Radioactive β-lactam (*see* **Notes 1** and **2**).

2.3 Sodium Dodecyl-Sulphate Polyacrylamide Gel Electrophoresis (SDS-PAGE)

1. Separating gel: 7.5% acrylamide separating gel, Persulfate 0.025%, TEMED 0.025%
2. Stacking gel: 5% acrylamide, ammonium persulfate 0.05%, TEMED 0.05% (use 30:0.8 = acrylamide:bisacrylamide which is commercially available; 10% persulfate solution can be stored in aliquots at –20°C)
3. Staining solution: 1 g Coomassie brilliant blue/Lsolution, 10% Methanol, 7.5% acetic acid.
4. Destaining solution: 30% Methanol, 7.5% acetic acid.
5. En^{3}Hance NEF-981-G (Du Pont de Nemours, Brussels, Belgium).
6. Kodak Royal X-Omat film.

3. Method

3.1. Preparation of Cell Lysates

1. Cultivate the bacteria in a suitable growth medium until middle to late exponential phase.
2. Determine the optical density (we use Nephelometry) and adjust to Nephelo (N) = 70–90. The maximum cell density is reached at approximately N = 110. We usually centrifuge 2 mL portions of the cell culture in large microcentrifuge tubes for 2–5 min (*see* **Note 3**).
3. Use a pipet to remove the supernatant completely and the longer centrifugation time. Cell pellets can be stored at –80°C for at least one year, generally we resuspend the cells in the appropriate amount of phosphate buffer prior to freezing.
4. Determine the volume you want to resuspend the cells. We use the equivalent of 1 mL culture at N = 20 per sample corresponding to 3×10^7 CFU when using the laboratory strain *S. pneumoniae* R6. Cells are resuspended in buffer without Triton so that 5 µL correspond to 1 sample.

   Example:

   2 mL cells harvested at N = 85
   resuspend in $2 \times 4.25 \times 5 = 42.5$ µL phosphate buffer
   use 5 µL cell suspension per sample

   You can store cells at –80°C for at least one year.

3.2 Lysis and Labeling with β-lactam (standard protocol).

Generally, cells are lysed and labeled with a β-lactam at the same time (*see* **Note 4**). Although in principle, Triton X100 could be added to the cells before freezing, we prefer to add the appropriate amount of Triton after the cell sample has been pipeted into the test tube, simply because pipeting is more accurate without Triton. If only short incubation with the β-lactam are used, cells should be incubated with Triton alone for approx 10 min to ensure cellular lysis, and labeled afterwards (*see* **Note 5**).

1. Remove resuspended cells from freezer, thaw them on ice.
2. Arrange test tubes and label them according to your protocol.
3. Prepare the β-lactam solutions needed for labeling.
4. Pipet 5 µL Triton X100 (0.4%) into each tube.
5. Add 5 µL of the resuspended cells directly into the Triton X100 drop.
6. Pipet the appropriate amount of the β-lactam; pipet to the wall of the test tube.
7. Centrifuge the droplets briefly (1 s) in the Eppendorf centrifuge.
8. Mix the sample.
9. Incubate immediately in the water bath.

3.3. Termination of the Labeling Reaction

1. Put samples on ice.
2. Add 20 µL SDS-sample buffer.
3. Put in boiling water bath for 2 min.
4. Centrifuge for 2 min in Eppendorf centrifuge to remove cellular debris and capsular material.
5. Load samples on gel (*see* **Note 4**).
6. Run the polyacrylamide gel (*see* **Note 5**).

3.4. Staining of the Gel

1. Incubate for 1 h in staining solution, shake at room temperature.
2. Incubate overnight with destaining solution, change frequently until background is clear.
3. Make a photographic record of the gel (*see* **Note 6**).
4. Soak gel in En^{3}Hance for 1 h, remove solution (can be reused).
5. Shake in cold water for 1 h.
6. Dry the gel.
7. Expose to film in the dark (*see* **Notes 7** and **8**).

4. Notes

1. Radioactive compounds used for PBP labeling. Commercially, only benzylpenicillin is available as radioactive β-lactam compounds; [^{3}H]-benzylpenicillin has a high specific activity and is recommended; [^{35}S]-benzylpenicillin: the relatively fast decay has to be considered; [^{14}C]-benzylpenicillin has a very low specific activity, and since several weeks of exposure of the film are needed, this compound is not very useful. A derivative of ampicillin can be synthesized using N-succinimidyl-[2,3-^{3}H]propionate (90–100 mmol, Amersham) ***(16)***. The specific radioactivity of the synthesized product cannot be easily determined, but can be estimated to be close to the radioactive N-succinimidyl-[2,3-^{3}H]propi-

onate, supposed that the separation of product [^{3}H]propionylampicillin ([^{3}H]PA) from the nonlabeled ampicillin used for its synthesis has been achieved.

In all cases it is advisable to portion the compound into aliquots suitable for labeling a given amount of samples and store it at –80°C to ensure comparable results.

2. Nonradioactive compounds. We have not tested these compounds on *S. pneumoniae*. Although some of the publications list *S. pneumoniae* as test organism, there is no guarantee that all PBPs are labeled with these compounds or whether the PBPs in complex with these compounds have altered electrophoretic mobilities ***(17–19)***.

   Anti-β-lactam antibodies. The advantage of using these antibodies lies in the fact that PBPs can be labeled with very high concentrations of nonradioactive β-lactams which are impossible to reach with the radioactive substances. Also, they can be used in combination with other antisera on Western blots thus allowing identification of low affinity PBP bands. The disadvantage is that not all PBPs can be detected this way although they are clearly labeled with the respective antibiotic ***(20,21)***, the reason of this is not clear. Since these antibodies are not commercially available, the reader is referred to the publications that explicitly list the experimental details.

   Anti-PBP antibodies. Specific antisera or monoclonal antibodies are helpful to identify the nature of the PBP. In resistant strains, the hmw PBPs are frequently not migrating at the same position compared to those of sensitive strains, and it is often not clear who is who. PBP1a and PBP2x are most variable in this respect; different mobilities in SDS gels have also been noted for PBP3, but this PBPs can be distinguished easily from all other PBPs independent on this property. Again, since the antibodies are not commercially available, the reader is referred to details description of the use of these antibodies in the following references ***(1,2,22)***.
3. Some clinical isolates do not pellet well, rather the cells form a light smear at the bottom of the tube which can be lost easily if you decant the supernatant.
4. In the context of determining low affinity variants it is also important to realize that one single point mutation generally confers only marginal resistance levels since the reduction in affinity for the β-lactam is not that high. Accordingly it is more difficult to trace a single point mutation since the difference in affinity to β-lactams is relatively small compared to that of the wild-type strain. For instance, the single point mutation in PBP2b Thr446Ala which appears in most of the low affinity PBP2b of clinical isolates ***(5)***, or the single point mutation in PBP3 Thr242Ile ***(10)***, result in only an approx 1.5-fold increase in resistance for piperacillin or cefotaxime, respectively, and single point mutations in PBP2x vary in their in vivo effect between a threefold to over 10-fold resistance increase ***(5)***.

   Concentrations of β-lactams and conditions during incubation with the β-lactam that have been successfully used to detect differences in affinity range between an estimated 0.02 to 0.05 μCi of [^{3}H]-PA in 15 μL sample, and incubation times as little as 2–5 min at 25°C.

5. To optimize the resolution of the PBP clusters use the following acrylamide:bis-acrylamide ratios in the separating gel:
   30:0.5 and 10% gels for better resolution of PBP 1 cluster (PBP1a and 1b) for better resolution of PBP 2 cluster (PBPx, 2a, and 2b).
6. If the gel bands are not straight and clear, apart from some error during mixing of the gel solutions common problems include insufficient centrifugation of the cell debris or too much material was loaded onto the gel.
7. The film has to be pre-exposed to guarantee quantitative blackening of the film *(15)*. This can be done either by preflashing the film using special filters that are mounted on the flash, or by exposing a pack of films to X-ray. The conditions may vary considerably in each laboratory, therefore the pre-exposure of the films should be monitored by OD measuring of developed film strips before using it for the gels.
8. You should expect to be able to see bands already after 2–3 d of exposure of the film. If you have used your own [^{3}H]-propionylampicillin for the first time, it is possible that is has not been separated sufficiently on the column from the nonradioactive compound. Possible problems include: the radioactive β-lactam used is too old and has decayed; you are dealing with a high level resistant strain where PBPs have very low affinity, then you may use 10-fold the concentration of the β-lactam used for labeling, if possible.

References

1. Hakenbeck, R., Briese, T., Chalkley, L., Ellerbrok, H., Kalliokoski, R., Latorre, C., Leinonen, M., and Martin, C. (1991) Variability of penicillin-binding proteins from penicillin-sensitive *Streptococcus pneumoniae. J. Infect. Dis.* **164,** 307–312.
2. Hakenbeck, R., Briese, T., Chalkley, L., Ellerbrok, H., Kalliokoski, R., Latorre, C., Leinonen, M., and Martin, C. (1991) Antigenic variation of penicillin-binding proteins from penicillin resistant clinical strains of *Streptococcus pneumoniae. J. Infect. Dis.* **164,** 313–319.
3. Hakenbeck, R. and Coyette, J. (1998) Resistant penicillin-binding proteins. *Cell. Mol. Life. Sci.* **54,** 332–340.
4. Goffin, C. and Ghuysen, J.-M. (1998) Multimodular penicillin-binding proteins: an enigmatic family of orthologs and paralogs. *Microb. Mol. Biol. Rev.* **62,** 1079–1081.
5. Grebe, T. and Hakenbeck, R. (1996) Penicillin-binding proteins 2b and 2x of *Streptococcus pneumoniae* are primary resistance determinants for different classes of β-lactam antibiotics. *Antimicrob. Agents Chemother.* **40,** 829–834.
6. Hakenbeck, R., S. Tornette and N.F. Adkinson (1987) Interaction of nonlytic β-lactams with penicillin-binding proteins in *Streptococcus pneumoniae. J Gen Microbiol* **133,** 755–760.
7. Muñóz, R., Dowson, C. G., Daniels, M., Coffey, T. J., Martin, C., Hakenbeck, R., and Spratt, B. G. (1992) Genetics of resistance to third-generation cephalosporins in clinical isolates of *Streptococcus pneumoniae. Mol. Microbiol.* **6,** 2461–2465.
8. Hakenbeck, R., König, A., Kern, I., van der Linden, M., Keck, W., Billot-Klein, D., Legrand, R., Schoot, B., and Gutmann, L. (1998) Acquisition of five high-M_r

penicillin-binding protein variants during transfer of high-level β-lactam resistance from *Streptococcus mitis* to *Streptococcus pneumoniae*. *J. Bacteriol.* **180,** 1831–1840.

9. van der Linden, M. and Hakenbeck, R. (1998) unpublished results.
10. Krauβ, J. and Hakenbeck, R. (1997) A mutation in the D,D-carboxypeptidase penicillin-binding protein 3 of *Streptococcus pneumoniae* contributes to cefotaxime resistance of the laboratory mutant C604. *Antimicrob. Agents Chemother.* **41,** 936–942.
11. Frère, J.-M. and Joris, B. (1985) Penicillin-sensitive enzymes in peptidoglycan biosynthesis. *Crit. Rev. Microbiol.* **11,** 299–396.
12. Adam, M., Damblon, C., Jamin, M., Zorzi, W., Dusart, V., Galleni, M., El Kharroubi, A., Piras, G., Spratt, B. G., Keck, W., Coyette, J., Ghuysen, J.-M., Nguyen-Distèche, M., and Frère, J.-M. (1991) Acyltransferase activities of the high-molecular-mass essential penicillin-binding proteins. *Biochem. J.* **279,** 601–604.
13. Krauβ, J., van der Linden, M., Frère, J.-M., Dideberg, O., and Hakenbeck, R. (1999) Penicillin-binding protein 2x of *Streptococcus pneumoniae*: remodeling of a penicillin target enzyme into a major resistance determinant, submitted.
14. Bonner, W. M. and Laskey, R. A. (1974) A film detection method for tritium-labeled proteins and nucleic acids in polyacrylamide gels. *Eur. J. Biochem.* **46,** 83–88.
15. Laskey, R. A. and Mills, A. D. (1975) Quantitative film dtection of 3H and 14C in polyacrylamide gels by fluorography. *Eur. J. Biochem.* **56,** 335–341.
16. Hakenbeck, R. and Kohiyama, M. (1982) Labelling of pneumococcal penicillin-binding proteins with [^{3}H]propionyl-ampicillin A rapid method for monitoring penicillin-binding activity. *FEMS Microbiol. Lett.* **14,** 241–245.
17. Zhao, G., Meir, T. I., Kahl, S. D., Gee, K. R., and Blaszczak, L. C. (1999) Bocillin FL, a sensitive and commercially available reagent for detection of penicillin-binding proteins. *Antimicrob. Agents Chemother.* **43,** 1124–1128.
18. Dargis, M. and Malouin, F. (1994) Use of biotinylated β-lactams and chemiluminescence for study and purification of penicillin-binding proteins in bacteria. *Antimicrob. Agents Chemother.* **38,** 973–980.
19. Weigel, L. M., Belisle, J. T., Radolf, J. D., and Norgard, M. V. (1994) Dioxigenin-ampicillin conjugate for detection of penicillin-binding proteins by chemiluminescence. *Antimicrob. Agents Chemother.* **38,** 330–336.
20. Hakenbeck, R., Briese, T., and Ellerbrok, H. (1986) Antibodies against the benzylpenicilloyl moiety as a probe for penicillin-binding proteins. *Eur. J. Biochem.* **157,** 101–106.
21. Briese, T., Ellerbrok, H., Schier, H.-M., and Hakenbeck, R. (1988) Reactivity of anti-β-lactam antibodies with β-lactam-penicillin-binding protein complexes, in *Antibiotic Inhibition of Bacterial Cell Surface Assembly and Function* (Actor, P., Daneo-Moore, L., Higgins, M. L., Salton, M. R. J., and Shockman, G. D., eds.), American Society for Microbiology, Washington, DC 20006, pp. 404–409.
22. Reichmann, P., König, A., Liñares, J., Alcaide, F., Tenover, F. C.,. McDougal, L., Swidsinski, S., and Hakenbeck, R. (1997) A global gene pool for high-level cephalosporin resistance in commensal *Streptococcus spp.* and *Streptococcus pneumoniae*. *J. Infect. Dis.* **176,** 1001–1012.

V

Transmission of Resistance

28

Mobilization of Transposons

Rationale and Techniques for Detection

Louis B. Rice

1. Introduction

The ability to share genetic information with other bacteria represents one of the most important adaptive mechanisms available to bacteria pathogenic for humans. The exchange of many different types of genetic information appears to occur frequently and exchange of determinants responsible for antimicrobial resistance is the best studied, since the movements of resistance determinants are easy to follow and the clinical importance of resistance dissemination is so great. The most common vehicles by which bacteria exchange resistance determinants are plasmids and transposons.

Plasmids are segments of DNA that replicate independently of the bacterial chromosome *(1)*. At a minimum, they must possess an origin of replication and genes that encode replication proteins. Many plasmids possess additional genes as well. Among the most common of these genes are genes encoding conjugation, mobilization, or antimicrobial resistance proteins. Occasionally, plasmids may also encode virulence genes. Plasmids that encode conjugation genes are called conjugative plasmids. Conjugative plasmids may transfer at high, intermediate, or low frequency, and may exhibit a broad or a narrow host range for replication. The functional and genetic analysis of plasmids is relatively straightforward, since the movement of phenotype (especially antibiotic resistance phenotype) can be followed, and since the entire replicon can be digested, cloned into a high-copy vector and sequenced with relative ease.

Transposons are mobile genetic elements that encode mobilization but not replicative functions. As a result, these elements must be integrated into replicative elements (the chromosome, plasmids) to survive. In order to be consid-

From: *Methods in Molecular Medicine, vol. 48: Antibiotic Resistance Methods and Protocols*
Edited by: S. H. Gillespie © Humana Press Inc., Totowa, NJ

ered a true transposon, a mobile element must be able to transpose to a separate replicon in the absence of host cell recombination. Some mobile elements encode only the genetic functions to facilitate movement. These are generally small (0.8–2.5 kb) and are referred to as insertion sequences *(2)*. Mobile elements that encode genes in addition to those responsible for movement (such as antibiotic resistance genes or virulence genes) are referred to as transposons. Transposons may owe their mobility to the presence of insertion sequences on their ends, or to the presence of transposition genes that interact in a specific way with the ends of the transposon to facilitate movement.

The genetic analysis of transposons is somewhat more complicated than for plasmids since these elements are always integrated within other replicative elements. As opposed to plasmids, which by virtue of their circular structure do not have true "ends," identification of the ends of transposons is critical to the definition of their structure. In addition, analysis of the ends of a transposon can often provide important insight into the nature of the element itself.

The clinical importance of transposons in the dissemination of antimicrobial resistance should not be underestimated. Many different types of transposons have been identified and characterized. In gram-positive bacteria, these transposons fall into one of three general categories. Conjugative transposons encode genes that mediate their own (and occasionally unrelated loci) transfer between a wide variety of genera *(3)*. Transposons of this class are widespread in nature and have recently been implicated in the transfer of VanB-type vancomycin resistance *(4)*. They transpose in a conservative fashion (an extra copy of the element does not result from transposition) and the prototype is the enterococcal transposon Tn*916*, generally encode resistance to tetracycline and minocycline. The second class of gram-positive transposons is the Tn*3*-family elements. These elements, of which the prototype is Tn*917*, an enterococcal erythromycin resistance-encoding transposon, are not conjugative by themselves but may be found on transferable plasmids *(5)*. They transpose in a replicative fashion, meaning that in addition to the transposed element, a second copy remains at the original site. Tn*3*-family elements have also been implicated in the mobilization of resistance to penicillin (β-lactamase-mediated) and vancomycin (VanA-type) in gram-positive bacteria *(6,7)*. The third class of transposons found in gram-positive bacteria are the composite transposons. These transposons owe their mobility to the presence of similar or identical copies of insertion sequences flanking a specific resistance determinant. It is generally presumed, although rarely demonstrated experimentally, that the transposition of these elements is replicative. In essence, any DNA segment between two functional and related IS elements can become a composite transposon. Perhaps the most prevalent of composite transposons in gram-positive bacteria are the Tn*4001*-like elements, originally described in *Staphylo-*

coccus aureus but now recognized to be widespread in gram-positive bacteria ***(8,9)***. This family of elements encodes resistance to a range of aminoglycosides (including gentamicin) by virtue of the presence of the *aac-6'-aph-2"* bifunctional aminoglycoside modifying enzyme gene between two inverted copies of the insertion sequence IS*256*. IS*256*-related composite transposons have also been implicated in the mobilization of resistance determinants for erythromycin, mercuric chloride, and vancomycin (VanB-type) ***(10,11)***.

The best way to define the limits of a mobile element is to mobilize it to a separate replicon, preferably one that has previously been well defined. Insertion into a known site allows a detailed evaluation of many different aspects of the transposon, including its total size, the nucleotide sequence of the ends of the element and a judgment about whether insertion is associated by the production of a duplication of the target sequence (target duplications of specific lengths are often characteristic of known classes of transposons). Replicons most commonly used for the mobilization of transposons are the conjugative plasmids.

In order to efficiently detect mobilization of a transposon, the transposon should be integrated within a nontransferable replicon, most commonly the bacterial chromosome or a nonconjugative, nonmobilizable plasmid. The transposable element should possess a phenotypically detectable marker, most conveniently an antimicrobial resistance gene. The conjugative plasmid to be used for mobilization should also contain a detectable marker. This is also often an antimicrobial resistance determinant, but may be another marker, such as a hemolysin gene. Also required is a plasmid-free recipient bacterial strain within which the conjugative plasmid can replicate. This recipient strain should also express one or two resistance determinants against antibiotics to which the donor strain is susceptible, in order to permit counter-selection of transconjugants. The frequency of plasmid conjugation should be very high—on the order of 10^{-1} transconjugants per recipient strain, in order to efficiently detect transposition. The rationale for the high frequency of transfer is simple—in most cases, transposition frequencies will be on the order of 10^{-7}–10^{-9} per mating event. Practically speaking, it is difficult to analyze more than 10^9 recipient CFU for a given mating. In order to obtain 10^8 transconjugants for a mating, highly conjugative plasmids are required (*see* **Note 1**). A schematic diagram using hemolysin plasmid pAD1 ***(12)*** to mobilize conjugative transposon Tn*5383* from one *Enterococcus faecalis* strain to another is shown in **Fig. 1**. A restriction digestion showing the results of such a mating is shown in **Fig. 2** ***(13)***.

The protocol listed below details the mating procedure used between CH116, a Tn*5383*-containing *E. faecalis* strain, with rifampin and fusidic acid-resistant *E. faecalis* recipient strain. The details are primarily derived from a paper published by Christie et al. ***(14)***.

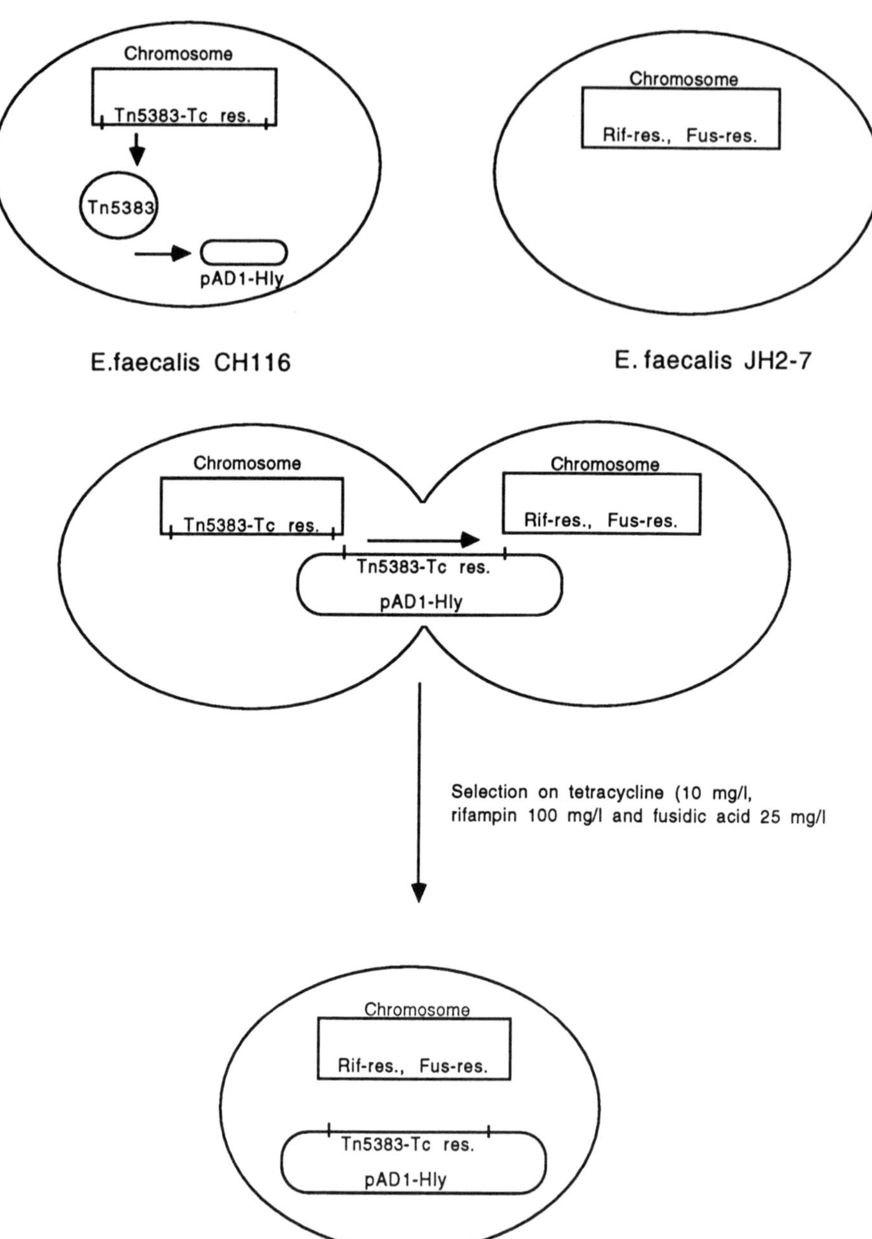

Fig. 1. Schematic diagram of the occurrences during mating to mobilize Tn*5381* from the chromosome of CH116. **(A)** Donor and recipient strain. Characteristics of chromosomal and plasmid determinants are indicated. Drawing depicts circularization of Tn*5383* within CH116, which is the first step of transposition of conjugative

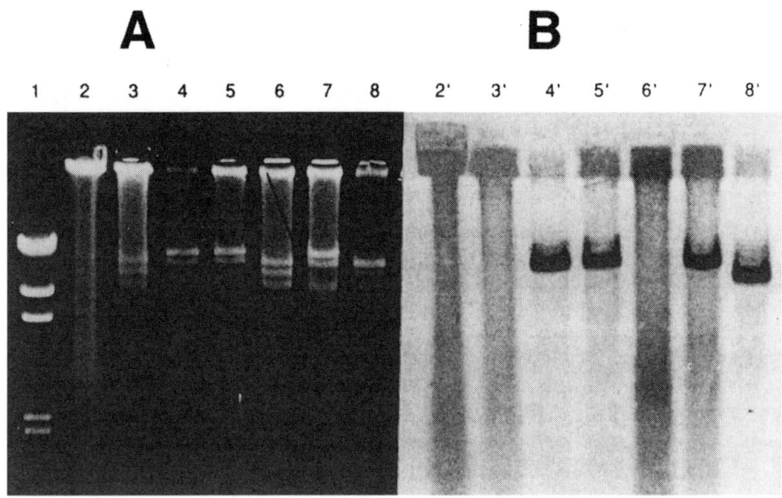

Fig. 2. **(A)** *Eco*RI digests of plasmid DNA from a mating between CH116 (pAD1) and JH2-7. Matings were performed in an effort to capture Tn*5383* onto pAD1. Lane 1: Bacteriophage lambda digested with *Hin*dIII (size standard - fragment sizes (kb) 23.03, 9.6, 6.6, 4.3, 2.3, 2.0); Lane 2: CH116 (plasmid free); Lane 3: CH116 (pAD1); Lanes 4–8: transconjugants resulting from the mating. **(B)** Hybridization of the DNA from the gel at left with a probe consisting of the 5 kb *Hin*cII fragment of Tn*916*, which contains the *tet*(M) tetracycline resistance gene. The lack of hybridization to a specific band in Lane 6' indicates that Tn*5383* has transferred from chromosome-to-chromosome, in conjunction with transfer of pAD1. From reference *(13)*.

2. Materials

1. Brain heart infusion agar.
2. Petri dishes.
3. Donor bacterial strains (*see* **Table 1**).
4. Recipient bacterial strains (*see* **Table 1**).
5. Antibiotics .
6. 4% defibrinated horse blood.
7. Sterile circular nitrocellulose filters (Whatman, S&S or any of several manufacturers).
8. 0.9% sterile saline.

---

transposons, prior to insertion in a second location, in this case within pAD1. **(B)** Mating event that occurs after insertion of Tn*5383* into pAD1. Plasmid:transposon cointegrate transfer to the recipient strain together. **(C)** After selection on plates containing tetracycline, rifampin and fusidic acid, transconjugants appear as tetracycline-, rifampin- and fusidic acid-resistant colonies. Insertion into the hemolysin region of pAD1 can be detected by selecting hyper-hemolytic or nonhemolytic colonies.

Table 1
Strains Used for Mobilization Protocol

Strain designation	Characteristics	Description
E. faecalis OGIX	Sm^r	Plasmid-free *E. faecalis* recipient strain ***(15)***
E. faecalis OGIX(pAD1)	Sm^r, Hly	Donor strain for pAD1 ***(16)***
E. faecalis CH116	βla+, Em^r, Gm^r, Sm^r, Tc^r, plasmid-free	Strain from which Tn*5383* to be mobilized ***(13)***
E. faecalis JH2-7	Rif^r, Fus^r	Plasmid-free *E. faecalis* recipient strain ***(17)***

βla+ β-lactamase-producing; Em^r-erythromycin-resistant; Gm^r-gentamicin-resistant; Rif^r-rifampin-resistant; Sm^r-streptomycin-resistant; Tc^r-tetracycline-resistant; Hly-hemolysin-producer

3. Method

Mobilization of conjugative transposons in *E. faecalis* to hemolysin-producing pheromone-responsive conjugative plasmid pAD1. These studies take advantage of the fact that insertion of conjugative transposons into the hemolysin determinant result in a loss of the hemolytic phenotype, whereas insertion into particular hot-spots upstream of the hemolysin determinant result in a hyper-hemolytic phenotype.

3.1. Conjugating pAD1 into CH116

1. Streak out OG1X(pAD1) on BHI agar plate containing 4% horse blood (*see* **Note 2**). Streak out CH116 on BHI agar plate containing gentamicin (500 µg/mL).
2. Select one hemolysin-producing colony from OG1X(pAD1) plate and one colony from the CH116 plate and inoculate one 5 mL test tube of BHI broth with each individually. Incubate overnight without shaking at 37°C.
3. Wash overnight cultures X 2 with sterile 0.9% saline.
4. Perform one 1:10 dilution in sterile saline of both washed cultures.
5. Place 50 µL aliquots of the different cultures onto sterile circular nitrocellulose membranes placed on nonselective BHI agar plate, allow to dry on bench top and incubate overnight at 37°C. Donor: recipient ratios should be 1:10, 1:1 and 10:1 (*see* **Notes 3** and **4**).
6. Place a 50 µL aliquot of donor alone, or recipient alone onto sterile nitrocellulose membranes placed on nonselective BHI agar plate, allow to dry and incubate overnight at 37°C.
7. Resuspend cells from nitrocellulose filters in 1 mL sterile saline. Perform serial 1:10 dilutions of the resuspensions in sterile saline.
8. Inoculate 100 µL aliquots of the diluted suspensions onto BHI agar plate containing gentamicin (500 µg/mL) and 4% defibrinated horse blood. Incubate overnight at 37°C.

9. Inoculate 100 µL aliquots of donor and recipient strains onto selective plates. Incubate overnight at 37°C. Plates inoculated with donor strains should not yield any colonies. Plates inoculated with recipient strains should not yield any hemolytic colonies. (These are the control plates.)
10. Colonies appearing on selective plates from the matings that are hemolytic should be CH116, now with pAD1. This fact can be conformed by plating these colonies onto plates containing other antibiotics (erythromycin, tetracycline) to which CH116 is resistant.

3.2. Mobilization of Tn5383

1. Select a single colony from the plate containing gentamicin (500 µg/mL) and 4% defibrinated horse blood and inoculate into 5 mL test tube of BHI broth overnight at 37°C. Select a single colony of *E. faecalis* JH2-7 from a BHI agar plate containing rifampin (100 µg/mL) and fusidic acid (25 µg/mL) and grow overnight in the same fashion.
2. Wash cells as described above.
3. Place aliquots onto nitrocellulose filters as described above and incubate on non-selective plates overnight at 37°C.
4. Resuspend cells from filters and perform serial dilutions in sterile saline as described above.
5. Inoculate 100 mL aliquots of mating filters and of control filters onto plates containing tetracycline (10 µg/mL), rifampin (100 µg/mL), fusidic acid (25 µg/mL).
6. Examine plates looking specifically for colonies that are tetracycline-resistant and hyper-hemolytic, or tetracycline-resistant and nonhemolytic. These colonies will predictably contain insertions of Tn*5383* in or around the pAD1 hemolysin gene.
7. Confirm insertion of Tn*5383* into pAD1 by performing secondary mating between presumed transconjugant and *E. faecalis* OG1X, with selection on plates containing streptomycin (200 µg/mL), tetracycline (10 µg/mL), and 4% defibrinated horse blood. If Tn*5383* is integrated into pAD1, transfer of tetracycline resistance should occur at a high frequency and correlate 1:1 with the donor hemolytic phenotype.
8. Confirm insertion of Tn*5383* into pAD1 by plasmid extraction, restriction digestion, and comparison with similarly-digested pAD1. Use these comparisons to identify the pAD1 restriction fragment within which the insertion occurred and to identify, through hybridization studies, the restriction fragments containing the ends of the transposon.

The above protocol addresses specifically the mobilization of conjugative transposons from *E. faecalis*, but its general strategy can be followed for mobilization of transposons in virtually any species, as long as highly conjugative plasmids can be identified and a suitable recipient strain is available. A useful conjugative plasmid for mobilization of transposons in *E. coli* and other gram-negative bacteria is pOX38Km, a kanamycin-resistant variant of the highly conjugative F plasmid ***(18)***.

Detailed functional and genetic analysis of transposons provides important insight into the mechanisms by which clinically important bacteria exchange genetic information containing antimicrobial resistance determinants, determinants that confer virulence characteristics, as well as untold other important pieces of genetic material. The ready availability of genetic tool to mobilize these elements, and the relatively low cost of these investigations should encourage investigators in many different areas to pursue these studies in their own laboratories.

4. Notes

1. If very low frequency events are being investigated, it may be important to "scale up" the procedure. We have been able to increase the number of CFU analyzed roughly 10–100-fold by using an entire plate as our "filter." We mix 50 µL aliquots of overnight cultures of donor and transconjugant in a microcentrifuge tube. This mixture is then spread over an entire nonselective agar plate (generally BHI agar, although Todd-Hewitt agar is acceptable for gram-positive bacteria and LB agar for gram-negative bacteria. The plate is incubated at 37°C overnight and the following day, the entire plate is scraped clean with a platinum loop and the entire inoculum spread over two plates containing the selective antibiotics. This strategy is obviously only feasible for resistance determinants for which inoculum effects are not important. It is therefore not feasible for selecting transfer of ampicillin resistance determinants in gram-negative bacteria.
2. If plasmids such as pAD1 are to be used, it must be recognized that the hemolysin encoded by this plasmid also serves as a bacteriocin, and will decrease the inoculum of the recipient strain in most cases. It is reasonable in this setting to use a 10-fold higher inoculum of recipients than donors.
3. A higher yield of transfer may be achieved by incubating the donor and recipient strain together in the overnight culture. This strategy is obviously to be avoided if the conjugative plasmid encodes a bacteriocin.
4. In order to determine frequency of transposition or frequency of transfer, it is important to calculate accurate counts of the numbers of donor and recipient bacterial CFU. These counts require serial dilution of the various mating mixtures. In order to save on laboratory resources, we employ a method in which small aliquots of the serial dilutions (10–25 µL) are placed on plates in duplicate. The number of colonies growing the following day for each dilution are counted, and the two numbers for each dilution are averaged. The number of colonies is then multiplied by the appropriate number to bring the volume of the calculation to 1 mL. This method allows us to determine the colony counts for a given species on a single plate.

References

1. Clewell, D. B. (1981) Plasmids, drug resistance and gene transfer in genus *Streptococcus. Microbiol. Rev.* **45,** 409–436.

2. Galas, D. J. and Chandler, M. (1989) Bacterial insertion sequences, i*n Mobile DNA*. Berg, D. E. and Howe, M. M., eds.), American Society for Microbiology, Washington, DC, pp. 109–162.
3. Rice, L. B. (1998) Tn*916*-family conjugative transposons and dissemination of antimicrobial resistance determinants. *Antimicrob. Agent Chemother.* **42,** 1871–1877.
4. Carias, L. L., Rudin, S. D., Donskey, C. J., and Rice, L. B. (1998) Genetic linkage and co-transfer of a novel, *vanB*-encoding transposon (Tn*5382*) and a low-affinity penicillin-binding protein 5 gene in a clinical vancomycin-resistant *Enterococcus faecium* isolate. *J. Bacteriol.* **180,** 4426–4434.
5. Shaw, J. H. and Clewell, D. B. (1985) Complete nucleotide sequence of macrolide-lincosamide-streptogramin B resistance transposon Tn*917* in *Streptococcus faecalis. J. Bacteriol.* **164,** 782–796.
6. Arthur, M., Molinas, C., Depardieu, F., and Courvalin, P. (1993) Characterization of Tn*1546*, a Tn*3*-related transposon conferring glycopeptide resistance by synthesis of depsipeptide peptidoglycan precursors in *Enterococcus faecium* BM4147. *J. Bacteriol.* **175,** 117–127.
7. Rowland, S. J. and Dyke, K. G. H. (1990) Tn*552*, a novel transposable element from *Staphylococcus aureus*. *Mol. Microbiol.* **4,** 961–975.
8. Lyon, B. R., May, J. W., and Skurray, R. A. (1984) Tn*4001*: a gentamicin and kanamycin resistance transposon in *Staphylococcus aureus*. *Mol. Gen. Genet.* **193,** 554–556.
9. Kaufhold, A., Podbielski, A., Horaud, T., and Ferrieri, P. (1992) Identical genes confer high-level resistance to gentamicin upon *Enterococcus faecalis*, *Enterococcus faecium*, and *Streptococcus agalactiae*. *Antimicrob. Agent Chemother.* **36,** 1215–1218.
10. Rice, L. B., Carias, L. L., and Marshall, S. H. (1995) Tn*5384*, a composite enterococcal mobile element conferring resistance to erythromycin and gentamicin whose ends are directly repeated copies of IS*256*. *Antimicrob. Agent Chemother.* **39,** 1147–1153.
11. Quintiliani, R., Jr. and Courvalin, P. (1996) Characterization of Tn*1547*, a composite transposon flanked by the IS*16* and IS*256*-like elements, that confers vancomycin resistance in *Enterococcus faecium* BM4281. *Gene* **172,** 1–8.
12. Ike, Y., Flannagan, S. E., and Clewell, D. B. (1992) Hyperhemolytic phenomena associated with insertions of Tn*916* into the hemolysin determinant of *Enterococcus faecalis* plasmid pAD1. *J. Bacteriol.* **174,** 1801–1809.
13. Rice, L. B., Marshall, S. H., and Carias, L. L. (1992) Tn*5381*, a conjugative transposon identifiable as a circular form in *Enterococcus faecalis*. *J. Bacteriol.* **174,** 7308–7315.
14. Christie, P. J., Korman, R. Z., Zahler, S. A., Adsit, J. C., and Dunny, G. M. (1987) Two conjugation systems associated with plasmid pCF10: identification of a conjugative transposon that transfers between *Streptococcus faecalis* and *Bacillus subtilis*. *J. Bacteriol.* **169,** 2529–2536.
15. Ike, Y., Craig, R. A., White, B. A., Yagi, Y., and Clewell, D. B. (1983) Modification of *Streptococcus faecalis* sex pheromones after acquisition of plasmid DNA. *Proc. Natl. Acad. Sci. USA*. **80,** 5369–5373.

16. Clewell, D. B., Tomich, P. K., Gawron-Burke, M. C., Franke, A. E., Yagi, Y., and An, F. Y. (1982) Mapping of *Streptococcus faecalis* plasmids pAD1 and pAD2 and studies relating to transposition of Tn*917*. *J. Bacteriol.* **152,** 1220–1230.
17. Jacob, A. E. and Hobbs, S. J. (1974) Conjugal transfer of plasmid-borne multiple antibiotic resistance in *Streptococcus faecalis* var. *zymogenes*. *J. Bacteriol.* **117,** 360–372.
18. Chandler, M. and Galas, D. J. (1983) Cointegrate formation mediated by Tn*9*. II. Activity of IS*1* is modulated by external DNA sequences. *J. Mol. Biol.* **170,** 61–91.

Index